Essentials of Biostatistics

Lisa M. Sullivan

Series Editor: Richard Riegelman

Essentials of Biostatistics

Lisa M. Sullivan, PhD

Chair, Department of Biostatistics
Boston University School of Public Health
Boston, Massachusetts

JONES AND BARTLETT PUBLISHERS

Sudbury, Massachusetts

BOSTON   TORONTO   LONDON   SINGAPORE

World Headquarters

Jones and Bartlett Publishers
40 Tall Pine Drive
Sudbury, MA 01776
978-443-5000
info@jbpub.com
www.jbpub.com

Jones and Bartlett Publishers
Canada
6339 Ormindale Way
Mississauga, Ontario
L5V 1J2
Canada

Jones and Bartlett Publishers
International
Barb House, Barb Mews
London W6 7PA
United Kingdom

Jones and Bartlett's books and products are available through most bookstores and online booksellers. To contact Jones and Bartlett Publishers directly, call 800-832-0034, fax 978-443-8000, or visit our website www.jbpub.com.

Substantial discounts on bulk quantities of Jones and Bartlett's publications are available to corporations, professional associations, and other qualified organizations. For details and specific discount information, contact the special sales department at Jones and Bartlett via the above contact information or send an email to specialsales@jbpub.com.

This publication is designed to provide accurate and authoritative information in regard to the Subject Matter covered. It is sold with the understanding that the publisher is not engaged in rendering legal, accounting, or other professional service. If legal advice or other expert assistance is required, the service of a competent professional person should be sought.

Library of Congress Cataloging-in-Publication Data

Sullivan, Lisa M. (Lisa Marie), 1961-
   Essentials of biostatistics in public health / Lisa M. Sullivan.
      p. ; cm.
   Includes bibliographical references and index.
   ISBN-13: 978-0-7637-3737-5 (pbk.)
   ISBN-10: 0-7637-3737-2 (pbk.)
   1. Public health--Statistical methods. 2. Medical statistics. I. Title.
   [DNLM: 1. Biometry--methods. 2. Public Health Practice. WA 950 S949e 2008]
   RA409.S73 2008
   362.1--dc22

                                              2007019656

6048

Production Credits

Publisher: Michael Brown
Associate Editor: Katey Birtcher
Production Director: Amy Rose
Production Editor: Tracey Chapman
Marketing Manager: Sophie Fleck
Manufacturing Buyer: Therese Connell
Composition: Graphic World
Cover Design: Kristin E. Ohlin
Cover Image: © Digital Vision/Getty Images
Printing and Binding: Malloy, Inc.
Cover Printing: John Pow Company

Printed in the United States of America
12 11 10 09 08   10 9 8 7 6 5 4 3 2

Table of Contents

Acknowledgments

I am very grateful to Professor Ralph D'Agostino Sr. for his constant guidance and support. I am also thankful to Dr. Richard Riegelman who was instrumental in providing invaluable insight from the development to the completion of the textbook. Special thanks to Lori Chibnik, Michelle Keyes, Michael Pencina, and Sharon Milewitz for their careful editing and reviewing. I thank my family for their constant support and most especially, I am thankful to Kimberly Dukes and Kevin Green for their unending love and support.

This textbook is dedicated to the memory of my cousin, Catherine Render. Catherine was a remarkable woman. She was a loving daughter, sister, wife, mother, cousin, and friend who excelled in every role. She lost a long battle with breast cancer in January 2006. She fought through many setbacks, always pushing forward optimistically, taking care of everyone around her, never asking why. She was and always will be an inspiration to her family and to so many others who were fortunate enough to know her.

Biostatisticians play an extremely important role in addressing important medical and public health problems. Unfortunately, there are many more problems than solutions. We must never lose sight of the fact that our work is important in improving health and well-being. We need qualified biostatisticians to work in research teams to address problems like breast cancer, cardiovascular disease, diabetes, and so many others.

Lisa M. Sullivan

Preface

Essentials of Biostatistics provides a fundamental and engaging background for students learning to apply and appropriately interpret biostatistical applications in the field of public health. The examples are real, important, and represent timely public health problems. The author aims to make the material relevant, practical and interesting for students. Throughout the textbook, the author uses data from the Framingham Heart Study and from clinical trials in a variety of major areas. The author presents example applications involving important risk factors such as blood pressure, cholesterol, smoking and diabetes and their relationships to incident cardiovascular and cerebrovascular disease throughout. Clinical trials investigating new drugs to lower cholesterol, to reduce pain and to promote healing following surgery are also considered. The author presents examples with relatively few subjects to illustrate computations while minimizing the actual computation time, as a particular focus is mastery of "by-hand" computations. All of the techniques are then applied to and illustrated on real data from the Framingham Study and large clinical trials. For each topic, the author discusses methodology—including assumptions, statistical computations and the appropriate interpretation of results. Key formulas are summarized at the end of each chapter.

Prologue

Learning to avoid being deceived by data is essential for all educated citizens. It is a key skill for future clinicians, public health practitioners, and health researchers. In *Essentials of Biostatistics*, Lisa Sullivan PhD has written a text that guides students through this maze. The text uses real and relevant examples drawn from her own experience working on the Framingham Heart Study and clinical trials.

Essentials of Biostatistics takes an intuitive, step-by-step, hands-on approach to walking students though statistical principles. The approach emphasizes understanding what questions to ask and what the answers mean.

Calculations are designed to enhance understanding. The accompanying Workbook utilizes Excel, making it familiar and engaging for students. The combination of text and workbook provides a solid foundation for future course work in statistics as well as the type of grounding needed to read and appreciate the health research literature.

Essentials of Biostatistics is a tried and true approach. Lisa Sullivan has spent 20 years teaching undergraduate students biostatistics and working with undergraduates as Assistant Dean for Undergraduate Education in Public Health at the Boston University School of Public Health. In these roles she has repeatedly won teaching awards for her skills and commitment to education in Biostatistics.

Dr. Sullivan possesses a unique combination of sophisticated biostatistics expertise with an engaging and articulate style—a rare combination indeed. Her recent appointment as Chair of the Department of Biostatistics confirms her expertise in biostatistics. Even a quick look at *Essentials of Biostatistics* will convince you of her skills in communication and education.

I am delighted that Lisa Sullivan has agreed to include her book and workbook in our Essential Public Health series. There is no better book to recommend for the anxious student first confronting the field of biostatistics. Students will find the book and workbook engaging and relevant. Just take a look and see for yourself.

Richard Riegelman MD, MPH, PhD
Series Editor—Essential Public Health series

CHAPTER 1

Introduction

Biostatistics is central to public health education and practice; it includes a set of principles and techniques that allows us to draw meaningful conclusions from information or data. Implementing and understanding biostatistical applications is a combination of art and science. Appropriately understanding statistics is important both professionally and personally, as we are faced with statistics every day.

For example, cardiovascular disease is the number one killer of men and women in the United States. The American Heart Association reports that more than 2600 Americans die every day of cardiovascular disease, which is approximately one American every 34 seconds. There are over 70 million adults in the United States living with cardiovascular disease, and the annual rates of development are estimated at 7 cases per 1000 in men aged 35–44 years and 68 cases per 1000 in men aged 85–94 years.[1] The rates in women are generally delayed about 10 years as compared to men.[2] Researchers have identified a number of risk factors for cardiovascular disease including blood pressure, cholesterol, diabetes, smoking, and weight. Smoking, and weight (specifically, overweight and obesity) are considered the most and second-most, respectively, preventable causes of cardiovascular disease death in the United States.[3,4] Family history, nutrition, and physical activity are also important risk factors for cardiovascular disease.[5]

The previous example describes cardiovascular disease, but similar statistics are available for many other diseases including cancer, diabetes, asthma, and arthritis. Much of what we know about cardiovascular and many other diseases comes from newspapers, news reports, or the Internet. Reporters describe or write about research studies on a daily basis. Nightly newscasts almost always contain a report of at least one research study. Some studies seem quite obvious, such as the positive effects of exercise on health, whereas other studies describe breakthrough medications that cure disease or prolong a healthy life. Newsworthy topics can include conflicting or contradictory results in medical research. One study might report that a new medical therapy is effective, whereas another study might suggest this new therapy is ineffectual; other studies may show vitamin supplements thought to be effective as being ineffective or even harmful. One study might demonstrate the effectiveness of a drug, and years later it is determined to be harmful due to some serious side effect. To understand and interpret these items requires knowledge of statistical principles and statistical thinking.

How are these studies conducted in the first place? For example, how is the extent of disease in a group or region quantified? How is the rate of development of new disease estimated? How are risk factors or characteristics that might be related to development or progression of disease identified? How is the effectiveness of a new drug determined? What could explain contradictory results? These questions are the essence of biostatistics.

1.1   WHAT IS BIOSTATISTICS?

Biostatistics is defined as the application of statistical principles in medicine, public health, or biology. Statistical principles are based in applied mathematics and include tools and techniques for collecting information or data and then summarizing, analyzing, and interpreting those results. These principles extend to making inferences and drawing conclusions that appropriately take uncertainty into account.

Biostatistical techniques can be used to address each of the aforementioned questions. In applied biostatistics, the objective is usually to make an inference about a specific population. By definition, this population is the collection of all individuals about whom we would like to make a statement. The population of interest might be all adults living in the United States or all adults living in the city of Boston. The definition of the population depends on the investigator's study question, which is the objective of the analysis. Suppose the population of interest is all adults living in the United States and we want to estimate the proportion of all adults with cardiovascular disease. To answer this question completely, we would examine every adult in the United States and assess whether they have cardiovascular disease. This would be an impossible task! A better and more realistic option would be to use a statistical analysis to estimate the desired proportion.

In biostatistics, we study samples or subsets of the population of interest. In this example, we would select a sample of adults living in the United States and assess whether each has cardiovascular disease or not. If the sample is representative of the population, then the proportion of adults in the sample with cardiovascular disease should be a good estimate of the proportion of adults in the population with cardiovascular disease. In biostatistics, we analyze samples and then make inferences about the population based on the analysis of the sample. This inference is quite a leap, especially if the population is large (e.g., the United States population of 300 million) and the sample is relatively small (for example, 5000 people). When we listen to news reports or read about studies, we often think about how results might apply to us personally. The vast majority of us have never been involved in a research study. We often wonder if we should believe results of research studies when we, or anyone we know, never participated in those studies.

1.2 WHAT ARE THE ISSUES?

Appropriately conducting and interpreting biostatistical applications requires attention to a number of important issues. These include, but are not limited to, the following:

- Clearly defining the objective or research question
- Choosing an appropriate study design (i.e., the way in which data are collected)
- Selecting a representative sample, and ensuring that the sample is of sufficient size
- Carefully collecting and analyzing the data
- Producing appropriate summary measures or statistics
- Generating appropriate measures of effect or association
- Quantifying uncertainty
- Appropriately accounting for relationships among characteristics
- Limiting inferences to the appropriate population

In this book, each of the preceding points will be addressed in turn. We will describe how to collect and summarize data and how to make appropriate inferences. To achieve these, we will use biostatistical principles that are grounded in mathematical and probability theory. A major goal will be to understand and interpret a biostatistical analysis. Let us now revisit our original questions and think about some of the issues previously identified.

How Is the Extent of Disease in a Group or Region Quantified?

Ideally, a sample of individuals in the group or region would be selected. That sample should be sufficiently large so that the results of the analysis of the sample will be adequately precise. (We will discuss techniques to determine the appropriate sample size in Chapter 8.) In general, a larger sample is preferable; however, we never want to sample more participants than are needed, for both financial and ethical reasons. The sample should also be representative of the population. For example, if the population is 60% women, ideally we would like the sample to be approximately 60% women. Once the sample is selected, each participant is assessed with regard to disease status. The proportion of the sample with disease can then be computed by taking the ratio of the number with disease to the total sample size. This proportion is an estimate of the proportion of the population with disease. Suppose the sample proportion is computed as 17% (i.e., 17% of those sampled have the disease). We would estimate the proportion of the population with disease to be approximately 17%. Because this is an estimate based on one sample, we must account for uncertainty, and this is reflected in what is called a *margin of error*. This might result in our estimating the proportion of the population with disease to be anywhere from 13% to 21%.

This study would likely be conducted at a single point in time; this type of study is commonly referred to as a *cross-sectional study*. Our estimate of the extent of disease refers only to the period under study. It would be inappropriate to make inferences about the extent of disease at future points based on this study. If we had selected adults living in Boston as our population, it would also be inappropriate to infer that the extent of disease in other cities or in other parts of Massachusetts would be the same as that observed in a sample of Bostonians. The task of estimating the extent of disease in a region or group seems straightforward on the surface. However, there are many issues that complicate things. For example, where do we get a list of the population, how do we decide who is in the sample, how do we ensure that specific groups are represented (e.g., women) in the sample, and how do we find the people we identify for the sample and convince them to participate? All of these questions must be addressed correctly to yield valid data and correct inferences.

How Is the Rate of Development of a New Disease Estimated?

To estimate the rate of development of a new disease—say, cardiovascular disease—we need a specific sampling strategy. For this analysis, we would sample only persons free of cardiovascular disease and follow them prospectively (going forward) in time to assess the development of the disease. A key issue in these types of studies is the follow-up period; the investigator must decide whether to follow participants for either one, five, or ten years or some other period for the development of the disease. If it is of interest to estimate the development of disease over ten years, it requires following each participant in the sample over ten years to determine their disease status. The ratio of the number of new cases of disease to the total sample size reflects the proportion or incidence of new disease over the predetermined follow-up period. Suppose we follow each of the participants in our sample for five years and find that 2.4% develop disease. Sometimes, this is reported as 24 cases per 1000 persons over five years, or as 24 per 5000 person-years (assuming a constant rate of disease development). Again, it is generally of interest to provide a range of plausible values for the proportion of new cases of disease; this is achieved by incorporating a margin of error to reflect the precision in our estimate. Incorporating the margin of error might result in an estimate of the rate of development of disease anywhere from 9 to 39 per 1000 persons over five years.

Epidemiology is a field of study focused on the study of health and illness in human populations, patterns of health or disease, and the factors that influence these patterns. The study described here is an example of an epidemiological study. Readers interested in learning more about epidemiology should see Magnus.[6]

How Are Risk Factors or Characteristics That Might Be Related to the Development or Progression of Disease Identified?

Suppose we hypothesize that a particular risk factor or exposure is related to the development of a disease. There are several different study designs or ways in which we might collect information to assess the relationship between a potential risk factor and disease onset. The most appropriate study design depends, among other things, on the distribution of both the risk factor and the outcome in the population of interest (e.g., how many participants are likely to have a particular risk factor or not). (We will discuss different study designs in Chapter 2 and which design is optimal in a specific situation.) Regardless of the specific design used, both the risk factor and

the outcome must be measured on each member of the sample. If we are interested in the relationship between the risk factor and the development of disease, we would again involve participants free of disease at the study's start and follow all participants for the development of disease. To assess whether there is a relationship between a risk factor and the outcome, we would estimate the proportion of participants with the risk factor who go on to develop disease and compare that to the proportion of participants who do not have the risk factor and go on to develop disease. There are several ways to make this comparison; it can be based on a difference in proportions or a ratio of proportions. (The details of these comparisons are discussed extensively in Chapter 6 and Chapter 7.)

Suppose that among those with the risk factor, 12% develop disease during the follow-up period, and among those free of the risk factor, 6% develop disease. The ratio of the proportions is called a *relative risk* and here it is equal to 0.12 / 0.06 = 2.0. The interpretation is that twice as many people with the risk factor develop disease as compared to people without the risk factor. The issue then is to determine whether this estimate, observed in one study sample, reflects an increased risk in the population. Accounting for uncertainty might result in an estimate of the relative risk anywhere from 1.1 to 3.2 times higher for persons with the risk factor. Because the range contains risk values greater than 1, the data reflect an increased risk (because a value of 1 suggests no increased risk).

Another issue in assessing the relationship between a particular risk factor and disease status involves understanding complex relationships among risk factors. Persons with the risk factor under study might be different from persons free of the risk factor; for example, they may be older and more likely to have other risk factors. There are methods that can be used to assess the association between the hypothesized risk factor and disease status while taking into account the impact of the other risk factors. These techniques involve statistical modeling. We will discuss how these models are developed and, more important, how results are interpreted in Chapter 9.

How Is the Effectiveness of a New Drug Determined?

The ideal study design from a statistical point of view is the *randomized controlled trial* or the *clinical trial*. (The term *clinical* means that the study involves people.) For example, suppose we want to assess the effectiveness of a new drug designed to lower cholesterol. Most clinical trials involve specific inclusion and exclusion criteria. For example, we might want to include only persons with total cholesterol levels exceeding 200 or 220, because the new medication would likely have the best chance to show an effect in persons with elevated cholesterol levels. We might also exclude persons with a history of cardiovascular disease. Once the inclusion and exclusion criteria are determined, we recruit participants. Each participant is randomly assigned to receive either the new experimental drug or a control drug. The randomization component is the key feature in these studies. Randomization theoretically promotes balance between the comparison groups. The control drug could be a *placebo* (an inert substance) or a cholesterol-lowering medication that is considered the current standard of care.

The choice of the appropriate comparator depends on the nature of the disease. For example, with a life-threatening disease, it would be unethical to withhold treatment, thus a placebo comparator would never be appropriate. In this example, a placebo might be appropriate as long as participants' cholesterol levels were not so high as to necessitate treatment. When participants are enrolled and randomized to receive either the experimental treatment or the comparator, they are not told to which treatment they are assigned. This is called *blinding* or *masking*. Participants are then instructed on proper dosing and after a predetermined time, cholesterol levels are measured and compared between groups. (Again, there are several ways to make the comparison and we will discuss different options in Chapter 6 and Chapter 7.) Because participants were randomly assigned to treatment groups, the groups should be comparable on all characteristics except the treatment received. If we find that the cholesterol levels are different between groups, the difference can likely be attributed to treatment.

Again, we must interpret the observed difference after accounting for chance or uncertainty. If we do observe a large difference in cholesterol levels between participants receiv-ing the experimental drug and the comparator, we can infer that the experimental drug is effective. However, inferences about the effect of the drug are only able to be generalized to the population from which participants were drawn—specifically, to the population defined by the inclusion and exclusion criteria. Clinical trials must be carefully designed and analyzed. There exist a number of issues that are specific to clinical trials, and we will discuss these in detail in Chapter 2.

Clinical trials are discussed extensively in the news, particularly recently. They are heavily regulated in the United States by the Food and Drug Administration (FDA).[7] Recent news reports discuss studies involving drugs that were granted approval for specific indications and later removed from the market due to safety concerns. We will review these studies and assess how they were conducted and, more important, why they are being reevaluated. For evaluating drugs, randomized controlled trials are considered the gold standard. Still, they can lead to controversy. Studies other than clinical trials are less ideal and are often more controversial.

What Could Explain Contradictory Results Between Different Studies of the Same Disease?

All statistical studies are based on analyzing a sample from the population of interest. Sometimes, studies are not designed appropriately and results may therefore be questionable. Sometimes, too few participants are enrolled, which could lead to imprecise and even inaccurate results. There are also instances where studies are designed appropriately, yet two different replications produce different results. Throughout this book, we will discuss how and when this might occur.

1.3   SUMMARY

In this book, we will investigate in detail each of the issues raised in this chapter. Understanding biostatistical principles is critical to public health education. Our approach will be through active learning: examples will be taken from the Framingham Heart Study and from clinical trials, which will be used throughout the book to illustrate concepts. Example applications involving important risk factors such as blood pressure, cholesterol, smoking, and diabetes and their relationships to incident cardiovascular and cerebrovascular disease will be discussed. Examples with relatively few subjects will help to illustrate computations while minimizing the actual computation time; a particular focus is mastery of "by-hand" computations. All of the techniques will then be applied to real data from the Framingham study and from clinical trials. For each topic, we will discuss methodology—including assumptions, statistical formulas, and the appropriate interpretation of results. Key formulas will be summarized at the end of each chapter. Examples will be selected to represent important and timely public health problems.

REFERENCES

1. American Heart Association. Available at *http://www.americanheart.org*.

2. Sytkowski, P.A., D'Agostino, R.B., Belanger, A., and Kannel, W.B. "Sex and time trends in cardiovascular disease incidence and mortality: The Framingham Heart Study, 1950–1989." *American Journal of Epidemiology*, 1996; 143(4): 338–350.

3. Wilson, P.W.F., D'Agostino, R.B., Levy, D., Belanger, A.M., Silbershatz, H., and Kannel, W.B. "Prediction of coronary heart disease using risk factor categories." *Circulation*, 1998; 97: 1837–1847.

4. The Expert Panel. "Expert panel on detection, evaluation, and treatment of high blood cholesterol in adults: summary of the second report of the NCEP expert panel (Adult Treatment Panel II)." *Journal of the American Medical Association*, 1993; 269: 3015–3023.

5. Kaikkonen, K.S., Kortelainen, M.L., Linna, E., and Huikuri, H.V. "Family history and the risk of sudden cardiac death as a manifestation of an acute coronary event." *Circulation*, 2006; 114(4): 1462–1467.

6. Magnus, M. *Essentials of Infectious Disease Epidemiology*. Sudbury, MA: Jones & Bartlett, 2007.

7. United States Food and Drug Administration. Available at *http://www.fda.gov*.

CHAPTER 2

Study Designs

Once a study objective or research question has been refined—which is no easy task, as it usually involves extensive discussion among investigators, a review of the literature and an assessment of ethical and practical issues—the next step is to choose the study design to most effectively and efficiently answer the question. The *study design* is the methodology that will be used to collect the information to address the research question. In Chapter 1, we raised a number of questions that might be of interest, including: How is the extent of a disease in a group or region quantified? How is the rate of development of a new disease estimated? How are risk factors or characteristics that might be related to the development or progression of a disease identified? How is the effectiveness of a new drug determined? To answer each of these questions, a specific study design must be selected. In this chapter, we will review a number of popular study designs. This review is not meant to be exhaustive but instead illustrative of some of the more popular designs for public health applications.

The studies we present can probably be best organized into two broad types: observational and randomized studies. In *observational* studies, we generally observe a phenomenon, whereas in *randomized* studies, we intervene and measure a response. Observational studies are sometimes called descriptive or associational studies, nonrandomized, or historical studies. In some cases, observational studies are used to alert the medical community to a specific issue, whereas in other instances, observational studies are used to generate hypotheses. We will later elaborate on other instances where observational studies are used to assess specific associations. Randomized studies are sometimes called analytic or experimental studies. They are used to test specific hypotheses or to evaluate the effect of an intervention (e.g., a behavioral or pharmacologic intervention).

Another way to describe or distinguish study types is on the basis of the time sequence involved in data collection. Some studies are designed to collect information at a point in time, others collect information on participants over time, and others evaluate data that has already been collected.

In biostatistical and epidemiologic research studies, we are often interested in the association between a particular exposure or risk factor (e.g., alcohol use, smoking) and an outcome (e.g., cardiovascular disease, lung cancer). In the following sections, we will discuss several observational study designs and several randomized study designs. We will describe each design, detail its advantages and disadvantages, and distinguish designs by the time sequence involved. We will then describe in some detail the Framingham Heart Study, which is an observational study and one of the world's most important studies of risk factors for cardiovascular disease.[1] We will then provide more detail on clinical trials, which are often considered the gold standard in terms of study design. At the end of this chapter, we will summarize the issues in selecting the appropriate study design. Before describing the specific design types, we present some key vocabulary terms that are relevant to study design.

2.1 VOCABULARY

- *Bias*—A systematic error that introduces uncertainty in estimates of effect or association
- *Blind/double blind*—The state whereby a participant is unaware of their treatment status (e.g., experimental drug or placebo). A study is said to be double blind when

both the participant and the outcome assessor are unaware of the treatment status (*masking* is used as an equivalent term to blinding).

• *Clinical trial*—A specific type of study involving human participants and randomization to the comparison groups

• *Cohort*—A group of participants who usually share some common characteristics and who are monitored or followed over time

• *Concurrent*—At the same time; optimally, comparison treatments are evaluated concurrently or in parallel

• *Confounding*—Complex relationships among variables that can distort relationships between the risk factors and the outcome

• *Cross-sectional*—At a single point in time

• *Incidence (of disease)*—The number of new cases of disease over a period of time

• *Intention-to-treat*—An analytic strategy whereby participants are analyzed in the treatment they were assigned regardless of whether they followed the study procedures completely (e.g., regardless of whether they took all of the assigned medication)

• *Matching*—A process of organizing comparison groups by similar characteristics

• *Per protocol*—An analytic strategy whereby only participants who adhered to the study protocol (i.e., the specific procedures given to them) are analyzed (in other words, an analysis of only those assigned to a particular group who followed all procedures for that group)

• *Placebo*—An inert substance designed to look, feel, and taste like the active or experimental treatment (e.g., saline solution would be a suitable placebo for a clear, tasteless liquid medication)

• *Prevalence (of disease)*—The proportion of individuals with a disease at a single point in time

• *Prognostic factor*—A characteristic that is strongly associated with an outcome (e.g., disease) such that it could be used to reasonably predict whether a person is likely to develop a disease or not

• *Prospective*—A study in which information is collected looking forward in time

• *Protocol*—A step-by-step plan for a study that details every aspect of the study design and data collection plan

• *Quasi-experimental design*—A design in which subjects are not randomly assigned to treatments

• *Randomization*—A process by which participants are assigned to receive different treatments (this is usually based on a probability scheme)

• *Retrospective*—A study in which information is collected looking backward in time

• *Stratification*—A process whereby participants are partitioned or separated into mutually exclusive or non-overlapping groups

2.2 OBSERVATIONAL STUDY DESIGNS

There are a number of observational study designs. We will describe some of the more popular designs from the simplest to the more complex.

2.2.1 The Case Report/Case Series

A *case report* is a very detailed report of the specific features of a particular participant or case. A *case series* is a systematic review of the interesting and common features of a small collection, or series, of cases. These types of studies are important in the medical field as they have historically served to identify new diseases. The case series does not include a control or comparison group (e.g., a series of disease-free participants). These studies are relatively easy to conduct but can be criticized as they are unplanned, uncontrolled, and not designed to answer a specific research question. They are often used to generate specific hypotheses, which are then tested with other larger studies. An example of an important case series was one published in 1981 by Gottleib et al., who reported on five young homosexual men who sought medical care with a rare form of pneumonia and other unusual infections.[2] The initial report was followed by more series with similar presentations, and in 1982 the condition being described was termed Acquired Immune Deficiency Syndrome (AIDS).

2.2.2 The Cross-Sectional Survey

A *cross-sectional survey* is a study conducted at a single point in time. The cross-sectional survey is an appropriate design when the research question is focused on the prevalence of a disease, a present practice, or an opinion. The study is non-randomized and involves a group of participants who are identified at a point in time and information is collected at that point in time. Cross-sectional surveys are useful for estimating the prevalence of specific risk factors or prevalence of the disease at a point in time. In some instances, it is of interest to make comparisons between groups of participants (e.g., between men and women, between participants under age 40, and those over age 40). However, inferences from the cross-sectional survey are limited to the time at which data are collected and do not generalize to future time points.

Cross-sectional surveys can be easy to conduct, are usually ethical, and are often large in size (i.e., involve many participants) to allow for estimates of risk factors, diseases, practices, or opinions in different subgroups of interest. However, a major limitation in cross-sectional surveys is the fact that both the exposure or development of a risk factor (e.g., hypertension) and the outcome have occurred. Because the study is conducted at a point in time (see Figure 2–1), it is not possible to assess temporal relationships, specifically whether the exposure or risk factor occurred prior to the outcome of interest. Another issue is related to non-response. While a large sample may be targeted, in some situations only a small fraction of participants approached agree to participate and complete the survey. Depending on the features of the participants and non-participants, non-response can introduce bias or limit generalizability.

In Figure 2.1, approximately one-third of the participants have the risk factor and two-thirds do not. Among those with the risk factor, almost half have the disease, as compared to a much smaller fraction of those without the risk factor. Is there an association between the risk factor and the disease?

2.2.3 The Cohort Study

A *cohort study* involves a group of individuals who usually meet a set of inclusion criteria at the start of the study. The cohort is followed and associations are made between a risk factor and a disease. For example, if we are studying risk factors for cardiovascular disease, we would ideally enroll a cohort of individuals free of cardiovascular disease at the start of the study. In a prospective cohort study, participants are enrolled and followed going forward in time (see Figure 2–2). In some

cases, the cohort is drawn from the general population, whereas in other cases a cohort is assembled. For example, when studying the association between a relatively common risk factor and an outcome, a cohort drawn from the general population will likely include sufficient numbers of individuals who have and do not have the risk factor of interest.

When studying the association between a rare risk factor and an outcome, special attention must be paid to constructing the cohort. In this instance, investigators might want to enrich the cohort to include participants with the risk factor (sometimes called a special exposure cohort). In addition, an appropriate comparison cohort would be included. The comparison group would include participants free of the risk factor but similar to the exposed cohort in other important characteristics. In a retrospective cohort study, the exposure or risk factor status of the participants is ascertained retrospectively, or looking back in time (see Figure 2–3 and the time of study start). For example, suppose we wish to assess the association between multivitamin use and neural tube defects in newborns. We enroll a cohort of women who delivered live born infants and ask each to report on their use of multivitamins before becoming pregnant. On the basis of these reports, we have an exposed and unexposed cohort. We then assess the outcome of the pregnancy for each woman. Retrospective cohort studies are often based on data gathered from medical records where risk factors and outcomes have occurred and been documented. A study is mounted and records are reviewed to assess risk factor and outcome status, both of which have already occurred.

The prospective cohort study is the more common cohort study design. These cohort studies have a major advantage in that they allow investigators to assess temporal relationships. It is also possible to estimate the incidence of a disease (i.e., the rate at which participants who are free of a disease develop that disease). We can also compare incidence rates between groups. For example, we might compare the incidence of cardiovascular disease between participants who smoke and participants who do not smoke as a means of quantifying the association between smoking and cardiovascular disease. Cohort studies can be difficult if the outcome or disease under study is rare or if there is a long latency period (i.e., it takes a long time for the disease to develop or be realized). When the disease is rare, the cohort must be sufficiently large so that adequate numbers of events (cases of disease) are observed. By adequate numbers, we mean specifically that there are sufficient numbers of events to produce stable, precise inferences employing meaningful statistical analyses. When the disease under study has a long latency

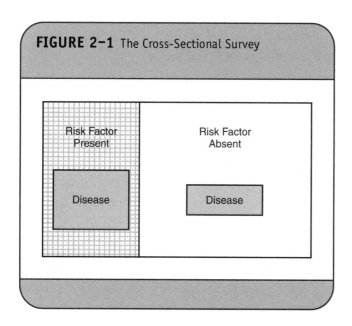

FIGURE 2–1 The Cross-Sectional Survey

Risk Factor Present

Risk Factor Absent

Disease

Disease

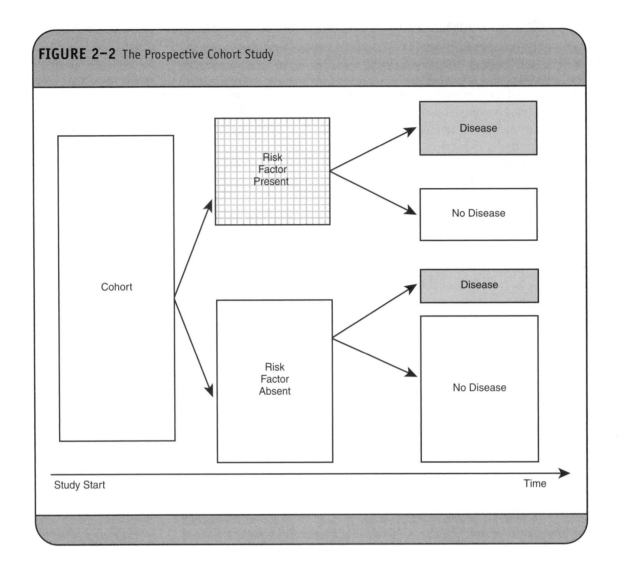

FIGURE 2–2 The Prospective Cohort Study

Cohort

Risk Factor Present

Risk Factor Absent

Disease

No Disease

Disease

No Disease

Study Start

Time

period, the study must be long enough in duration so that sufficient numbers of events are observed. However, this can introduce another difficulty in a loss of participant follow-up over a longer study period.

Cohort studies can also be complicated by confounding. *Confounding* is a distortion of the effect of an exposure or risk factor on the outcome by other characteristics. For example, suppose we wish to assess the association between smoking and cardiovascular disease. We may find that smokers in our cohort are much more likely to develop cardiovascular disease. However, it may also be the case that the smokers are less likely to exercise, have higher cholesterol levels, and so on. These complex relationships among the variables must be reconciled by statistical analyses. In Chapter 9, we will describe in detail the methods used to handle confounding.

2.2.4   The Case-Control Study

The *case-control study* is a study often used in epidemiologic research where again the question of interest is whether there is an association between a particular risk factor or exposure and an outcome. Case-control studies are particularly useful when the outcome of interest is rare. As noted previously, cohort studies are not efficient in this setting as they would require that large numbers of participants be enrolled in the study to realize a sufficient number of outcome events. In a case-control study, participants are identified on the basis of their outcome status. Specifically, we select a set of cases, or persons with the outcome of interest. We then select a set of controls, who are persons similar to the cases except for the fact that they are free of the outcome of interest. We then assess exposure or risk factor status retrospectively (see Figure 2–4).

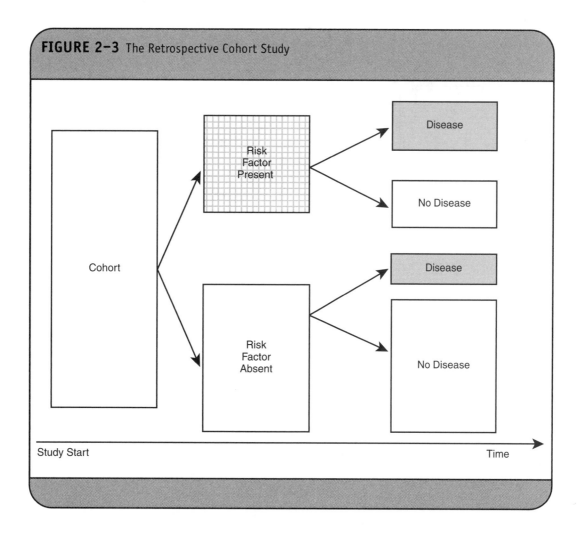

FIGURE 2-3 The Retrospective Cohort Study

Cohort

Risk Factor Present

Risk Factor Absent

Disease

No Disease

Disease

No Disease

Study Start

Time

We hypothesize that the exposure is related to the disease and evaluate this by comparing the cases and controls with respect to the proportions that are exposed; that is, we draw inferences about the relationship between exposure or risk factor status and disease. There are a number of important issues that must be addressed in designing case-control studies. We will detail some of the most important ones.

First, cases must be selected very carefully. An explicit definition is needed to identify cases so that the cases are as homogeneous as possible. The explicit definition of a case must be established before any participants are selected or data collected. Diagnostic tests to confirm disease status should be included whenever possible to minimize the possibility of incorrect classification.

Controls must also be selected carefully. The controls should be comparable to the cases in all respects except for the fact that they do not have the disease of interest. In fact, the controls should represent non-diseased participants who would have been included as cases if they had the disease.

The same diagnostic tests used to confirm disease status in the cases should be applied to the controls to confirm non-disease status.

Usually, there are many more controls available for inclusion in a study than cases, so it is often possible to select several controls for each case, thereby increasing the sample size for analysis. Investigators have shown that taking more than four controls for each case does not substantially improve the precision of the analysis.[3] (This result will be discussed in subsequent chapters.) In many instances, two controls per case are selected and are denoted as a 2:1 ("two to one") control to case ratio.

The next issue is to assess exposure or risk factor status, and this is done retrospectively. Because the exposure or risk factor might have occurred long ago, studies that can establish risk factor status based on documentation or records are preferred over those that rely on a participant's memory of past events. Sometimes, such data are not documented, so participants are queried with regard to risk

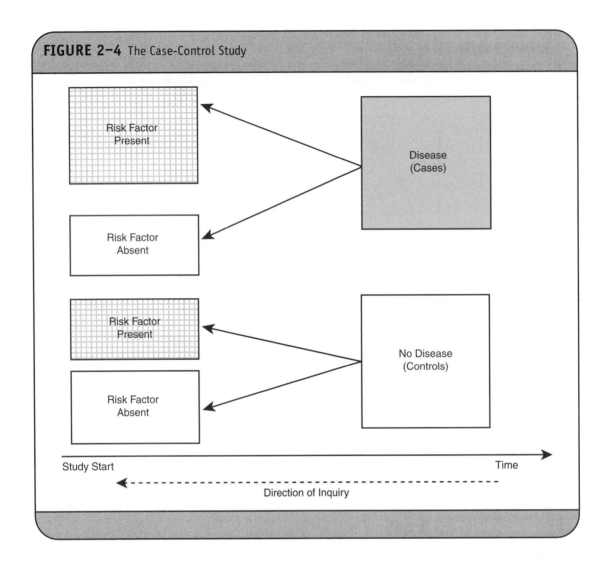

FIGURE 2-4 The Case-Control Study

factor status. This must be done in a careful and consistent manner for all participants, regardless of their outcome status—assessment of exposure or risk factor status must be performed according to the same procedures or protocol for cases and controls. In addition, the individual collecting exposure data should not be aware of the participant's outcome status (i.e., they should be blind to whether the participant is a case or a control).

Case-control studies have several positive features. They are cost- and time-efficient for studying rare diseases. With case-control studies, an investigator can ensure that a sufficient number of cases are included. Case-control studies are also efficient when studying diseases with long latency periods. Because the study starts after the disease has been diagnosed, investigators are not waiting for the disease to occur during the study period. Case-control studies are also useful when there are several potentially harmful exposures under consideration; data can be collected on each exposure and evaluated.

The challenges of the case-control study center mainly around bias. We will discuss several of the more common sources of bias here; there are still other sources of bias to consider. Misclassification bias can be an issue in case-control studies and refers to the incorrect classification of outcome status (case or control) or the incorrect classification of exposure status. If misclassification occurs at random—meaning there is a similar extent of misclassification in both groups—then the association between the risk factor and the outcome can be dampened (underestimated). If misclassification is not random—for example, if more cases are incorrectly classified as having the exposure or risk factor—then the association can be exaggerated (overestimated). Another source of bias is called selection bias, and it can result in a distortion of the association (over- or underestimation of the true association) between exposure and outcome status resulting from the selection of cases and controls. Specifically, the relationship between exposure status and disease may be different in those individuals who chose to participate in the study as compared to those who did not. Yet another source of bias is called recall bias, and again, it can result in adistortion of the association between exposure and outcome. It occurs when cases or controls differentially recall exposure status. It is possible that persons with a disease (cases) might be more likely to recall prior exposures than persons free of the disease. The latter might not recall the same information as readily. With case-control studies, it is also not always possible to establish a temporal relationship between exposure and outcome. For example, in the present example both the exposure and outcome are measured at the time of data collection. Finally, because of the way we select participants (on the basis of their outcome status) in case-control studies, we cannot estimate incidence (i.e., the rate at which a disease develops).

2.2.5 The Nested Case-Control Study

The *nested case-control study* is a specific type of case-control study that is usually designed from a cohort study. For example, suppose a cohort study involving 1000 participants is run to assess the relationship between smoking and cardiovascular disease. In the study, suppose that 20 participants develop myocardial infarction (MI, i.e., heart attack) and we are interested in assessing whether there is a relationship between body mass index (measured as the ratio of weight in kilograms to height in meters squared) and MI. With so few participants suffering this very specific outcome, it would be difficult analytically to assess the relationship between body mass index and MI because there are a number of confounding factors that would need to be taken into account. This process generally requires large samples (specifics will be discussed in Chapter 9). A nested case-control study could be designed to select suitable controls for the 20 cases that are similar to the cases except that they are free of MI. To facilitate the analysis, we would carefully select the controls and might match the controls to cases on gender, age, and other risk factors known to affect MI, such as blood pressure and cholesterol. Matching is one way of handling confounding. The analysis would then focus specifically on the association between body mass index and MI.

2.3 RANDOMIZED STUDY DESIGNS

Cohort and case-control studies often address the question: Is there an association between a risk factor or exposure and an outcome (e.g., a disease)? Each of these observational study designs has its advantages and disadvantages. In the cohort studies, we compare incidence between the exposed and unexposed

groups, whereas in the case-control study we compare exposure between those with and without a disease. These are different comparisons, but in both scenarios, we make inferences about associations. (In Chapter 6 and Chapter 7, we will detail the statistical methods used to estimate associations and to make statistical inferences.) As we described, observational studies can be subject to bias and confounding. In contrast, randomized studies are considered to be the gold standard of study designs as they minimize bias and confounding. The key feature of randomized studies is the random assignment to the comparison groups. In theory, randomizing makes the groups comparable in all respects except the way the participants are treated (e.g., treated with an experimental medication or a placebo, treated with a behavioral intervention, or not). We will describe two popular randomized designs in detail.

2.3.1 The Randomized Controlled Trial (RCT) or Clinical Trial

The *randomized controlled trial* (RCT) is a design with a key and distinguishing feature—the randomization of participants to one of several comparison treatments or groups. In pharmaceutical trials, there are often two comparison groups; one group gets an experimental drug and the other a control drug. If ethically feasible, the control might be a placebo. If a placebo is not ethically feasible (e.g., it is ethically inappropriate to use a placebo because participants need medication), then a medication currently available and considered the standard of care would be an appropriate comparator. This is called an active-controlled trial as opposed to a placebo-controlled trial. In clinical trials, data are collected prospectively (see Figure 2–5).

The idea of randomization is to balance the groups in terms of known and unknown prognostic factors (i.e., characteristics that might affect the outcome), which minimizes confounding. Because of the randomization feature, the comparison groups—in theory—differ only in the treatment received. One group receives the experimental treatment and the other does not. With clinical trials, we can make much stronger inferences than we can with observational studies. Specifically, with clinical trials, inferences are made with regard to the effect of treatments on outcomes, whereas with observational studies, inferences are limited to associations between risk factors and outcomes.

It is important in clinical trials that the comparison treatments are evaluated concurrently. In the study depicted in Figure 2.5, the treatments are administered at the same point in time, generating parallel comparison groups. Consider a clinical trial evaluating an experimental treatment for allergies. If the experimental treatment is given during the spring

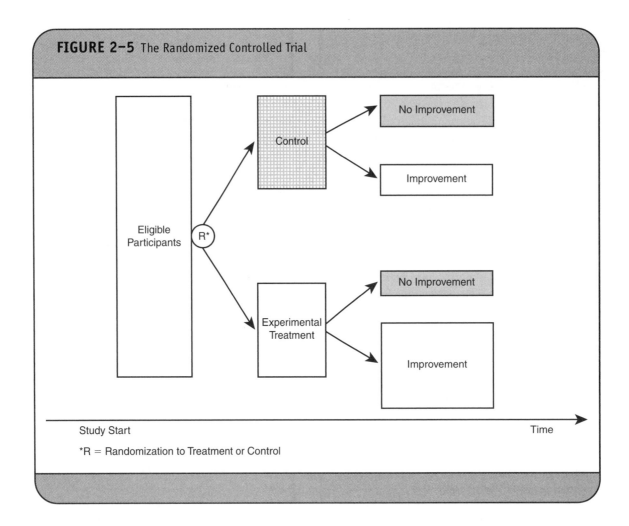

FIGURE 2–5 The Randomized Controlled Trial

and the control is administered during the winter, we might see very different results simply because allergies are highly dependent on the season or the time of year.

It is also important in clinical trials to include multiple study centers, often referred to as multicenter trials. The reason for including multiple centers is to promote generalizability. If a clinical trial is conducted in a single center and the experimental treatment is shown to be effective, there may be a question as to whether the same benefit would be seen in other centers. In multicenter trials, the homogeneity of the effect across centers can be analyzed directly.

Ideally, clinical trials should be double blind. Specifically, neither the investigator nor the participant should be aware of the treatment assignment. However, sometimes it is impossible or unethical to blind the participants. For example, consider a trial comparing a medical and a surgical procedure. In this situation, the participant would definitely know whether they underwent a surgical procedure. In some very rare situations, sham surgeries are performed but these are highly unusual, as participant safety is always of the utmost concern. It

is critical that the outcome assessor is blind to the treatment assignment.

There are many ways to randomize participants in clinical trials. Simple randomization involves essentially flipping a coin and assigning each participant to either the experi-mental or the control treatment on the basis of the coin toss. In multicenter trials, separate randomization schedules are usually developed for each center. This ensures a balance in the treatments within each center and does not allow for the possibility that all patients in one center get the same treatment. Sometimes, it is important to minimize imbal-ance between groups with respect to other characteristics. For example, suppose we wanted to be sure we had participants of similar ages in each of the comparison groups. We could develop separate or stratified randomization schedules for participants less than 40 years of age and participants 40 years of age and older within each center. There are many ways to perform the randomization and the appropriate procedure depends on many factors, including the relationship between important prognostic factors and the outcome, the number of centers involved, and so on.

The major advantage of the clinical trial is that it is the cleanest design from an analytic point of view. Randomization minimizes bias and confounding so, theoretically, any benefit (or harm) that is observed can be attributed to the treatment. However, clinical trials are often expensive and very time-consuming. Clinical trials designed around outcomes that are relatively rare require large numbers of participants to demonstrate a significant effect. This increases the time and cost of conducting the trial. There are often a number of challenges in clinical trials that must be faced. First, clinical trials can be ethically challenging. Choosing the appropriate control group requires careful assessment of ethical issues. For example, in cancer trials it would never be possible to use a placebo comparator, as this would put participants at unnecessary risk. Next, clinical trials can be difficult to set up. Recruitment of centers and participants can be difficult. For example, participants might not be willing to participate in a trial because they cannot accept the possibility of being randomly assigned to the control group. Careful monitoring of participants is also a crucial aspect of clinical trials. For example, investigators must be sure that participants are taking the assigned drug as planned and are not taking other medications that might interfere with the study medications (called concomitant medications). Most clinical trials require frequent follow-up with participants—for example, every 2 weeks for 12 weeks. Investigators must work to minimize loss to follow-up to ensure that important study data are collected at every time point during the study. Subject retention and adherence to the study protocol are essential for the success of a clinical trial.

In some clinical trials, there are very strict inclusion and exclusion criteria. For example, suppose we are evaluating a new medication hypothesized to lower cholesterol. To allow the medication its best chance to demonstrate benefit, we might include only participants with very high total cholesterol levels. This means that inferences about the effect of the medication would then be limited to the population from which the participants were drawn. Clinical trials are sometimes criticized for being too narrow or restrictive. In designing trials, investigators must weigh the impact of the inclusion and exclusion criteria on the observed effects and on their generalizability.

Designing clinical trials can be very complex. There are a number of issues that need careful attention, including: refining the study objective so that it is clear, concise, and answerable; determining the appropriate participants for the trial (detailing inclusion and exclusion criteria explicitly); determining the appropriate outcome variable; deciding on the appropriate control group; developing and implementing a strict monitoring plan; determining the number of participants to enroll; and detailing the randomization plan. While achieving these goals is challenging, a successful randomized clinical trial is considered the best means of establishing the effectiveness of a medical treatment.

2.3.2 The Crossover Trial

The *crossover trial* is a clinical trial where each participant is assigned to two or more treatments sequentially. When there are two treatments (e.g., an experimental and a control), each participant receives both treatments. For example, half of the participants are randomly assigned to receive the experimental treatment first and then the control; the other half receive the control first and then the experimental treatment. Outcomes are assessed following the administration of each treatment in each participant (see Figure 2–6). Participants receive the randomly assigned treatment in Period 1. The outcome of interest is then recorded for the Period 1 treatment. In most crossover trials, there is then what is a called a wash-out period where no treatments are given. The wash-out period is included so that any therapeutic effects of the first treatment are removed prior to administering the second treatment in Period 2. In a trial with an experimental and a control treatment, Period 2 participants who received the control treatment during Period 1 receive the experimental treatment in Period 2 and vice versa.

There are several ways in which participants can be assigned to treatments in a crossover trial. The two most popular schemes are called random and fixed assignment. In the random assignment scheme (already mentioned), participants are randomly assigned to the experimental treatment or the control. Participants are then assigned the other treatment in Period 2. In a fixed assignment strategy, all participants are assigned the same treatment sequence. For example, everyone gets the experimental treatment first, followed by the control treatment or vice versa. There is an issue with the fixed scheme in that investigators must assume that the outcome observed on the second treatment (and subsequent treatments, if there are more than two) would be equivalent to the outcome that would be observed if that treatment were assigned first (i.e., that there are no carry-over effects). Randomly varying the order in which the treatments are given allows the investigators to assess whether there is any order effect.

The major advantage to the crossover trial is that each participant acts as their own control; therefore, we do not need to worry about the issue of treatment groups being comparable with respect to baseline characteristics. In this study design, fewer participants are required to demonstrate an effect. A disadvantage is that there may be carry-over effects such that the outcome assessed following the second treatment

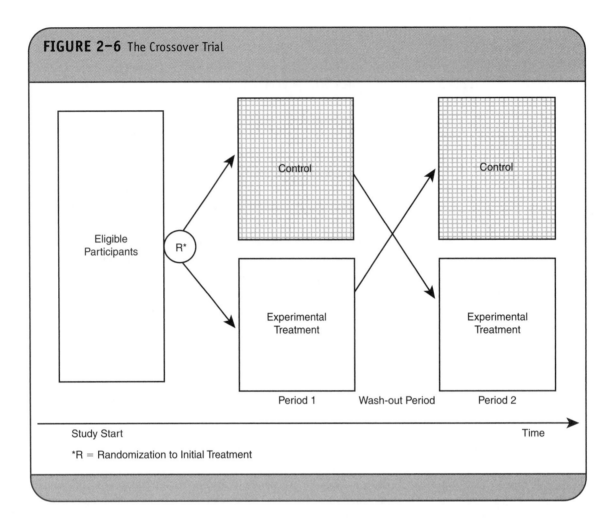

FIGURE 2–6 The Crossover Trial

Control

Control

Eligible
Participants

R*

Experimental
Treatment

Experimental
Treatment

Period 1   Wash-out Period   Period 2

Study Start   Time

*R = Randomization to Initial Treatment

is affected by the first treatment. Investigators must be careful to include a wash-out period that is sufficiently long to minimize carry-over effects. A participant in Period 2 may not be at the same baseline as they were in Period 1, thus destroying the advantage of the crossover. In this situation, the only useful data may be from Period 1. The wash-out period must be short enough so that participants remain committed to completing the trial. Because participants in a crossover trial receive each treatment, loss to follow-up or dropout is critical because losing one participant means losing outcome data on both treatments.

Crossover trials are best suited for short-term treatments of chronic, relatively stable conditions. A crossover trial would not be efficient for diseases that have acute flare-ups because these could influence the outcomes that are observed yet have nothing to do with treatment. Crossover trials are also not suitable for studies with death or another serious condition considered as the outcome.

Similar to the clinical trial described previously, adherence or compliance to the study protocol and study medication

in the crossover trial is critical. Participants are more likely to skip medication or drop out of a trial if the treatment is unpleasant or if the protocol is long or difficult to follow. Every effort must be made on the part of the investigators to maximize adherence and to minimize loss to follow-up.

2.4   THE FRAMINGHAM HEART STUDY

We now describe one of the world's most well-known studies of risk factors for cardiovascular disease. The Framingham Heart Study started in 1948 with the enrollment of a cohort of just over 5000 individuals free of cardiovascular disease who were living in the town of Framingham, Massachusetts.[1] The Framingham Heart Study is a longitudinal cohort study that involves repeated assessments of the participants approximately every two years. The study celebrated its fiftieth anniversary in 1998 and it still continues today. The original cohort has been assessed 28 times. At each assessment, complete physical examinations are conducted (e.g., vital signs, blood pressure, medication history), blood samples are taken to measure lipid levels and novel risk factors, participants also have echocardiograms in addition to other assessments of cardiovascular functioning. In the early 1970s, approximately 5000 offspring of the original cohort and their spouses were enrolled into what was called the Framingham Offspring cohort (the second generation of the original cohort). These participants have been followed approximately every four years and have been assessed over eight times. In the early 2000s, a third generation of over 4000 participants was enrolled and they will be followed approximately every four years.

Over the past 50 years, hundreds of papers have been published from the Framingham Heart Study identifying important risk factors for cardiovascular disease such as smoking, blood pressure, cholesterol, physical inactivity, and diabetes. This study also identified risk factors for stroke, heart failure, and peripheral artery disease. Researchers have identified psychosocial risk factors for heart disease and now with three generations of participants in the Framingham Study, investigators are assessing genetic risk factors for obesity, diabetes, and cardiovascular disease. More details on the Framingham Heart Study, its design, investigators, research milestones, and publications can be found at *http://www.nhlbi.nih.go v/about/ framingham* and at *http://www.bu.edu/alumni/bostonia/2005/ summer/pdfs/heart.pdf*.

2.5   MORE ON CLINICAL TRIALS

Clinical trials are extremely important, particularly in medical research. In Section 2.3, we outlined clinical trials from a design standpoint but there are many more aspects of clinical trials that should be mentioned. First, clinical trials must be conducted at the correct time in the course of history. For example, suppose we ask the research question: Is the Polio vaccine necessary today? To test this hypothesis, a clinical trial could be initiated in which some children receive the vaccine while others do not. The trial would not be feasible today because it would be unethical to withhold the vaccine from some children. No one would risk the consequences of the disease to study whether the vaccine is necessary.

As noted previously, the design of a clinical trial is extremely important to ensure the generalizability and validity of the results. Well-designed clinical trials are very easy to analyze, whereas poorly designed trials are extremely difficult, sometimes impossible, to analyze. The issues that must be considered in designing clinical trials are outlined here. Some have been previously identified but are worth repeating.

The number of treatments involved. If there are two treatments involved, statistical analyses are straightforward because only one comparison is necessary. If more than two treatments are involved, then more complicated statistical analyses are required and the issue of multiple comparisons must be addressed (these issues will be discussed in Chapter 7 and Chapter 9). The number of treatments involved in a clinical trial should always be based on substantive criteria and not be reduced to simplify statistical analysis.

The control treatment. In clinical trials, an experimental (or newly developed) treatment is compared against a control treatment. The control treatment may be a treatment that is currently in use and considered the standard care, or the control treatment may be a placebo. If a standard treatment exists, it should be used as the control because it would be unethical to offer patients a placebo when a conventional treatment is available. (While clinical trials are considered the gold standard design to evaluate the effectiveness of an experimental treatment, there are instances where a control group is not available. Techniques to evaluate effectiveness in the absence of a control group are described in D'Agostino and Kwan.[4])

Outcome measures. The outcome or outcome measures of interest must be clearly identified in the design phase of the clinical trial. The primary outcome is the one specified in the planned analysis and is used to determine the sample size required for the trial (this is discussed in detail in Chapter 8). Primary outcomes are usually more objective than subjective in nature. It is appropriate to specify secondary outcomes, and results based on secondary outcomes should be reported as such. Analyses of secondary outcomes can provide important information and, in some cases, enough evidence for a follow-up trial in which the secondary outcomes become the primary outcomes.

Blinding. Blinding refers to the fact that patients are not aware of which treatment (experimental or control) they are receiving in the clinical trial. A single blind trial is one in which the investigator knows which treatment a patient is receiving but the patient does not. Double blinding refers to the situation in which both the patient and the investigator are not aware of which treatment is assigned. In many clinical trials, only the statistician knows which treatment is assigned to each patient. In all cases, the investigator measuring the outcome should be unaware of the treatment assignment.

Single versus multicenter trials. Some clinical trials are conducted at a single site or clinical center, whereas others are conducted—usually simultaneously—at several centers. There are advantages to including several centers, such as increased generalizability and an increased number of available patients. There are also disadvantages to including multiple centers, such as needing more resources to manage the trial and the introduction of center-specific characteristics (e.g., expertise of personnel, availability or condition of medical equipment, specific characteristics of participants) that could affect the observed outcomes.

Randomization. Randomization is a critical component of clinical trials. There are a number of randomization strategies that might be implemented in a given trial. The exact strategy depends on the specific details of the study protocol.

Sample size. The number of patients required in a clinical trial depends on the variation in the primary outcome and the expected difference in outcome scores between the treatment and control patients.

Population and sampling. The study population should be explicitly defined by the study investigators (patient inclusion and exclusion criteria). A strategy for patient recruitment must be carefully determined and a system for checking inclusion and exclusion criteria for each potential enrollee must be developed and followed.

Ethics. Ethical issues often drive the design and conduct of clinical trials. There are some ethical issues that are common to all clinical trials, such as the safety of the treatments involved. There are other issues that relate only to certain trials. Most institutions have Institutional Review Boards (IRBs) that are responsible for approving research study protocols. Research protocols are evaluated on the basis of scientific accuracy and with respect to potential risks and benefits to participants. All participants in clinical trials must provide informed consent, usually on consent forms approved by the appropriate IRB.

Protocols. Each clinical trial should have a manual of operations or procedures in which every aspect of the trial is clearly defined. The protocol details all aspects of subject enrollment, treatment assignment, data collection, monitoring, data management, and statistical analysis. The protocol ensures consistency in the conduct of the trial and is particularly important when a trial is conducted at several clinical centers (i.e., in a multicenter trial).

Monitoring. Monitoring is a critical aspect of all clinical trials. Specifically, participants are monitored with regard to their adherence to all aspects of the study protocol (e.g., attending all scheduled visits, completing study assessments, taking the prescribed medications or treatments). Participants are also carefully monitored for any side effects or adverse events. Protocol violations (e.g., missing scheduled visits) are summarized at the completion of a trial, as are the frequencies of adverse events.

Data management. Data management is a critical part of any study and is particularly important in clinical trials. Data management includes tracking subjects (ensuring that subjects complete each aspect of the trial on time), data entry, quality control (examining data for out-of-range values or inconsistencies), data cleaning, and constructing analytic databases. In most studies, a data manager is assigned to supervise all aspects of data management.

The statistical analysis in a well-designed clinical trial is straightforward. Assuming there are two treatments involved (an experimental treatment and a control), there are essentially three phases of analysis:

- Baseline comparisons, in which the patients assigned to the experimental treatment group are compared to the patients assigned to the control group with respect to relevant characteristics measured at the baseline. These analyses are used to check that the randomization was successful in generating balanced groups.
- Crude analysis, in which outcomes are compared between patients assigned to the experimental and control treatments. In the case of a continuous outcome (e.g., weight), the difference in means is estimated; in the case of a dichotomous outcome (e.g., development of disease or not), relative risks are estimated; and in the case of time-to-event data (e.g., time to a heart attack), survival curves are estimated. (The specifics of these analyses are discussed in detail in Chapter 6 and Chapter 7.)
- Adjusted analyses are then performed, similar to the crude analysis, which incorporate important covariates (i.e., variables that are associated with the outcome) and confounding variables. (The specifics of statistical adjustment are discussed in detail in Chapter 9.)

There are several analytic samples considered in statistical analysis of clinical trials data. The first is the Intent to Treat (ITT) analysis sample. It includes all patients who were randomized. The second is the Per Protocol analysis sample, and it includes only patients who completed the treatment (i.e., followed the treatment protocol as designed). The third is the Safety analysis sample, and it includes all patients who took at least one dose of the assigned treatment even if they did not complete the treatment protocol. All aspects of the design, conduct, and analysis of a clinical trial should be carefully documented. Complete and accurate records of the clinical trial are essential for applications to the Food and Drug Administration (FDA).[5]

Clinical trials are focused on safety and efficacy. Safety is assessed by the nature and extent of adverse events (side effects). Adverse events may or may not be due to the drug under testing. In most clinical trials, clinicians indicate whether the adverse event is likely due to the drug or not. Efficacy is assessed by improvements in symptoms or other aspects of the indication or disease that the drug was designed to address.

There are several important stages in clinical trials. Preclinical studies are studies of safety and efficacy in animals.

Clinical studies are studies of safety and efficacy in humans. There are three phases of clinical studies, described here.

Phase I: First Time in Humans Study. The main objectives in a Phase I study are to assess the toxicology and safety of the proposed treatment in humans and to assess the pharmacokinetics (how fast the drug is absorbed in, flows through, and is secreted from the body) of the proposed treatment. Phase I studies are not generally focused on efficacy (how well the treatment works); instead, safety is the focus. Phase I studies usually involve 10 to 15 patients, and many Phase I studies are performed in healthy, normal volunteers to assess side effects and adverse events. In Phase I studies, one goal is to determine the maximum tolerated dose (MTD) of the proposed drug in humans. Investigators start with very low doses and work up to higher doses. Investigations usually start with three patients, and three patients are added for each elevated dose. Data are collected at each stage to assess safety, and some Phase I studies are placebo-controlled. Usually, two or three separate Phase I studies are conducted.

Phase II: Feasibility or Dose-Finding Study. The focus of a Phase II study is still on safety, but of primary interest are side effects and adverse events (which may or may not be directly related to the drug). Another objective in the Phase II study is efficacy, but the efficacy of the drug is based on descriptive analyses in the Phase II study. In some cases, investigators do not know which specific aspects of the indication or disease the drug may affect or which outcome measure best captures this effect. Usually, investigators measure an array of outcomes to determine the best outcome for the next phase. In Phase II studies, investigators determine the optimal dosage of the drug with respect to efficacy (e.g., lower doses might be just as effective as the MTD). Phase II studies usually involve 50 to 100 patients who have the indication or disease of interest. Phase II studies are usually placebo-controlled or compared to a standard, currently available treatment. Subjects are randomized and studies are generally double blind. If a Phase II study indicates that the drug is safe but not effective, investigation cycles back to Phase I. Most Phase II studies proceed to Phase III based on observed safety and efficacy.

Phase III: Confirmatory Clinical Trial. The focus of the Phase III trial is efficacy, although data are also collected to monitor safety. Phase III trials are designed and executed to confirm the effect of the experimental treatment. Phase III trials usually involve two treatment groups, an experimental treatment at the determined optimal dose and a placebo or standard of care treatment. Some Phase III trials involve three groups: placebo, standard care, and experimental treatment. Sample sizes can range from 200 to 500 patients, depending on what is determined to be a clinically significant effect. (The exact number is deter-

mined by specific calculations that are described in Chapter 8.) At least two successful clinical trials performed by independent investigators at different clinical centers are required in Phase III studies to assess whether the effect of the treatment can be replicated by independent investigators in at least two different sets of participants. More details on the design and analysis of clinical trials can be found in Chow and Liu.[6]

Investigators need positive results (statistically proven efficacy) in at least two separate trials to submit an FDA application for drug approval. The FDA also requires clinical significance in two trials, with clinical significance specified by clinical investigators in the design phase when the number of subjects is determined (see Chapter 8).

The FDA New Drug Application (NDA) contains a summary of results of Phase I, Phase II, and Phase III studies. The FDA reviews an NDA within six months to one year after submission and grants approval or not. If a drug is approved, the sponsor may conduct Phase IV trials, also called post-marketing trials, that can be retrospective (e.g., based on medical record review) or prospective (e.g., a clinical trial involving many patients to study rare adverse events). These studies are often undertaken to understand the long-term effects (efficacy and safety) of the drug.

2.6   SAMPLE SIZE IMPLICATIONS

Biostatisticians have a critical role in designing studies, not only to work with investigators to select the most efficient design to address the study hypotheses but also to determine the appropriate number of participants to involve in the study. In Chapter 8, we provide formulas to compute the sample sizes needed to appropriately answer research questions. The sample size needed depends on the study design, the anticipated effect of the drug (e.g., the difference between the experimental and control drugs) and also on the statistical analysis that will be used to answer the study questions. The sample size should not be too small such that an answer about the drug under investigation is not possible because in this instance, both participants and the investigators have wasted time and money. Alternatively, a sample size should not be too large because again time and money would be wasted but, in addition, participants may have been placed at unnecessary risk. Both scenarios are unacceptable from an ethical standpoint, and therefore careful attention must be paid when determining the appropriate sample size for any study or trial.

2.7   SUMMARY

To determine which study design is most efficient for a specific application, investigators must have a specific, clearly defined study question. It is also important to understand current research on the topic under investigation. The most efficient design depends on the expected association or effect, the prevalence or incidence of outcomes, the prevalence of risk factors or exposures, and the expected duration of the study. Also important are practical issues, costs and—most important—ethical issues.

Choosing the appropriate study design to address a research question is critical. Whenever possible, prior to mounting a planned study, investigators should try to run a pilot or feasibility study, which is a smaller-scale version of the planned study, as a means to identify potential problems and issues. Whereas pilot studies can be time-consuming and costly, they are usually more than worthwhile.

2.8 PRACTICE PROBLEMS

1. An investigator wants to assess whether smoking is a risk factor for pancreatic cancer. Electronic medical records at a local hospital will be used to identify 50 patients with pancreatic cancer. One hundred patients who are similar but free of pancreatic cancer will also be selected. Each participant's medical record will be analyzed for smoking history. Identify the type of study proposed and indicate its specific strengths and weaknesses.

2. What is the most likely source of bias in the study described in Problem 1?

3. An investigator wants to assess whether the use of a specific medication given to infants born prematurely is associated with developmental delay. Fifty infants who were given the medication and 50 comparison infants who were also born prematurely but not given the medication will be selected for the analysis. Each infant will undergo extensive testing at age 2 for various aspects of development. Identify the type of study proposed and indicate its specific strengths and weaknesses.

4. Is bias or confounding more of an issue in the study described in Problem 3? Give an example of a potential source of bias and a potential confounding factor.

5. A study is planned to assess the effect of a new surgical intervention for gall bladder disease. One hundred patients with gall bladder disease will be randomly assigned to receive either the new surgical intervention or the standard surgical intervention. The efficacy of the new surgical intervention will be measured by the time a patient takes to return to normal activities, recorded in days. Identify the type of study proposed and indicate its specific strengths and weaknesses.

6. An investigator wants to assess the association between caffeine consumption and impaired glucose

tolerance, a precursor to diabetes. A study is planned to include 70 participants. Each participant will be surveyed with regard to their daily caffeine consumption. In addition, each participant will submit a blood sample that will be used to measure their glucose level. Identify the type of study proposed and indicate its specific strengths and weaknesses.

7. Could the study described in Problem 6 be designed as a randomized clinical trial? If so, briefly outline the study design; if not, describe the barriers.

8. A study is planned to compare two weight-loss programs in patients who are obese. The first program is based on restricted caloric intake and the second is based on specific food combinations. The study will involve 20 participants and each participant will follow each program. The programs will be assigned in random order (i.e., some participants will first follow the restricted-calorie diet and then follow the food-combination diet, whereas others will first follow the food-combination diet and then follow the restricted-calorie diet). The number of pounds lost will be compared between diets. Identify the type of study proposed and indicate its specific strengths and weaknesses.

9. An orthopedic surgeon observes that many of his patients coming in for total knee replacement surgery played organized sports before the age of 10. He plans to collect more extensive data on participation in organized sports from four patients undergoing knee replacement surgery and to report the findings. Identify the type of study proposed and indicate its specific strengths and weaknesses.

10. Suggest an alternative design to address the hypothesis in Problem 9. What are the major issues in addressing this hypothesis?

REFERENCES

1. D'Agostino, R.B. and Kannel, W.B. "Epidemiological background and design: The Framingham Study." *Proceedings of the American Statistical Association Sesquicentennial Invited Paper Sessions*, 1989: 707–719.

2. Gottlieb, M.S., Schroff, R., Scganker, H.M., Weisman, J.D., Fan, P.T., Wolf, R.A., and Saxon, A. "*Pneumocystis carinii* pneumonia and *mucosal candidiasis* in previously healthy homosexual men: Evidence of a new acquired cellular immunodeficiency." *New England Journal of Medicine*, 1981; 305(24): 1425–1431.

3. Schelesselman, J.J. *Case-Control Studies: Design, Conduct, Analysis*. New York: Oxford University Press, 1982.

4. D'Agostino, R.B. and Kwan, H. "Measuring effectiveness: What to expect without a randomized control group." *Medical Care*, 1995; 33(4 Suppl.): AS95–105.

5. United States Food and Drug Administration. Available at *http://www.fda.gov*.

6. Chow, S.C. and Lie, J.P. *Design and Analysis of Clinical Trials: Concepts and Methodologies*. New York: John Wiley & Sons, 1998.

CHAPTER 3

Quantifying the Extent of Disease

In Chapter 2, we presented several different study designs that are popular in public health research. In subsequent chapters, we discuss statistical procedures to analyze data collected under different study designs. In statistical analyses, we first describe information we collect in our study sample and then estimate or make generalizations about the population based on data observed in the sample. The first step is called *descriptive statistics* and the second is called *inferential statistics*. Our goal is to present techniques to describe samples and procedures for generating inferences that appropriately account for variability in our estimates. Remember that we analyze only a fraction or subset, called a sample, of the entire population, and based on that sample we make inferences about the larger population. Before we get to those procedures, we will focus on some important measures for quantifying disease. Two quantities that are often used in epidemiological and biostatistical analysis are prevalence and incidence. We will describe each in turn and then discuss measures that are used to compare groups in terms of prevalence and incidence of disease.

3.1 PREVALENCE

Prevalence refers to the proportion of participants with a disease at a particular point in time. Consider the prospective cohort study we described in Chapter 2 where a cohort of participants is enrolled at a specific time. We call the initial point or starting point of the study the baseline time point. Suppose in our cohort study each individual undergoes a complete physical examination at baseline. At this initial examination, we determine—among other things—whether each participant has a history of (i.e., has been previously diagnosed with) cardiovascular disease (CVD). An estimate of

the prevalence of CVD is computed by taking the ratio of the number of existing cases of CVD to the total number of participants examined. This is called the point prevalence (PP) of CVD as it refers to the extent of disease at a specific point in time (i.e., at baseline in our example).

$$\text{Point prevalence} = \frac{\text{Number of persons with disease}}{\text{Number of persons examined at baseline}}$$

Example 3.1. The fifth examination of the offspring in the Framingham Heart Study was conducted between 1991 and 1995. A total of $n = 3799$ participants participated in the fifth examination. Table 3–1 shows the numbers of men and women with diagnosed CVD at the fifth examination. The point prevalence of CVD among all participants attending the fifth examination of the Framingham Offspring Study is $379 / 3799 = 9.98\%$. The point prevalence of CVD among men is $244 / 1792 = 13.62\%$, and the point prevalence of CVD among women is $135 / 2007 = 6.73\%$.

Table 3–2 contains data on prevalent CVD among participants who were currently smoking cigarettes at the time of the fifth examination of the Framingham Offspring Study. Almost 20% ($744 / 3799$) of the participants attending the fifth

TABLE 3–1 Men and Women with Diagnosed CVD

	Free of CVD	History of CVD	Total
Men	1548	244	1792
Women	1872	135	2007
Total	3420	379	3799

TABLE 3-2 Men and Women Currently Smoking

	Free of CVD	History of CVD	Total
Non-smoker	2757	298	3055
Current smoker	663	81	744
Total	3420	379	3799

examination of the Framingham Offspring study reported that they were current smokers at the time of the exam. The point prevalence of CVD among nonsmokers was 298 / 3055 = 9.75%, and the point prevalence of CVD among current smokers was 81 / 744 = 10.89%.

3.2   INCIDENCE

In epidemiological studies, we are often more concerned with estimating the likelihood of developing disease rather than the proportion of people who have a disease at a point in time. The latter reflects prevalence, whereas *incidence* reflects the likelihood of developing a disease among a group of participants free of the disease who are considered at risk of developing the disease over a specified observation period. Consider the study described previously and suppose we remove participants with a history of CVD from our fixed cohort at baseline so that only participants free of CVD are included (i.e., those who are truly "at risk" of developing a disease). We follow these participants prospectively for 10 years and record, for each individual, whether or not they develop CVD during this follow-up period. If we are able to follow each individual for 10 years and can ascertain whether or not each develops CVD, then we can directly compute the likelihood or risk of developing CVD over 10 years. Specifically, we take the ratio of the number of new cases of CVD to the total number of participants free of disease at the outset. This is referred to as cumulative incidence (CI):

Cumulative incidence =

$$\frac{\text{Number of persons who develop a disease during a specified period}}{\text{Number of persons at risk (at baseline)}}$$

Cumulative incidence reflects the proportion of participants who become diseased during a specified observation period. The total number of persons at risk is the same as the total number of persons included at baseline who are disease-free. The computation of cumulative incidence assumes that all of these individuals are followed for the entire observation period. This may be possible in some applications—for example, during an acute disease outbreak with a short follow-up or observation period. However, in longer studies it can be difficult to follow every individual for the development of disease because some individuals may relocate, may not respond to investigators, or may die during the study. In this example, the cohort is older (as is the case in most studies of cardiovascular disease, as well as in studies of any other diseases that occur more frequently in older persons) and the follow-up period is long (10 years), making it difficult to follow every individual. Methods to handle incomplete follow-up are described later.

3.2.1   Problems Estimating the Cumulative Incidence

There are a number of problems that can arise that make estimating the cumulative incidence of disease difficult. Because studies of incidence are by definition longitudinal (e.g., 5 or 10 years of follow-up), some study participants may be lost over the course of the follow-up period. Some participants might choose to drop out of the study, others might relocate, and others may die during the follow-up period. Different study designs could also allow for participants to enter at different times (i.e., all participants are not enrolled at baseline but instead, there is a rolling or prolonged enrollment period). For these and other reasons, participants are often followed for different lengths of time. We could restrict attention to only those participants who completed the entire follow-up; however, this would result in ignoring valuable information. A better approach involves accounting for the varying follow-up times as described here.

3.2.2   Person-Time Data

Again, in epidemiological studies we are generally interested in estimating the probability of developing disease (incidence) over a particular time period (e.g., 10 years). The cumulative incidence assumes that the total population at risk is followed for the entire observation period and that the disease status is ascertained for each member of the population. For the reasons stated previously, it is not always possible to follow each individual for the entire observation period.

Making use of the varying amounts of time that different participants contribute to the study results in changing the unit of analysis from the person or study participant to one of person-time, which is explicitly defined. The time unit might be months or years (e.g., person-months or person-years). For example, suppose that an individual enters a study in 1990 and is followed until 2000, at which point they are determined to be disease-free. A second individual enters the same study in

1995 and develops the disease under study in 2000. The first individual contributes 10 years of disease-free follow-up time, whereas the second individual contributes five years of disease-free follow-up time and then contracts the disease. We would want to use all of this information to estimate the incidence of the disease. Together, these two participants contribute 15 years of disease-free time.

3.2.3　Incidence Rate

The *incidence rate* uses all available information and is computed by taking the ratio of the number of new cases to the total follow-up time (i.e., the sum of all disease-free person-time). Rates are estimates that attempt to deal with the problem of varying follow-up times and reflect the likelihood of an individual changing disease status (e.g., developing disease) in a specified unit of time. The denominator is the sum of all of the disease-free follow-up times, specifically time during which participants were considered at risk for developing the disease. Rates are based on a specific time period (e.g., 5 years, 10 years) and are usually expressed as an integer value per a multiple of participants over a specified time (e.g., the incidence of disease is 12 per 1000 person-years).

The incidence rate (IR), also called the incidence density (ID), is computed by taking the ratio of the number of new cases of disease to the total number of person-time units available. These person-time units may be person-years (e.g., one individual may contribute 10 years of follow-up, whereas another may contribute five years of follow-up) or person-months (e.g., 360 months, 60 months). The denominator is the sum of all of the participants' time at risk (i.e., disease-free time). The IR or ID is reported as a rate relative to a specific time interval (e.g., 5 per 1000 person-years). The incidence rate is given as:

Incidence Rate =

$$\frac{\text{Number of persons who develop disease during a specified period}}{\text{Sum of the lengths of time during which persons are disease-free}}$$

For presentation purposes, the incidence rate is usually multiplied by some multiple of 10 (e.g., 100, 1000, 10,000) to produce an integer value (see Example 3.2).

Example 3.2. Consider again the fifth examination of the offspring in the Framingham Heart Study. As described in Example 3.1, a total of $n = 3799$ participants attended the fifth examination, and 379 had a history of CVD. This leaves a total of $n = 3420$ participants free of CVD at the fifth examination. Suppose we follow each participant for the development of CVD over a 10-year period. Table 3–3 shows the numbers of men and women who develop CVD over a 10-year follow-up period.

TABLE 3–3 Men and Women who Develop CVD

	Developed		
	No CVD	**CVD**	**Total**
Men	1358	190	1548
Women	1753	119	1872
Total	3111	309	3420

TABLE 3–4 Total Disease-Free Time in Men and Women

	Developed CVD	Total Follow-Up Time (years)	IR
Men	190	9984	0.01903
Women	119	12153	0.00979
Total	309	22137	0.01396

Because each participant was not followed for the full 10-year period (the mean follow-up time was 7 years), we cannot correctly estimate cumulative incidence using the previous data. The estimate of the cumulative incidence assumes that each of the 3111 persons free of CVD is followed for 10 years. Because this was not the case, our estimate of cumulative incidence would be incorrect; instead, we must sum all of the available follow-up time and estimate an incidence rate. Table 3–4 displays the total disease-free follow-up times for men and women along with the incidence rates. The incidence rates could be reported as 190 per 10,000 person-years for men and 98 per 10,000 person-years for women; equivalent to this is 19 per 1000 men per 10 years and 9.8 per 1000 women per 10 years.

The denominator of the incidence rate accumulates disease-free time over the entire observation period, and the unit of analysis is person-time (e.g., person-years in Example 3.2). In comparison, the denominator of the cumulative incidence is measured at the beginning of the study (baseline) and the unit of analysis is the person. It is worth noting that rates have dimensions (number of new cases per person-time units) and are often confused with probabilities or proportions, which are dimensionless. Example 3.3 illustrates the difference between the prevalence, cumulative incidence, and incidence rate. It is important to note that the time component is an integral part of the denominator of the incidence rate, whereas with the cumulative incidence the time component is only part of the interpretation.

Example 3.3. Consider a prospective cohort including six participants. Each participant is enrolled at baseline, and the goal of the study is to follow each participant for 10 years. Over the course of the follow-up period, some participants develop CVD and some die. Figure 3–1 displays the course of follow-up for each participant. In this example, Participant 1 develops CVD six years into the study, Participant 2 dies nine years into the study but is free of CVD, Participant 3 survives the complete follow-up period disease-free, Participant 4 develops CVD two years into the study and dies after eight years, Participant 5 drops out of the study after seven disease-free years, and Participant 6 develops CVD five years into the study.

Using the data in Example 3.3, we will now compute prevalence, cumulative incidence, and incidence rate.

$$\text{Prevalence of CVD at baseline} = 0/6 = 0\%$$

$$\text{Prevalence of CVD at 5 years} = 2/6 = 33\%$$

$$\text{Prevalence of CVD at 10 years} = 2/3 = 67\%$$

(Note that we can only assess disease status in Participants 1, 3, and 6.)

$$\text{Cumulative incidence of CVD at 5 years} = 2/6 = 33\%$$

$$\text{Cumulative incidence of CVD at 10 years} = 3/6 = 50\%$$

$$\text{10-year incidence rate of CVD} =$$
$$3/(6+9+10+2+7+5) = 3/39 = 0.0769$$

We could report this as an incidence rate of CVD of 7.7 per 100 persons over 10 years (or as 7.7 per 1000 person-years).

$$\text{Incidence rate of death per person-year} = 2/(10+9+10+$$
$$8+7+10) = 2/54 = 0.037$$

We could report this as an incidence rate of death of 37 per 1000 person-years (or 3.7 per 100 persons over 10 years).

Notice that the prevalence and cumulative incidence are shown as percents (these could also be shown as proportions or probabilities), whereas the incidence rates are reported as the number of events per person-time.

3.3 RELATIONSHIPS BETWEEN PREVALENCE AND INCIDENCE

The prevalence (proportion of the population with a disease at a point in time) of a disease depends on the incidence (risk of developing disease within a specified time) of the disease as well as the duration of the disease. If the incidence is high but the duration is short, the prevalence (at a point in time) will be low by comparison. In contrast, if the incidence is low but the duration of the disease is long, the prevalence will be

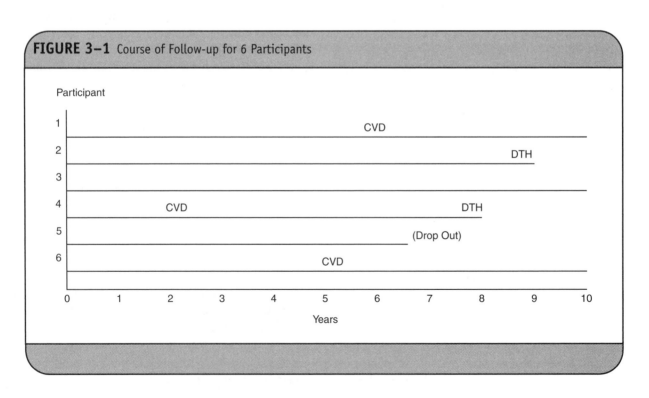

FIGURE 3–1 Course of Follow-up for 6 Participants

high. When the prevalence of disease is low (less than 1%), the prevalence is approximately equal to the product of the incidence and the mean duration of the disease (assuming that there have not been major changes in the course of the disease or its treatment).[1] Hypertension is an example of a disease with a relatively high prevalence and low incidence (due to its long duration). Influenza is an example of a condition with low prevalence and high incidence (due to its short duration).

The incidence rate is interpreted as the instantaneous potential to change the disease status (i.e., from non-diseased to diseased, also called the hazard) per unit time. An assumption that is implicit in the computation of the IR or ID is that the risk of disease is constant over time. This is not a valid assumption for many diseases because the risk of disease can vary over time and among certain subgroups (e.g., persons of different ages have different risks of disease). It is also very important that only persons who are at risk of developing the disease of interest are included in the denominator of the estimate of incidence. For example, if a disease is known to affect only people over 65 years of age, then including disease-free follow-up time measured on study participants less than 65 years of age will underestimate the true incidence. Person-times measured in these participants should not be included in the denominator as they are not truly at risk of developing the disease prior to age 65.

3.4   COMPARING THE EXTENT OF DISEASE BETWEEN GROUPS

It is often of interest to compare groups with respect to their likelihood of developing a disease. These groups might be defined by an exposure to a potentially harmful agent (e.g., exposed or not), by a particular socio-demographic characteristic (e.g., men or women) or by a particular risk factor (e.g., current smoker or not). Popular comparative measures are generally categorized as difference measures or ratios. Differences or ratios can be constructed to compare prevalence measures or incidence measures between comparison groups.

3.4.1   Difference Measures: Risk Difference and Population Attributable Risk

The *risk difference* (RD), also called excess risk, measures the absolute effect of the exposure or the absolute effect of the risk factor of interest on prevalence or cumulative incidence. The risk difference is defined as the difference in point prevalence or cumulative incidence between groups and is given by the following:

$$\text{Risk difference} = PP_{exposed} - PP_{unexposed}$$

In Example 3.1, we computed the point prevalence of CVD for smokers and nonsmokers. Exposed persons are those who reported smoking at the fifth examination of the Framingham Offspring Study. Using data from Example 3.1, the risk difference in CVD for smokers as compared to nonsmokers is computed by subtracting the point prevalence for nonsmokers from the point prevalence for smokers. The risk difference is $0.1089 - 0.0975 = 0.0114$, and this indicates that the absolute risk of CVD is 0.0114 higher among smokers as compared to nonsmokers. The risk difference can also be computed by taking the difference in cumulative incidences between comparison groups. The risk difference represents the excess risk associated with exposure to the risk factor, and the range of possible values is −1 to +1. The risk difference is positive when the risk for those exposed is greater than that for those unexposed. The risk difference can be negative if the risk for those exposed is less than the risk for those unexposed. If exposure to the risk factor is unrelated to the risk of disease, then the risk difference will be 0. A value of 0 is the null or no-difference value of the risk difference.

The *population attributable risk* (PAR) is another difference measure that quantifies the association between a risk factor and the prevalence or cumulative incidence of disease. The population attributable risk is computed as follows:

$$\text{Population attributable risk} = \frac{PP_{overall} - PP_{unexposed}}{PP_{overall}}$$

The population attributable risk is computed by first assessing the difference in overall risk (exposed and unexposed persons combined) and the risk of those unexposed. This difference is then divided by the overall risk and is usually presented as a percentage. Using data presented in Example 3.1, the risk of CVD for all participants attending the fifth examination of the Framingham Offspring Study is 379 / 3799 = 0.0998. The population attributable risk is computed as (0.0998 − 0.0975) / 0.0998 = 0.023 = 2.3%. The population attributable risk ranges from 0% to 100%. The magnitude of the population attributable risk is interpreted as the percentage of risk associated with, or attributable to, the risk factor. If exposure to the risk factor is unrelated to the risk of disease, then the population attributable risk is 0% (i.e., none of the risk is associated with exposure to the risk factor). The population attributable risk is also interpreted as the percentage of the risk that could be eliminated if the exposure or risk factor were removed.

3.4.2 Ratios: Relative Risk, Odds Ratio, and Rate Ratio

The *relative risk* (RR), also called the risk ratio, is a useful measure to compare the prevalence or cumulative incidence of disease between two groups. It is computed by taking the ratio of the respective prevalences or cumulative incidences. Generally, the reference group (e.g., unexposed persons, persons without the risk factor, or persons assigned to the control group in a clinical trial setting) is considered in the denominator:

$$\text{Relative risk} = \frac{PP_{exposed}}{PP_{unexposed}}$$

The relative risk is often felt to be a better measure of the strength of the effect than the risk difference (or attributable risk) because it is relative to a baseline (or comparative) level. Using data presented in Example 3.1, the relative risk of CVD for smokers as compared to nonsmokers is 0.1089 / 0.0975 = 1.12; that is, the prevalence of CVD is 1.12 times higher among smokers as compared to nonsmokers. The range of the relative risk is 0 to infinity. If exposure to the risk factor is unrelated to the risk of disease, then the relative risk will be 1. A value of 1 is considered the null or no-effect value of the relative risk.

Under some study designs (e.g., the case control study described in Chapter 2), it is not possible to compute a relative risk. Instead, an *odds ratio* is computed as a measure of effect. Suppose in a case-control study that we want to assess the relationship between exposure to a particular risk factor and disease status. Recall that in a case-control study, we select participants on the basis of their outcome—some have the condition of interest (cases) and some do not (controls).

Example 3.4. Table 3–5 shows the relationship between prevalent hypertension and prevalent cardiovascular disease at the fifth examination of the offspring in the Framingham Heart Study. The probability that a person with hypertension has CVD is 181 / 840 = 0.216. The probability that a person free of hypertension has CVD is 188 / 2942 = 0.064. Odds are different from probabilities in that odds are computed as the ratio of the number of events to the number of nonevents, whereas a probability is the ratio of the number of events to the total sample size. The odds that a person with hypertension has CVD are 181 / 659 = 0.275. The

odds that a person free of hypertension has CVD are 188 / 2754 = 0.068. The relative risk of CVD for persons with as compared to without hypertension is 0.216 / 0.064 = 3.38, or persons with hypertension are 3.38 times more likely to have prevalent CVD than persons without hypertension. The *odds ratio* is computed in a similar way but based on the ratio of odds. The odds ratio is 0.275 / 0.068 = 4.04 and is interpreted as: The odds of developing CVD are 4.04 times higher in people with hypertension as compared to people without hypertension.

Perhaps the most important characteristic of an odds ratio is its invariance property. Using the previous data, the odds that a person with CVD has hypertension are 181 / 188 = 0.963. The odds that a person free of CVD has hypertension are 659/ 2754 = 0.239. The odds ratio for hypertension is therefore 0.963 / 0.239 = 4.04. This property does not hold for a relative risk. For example, the probability that a person with CVD has hypertension is 181 / 369 = 0.491. The probability that a person free of CVD has hypertension is 659 / 3413 = 0.193. The relative risk for hypertension is 0.491 / 0.193 = 2.54.

The invariance property of the odds ratio makes it an ideal measure of association for a case-control study. For example, suppose we conduct a case-control study to assess the association between cigarette smoking and a rare form of cancer (e.g., a cancer that is thought to occur in less than 1% of the general population). The cases are individuals with the rare form of cancer and the controls are similar to the cases but free of the rare cancer. Suppose we ask each participant whether they formerly smoked or are currently smoking cigarettes. The data are shown in Table 3–6.

Using these data, we cannot calculate the incidence of cancer in the total sample or the incidence of cancer in smokers or in nonsmokers because of the way in which we collected the data. In this sample, 40 / 69 = 0.58 = 58% of the smokers have cancer and 10 / 31 = 0.32 = 32% of the nonsmokers have cancer—yet this is a rare cancer. These estimates do not reflect reality because the sample was

TABLE 3–5 Prevalent Hypertension and Prevalent CVD

	No CVD	CVD	Total
No hypertension	2754	188	2942
Hypertension	659	181	840
Total	3413	369	3782

specifically designed to include an equal number of cases and controls. Had we sampled individuals at random from the general population (using a cohort study design), we might have needed to sample more than 10,000 individuals to realize a sufficient number of cases for analysis. With this case-control study, we can estimate an association between smoking and cancer using the odds ratio. The odds of cancer in smokers are 40 / 29 = 1.379 and the odds of cancer in nonsmokers are 10 / 21 = 0.476. The odds ratio is 1.379 / 0.476 = 2.90, suggesting that smokers are 2.9 times more likely to have cancer than nonsmokers. Note that this is equal to the odds ratio of smoking in cases versus controls, i.e., (40 / 10) / (29 / 21) = 4 / 1.39 = 2.9.

The fact that we can estimate an odds ratio in a case-control study is a useful and important property. The odds ratio estimated in a study using a prospective sampling scheme (i.e., sampling representative groups of smokers and non-smokers and monitoring for cancer incidence) is equivalent to the odds ratio based on a retrospective sampling scheme (i.e., sampling representative groups of cancer and patients free of cancer and recording smoking status).

The odds can also be computed by taking the ratio of the point prevalence (PP) or cumulative incidence (CI) of disease to (1 − PP) or (1 − CI), respectively. The odds ratio is the ratio of the odds of developing disease for persons exposed as compared to those unexposed. Using cumulative incidences, the odds ratio is defined as:

$$\text{Odds ratio} = \frac{CI_{exposed}/1\text{-}CI_{exposed}}{CI_{unexposed}/1\text{-}CI_{unexposed}}$$

The odds ratio will approximate the relative risk when the disease under study is rare, usually defined as a prevalence or cumulative incidence less than 10%. For this reason, the interpretation of an odds ratio is often taken to be identical to that of a relative risk when the prevalence or cumulative incidence is low.

TABLE 3–6 Smoking and Cancer

	Cancer (Case)	No Cancer (Control)	Total
Smoker	40	29	69
Nonsmoker	10	21	31
Total	50	50	100

The *rate ratio* is a useful measure to compare incidence rates between two groups. It is computed by taking the ratio of the respective incidence rates. The rate ratio is similar to the risk ratio described previously, which was used to compare prevalences or cumulative incidences between groups, except that the rate ratio is based on person-time data rather than individual-level data.

3.4.3   Issues with Person-Time Data

There are some special characteristics of person-time data that need attention, one of which is censoring. *Censoring* occurs when the event of interest (e.g., disease status) is not observed on every individual, usually due to time constraints (e.g., the study follow-up period ends, subjects are lost to follow-up, or they withdraw from the study). In epidemiological studies, the most common type of censoring that occurs is called right censoring. Suppose that we conduct a longitudinal study and monitor subjects prospectively over time for the development of CVD. For participants who develop CVD, their time to event is known; for the remaining subjects, all we know is that they did not develop the event during the observation period. For these participants, their time-to-event (also called their survival time) is longer than the observation time. For analytic purposes, these times are censored and are called Type I censored or right-censored times. Methods to handle survival time, also called time-to-event data, are discussed in detail in Allison.[2]

3.5   SUMMARY

Prevalence and incidence measures are important measures that quantify the extent of disease in study populations. Understanding the difference between prevalence and incidence is critical. Prevalence refers to the extent of a disease at a point in time, whereas incidence refers to the development of disease over a specified time. Because it can be difficult to ascertain disease status in every participant in longitudinal studies—particularly when the follow-up period is long—measures that take into account all available data are needed. Incidence rates that account for varying follow-up times are useful measures in epidemiological analysis.

The formulas to estimate and compare prevalence and incidence are summarized in Table 3–7. In the next chapter, we will present descriptive statistics. Specifically, we will discuss how to estimate prevalence and incidence in study samples. We will then move into statistical inference procedures, where we will discuss estimating unknown population parameters based on sample statistics.

TABLE 3–7 Summary of Key Formulas

Measure	Formula
Point prevalence (PP)*	$\dfrac{\text{Number of persons with disease}}{\text{Number of persons examined at baseline}}$
Cumulative incidence (CI)*	$\dfrac{\text{Number of persons who develop disease during a specified period}}{\text{Number of persons at risk (at baseline)}}$
Incidence rate (IR)	$\dfrac{\text{Number of persons who develop disease during a specified period}}{\text{Sum of the lengths of time during which persons are disease-free}}$
Risk difference (RD)	$PP_{exposed} - PP_{unexposed}$
Population attributable risk (PAR)	$\dfrac{PP_{overall} - PP_{unexposed}}{PP_{overall}}$
Relative risk (RR)	$\dfrac{PP_{exposed}}{PP_{unexposed}}$
Odds ratio (OR)	$\dfrac{PP_{exposed}/(1-PP_{exposed})}{PP_{unexposed}/(1-PP_{unexposed})}$

* Can also be expressed as a percentage.

3.6   PRACTICE PROBLEMS

1. A cohort study is conducted to assess the association between clinical characteristics and the risk of stroke. The study involves $n = 1250$ participants who are free of stroke at the study start. Each participant is assessed at study start (baseline) and every year thereafter for five years. Table 3–8 displays data on hypertension status measured at baseline and hypertension status measured two years later.

    a. Compute the prevalence of hypertension at baseline.

    b. Compute the prevalence of hypertension at two years.

    c. Compute the incidence of hypertension over two years.

2. The data shown in Table 3–9 were collected in the study described in Problem 1 relating hypertensive status measured at baseline to incident stroke over five years.

    a. Compute the cumulative incidence of stroke in this study.

    b. Compute the cumulative incidence of stroke in patients classified as hypertensive at baseline.

    c. Compute the cumulative incidence of stroke in patients free of hypertension at baseline.

TABLE 3–8 Hypertension at Baseline and Two Years later

	Two Years Later: Not Hypertensive	Two Years Later: Hypertensive
Baseline: Not hypertensive	850	148
Baseline: hypertensive	45	207

TABLE 3–9 Hypertension at Baseline and Stroke Five Years Later

	Free of Stroke at Five Years	Stroke
Baseline: Not hypertensive	952	46
Baseline: Hypertensive	234	18

d. Compute the risk difference of stroke for patients with hypertension as compared to patients free of hypertension.

e. Compute the relative risk of stroke for patients with hypertension as compared to patients free of hypertension.

f. Compute the population attributable risk of stroke due to hypertension.

3. A case-control study is conducted to assess the relationship between heavy alcohol use during the first trimester of pregnancy and miscarriage. Fifty women who suffered miscarriage are enrolled, along with 50 who delivered full-term. Each participant's use of alcohol during pregnancy is ascertained. Heavy drinking is defined as four or more drinks on one occasion. The data are shown in Table 3–10.

a. Compute the odds of miscarriage in women with heavy alcohol use during pregnancy.

b. Compute the odds of miscarriage in women with no heavy alcohol use during pregnancy.

c. Compute the odds ratio for miscarriage as a function of heavy alcohol use.

4. A randomized trial is conducted to evaluate the efficacy of a new cholesterol-lowering medication. The primary outcome is incident coronary artery disease. Participants are free of coronary artery disease at the start of the study and randomized to receive either the new medication or a placebo. Participants are followed for a maximum of 10 years for the development of coronary artery disease. The observed data are shown in Table 3–11.

a. Compute the relative risk of coronary artery disease for patients receiving the new cholesterol medication as compared to those receiving a placebo.

b. Compute the odds ratio of coronary artery disease for patients receiving the new cholesterol medication as compared to those receiving a placebo.

c. Which measure is more appropriate in this design, the relative risk or odds ratio? Justify briefly.

TABLE 3–10 Alcohol Use and Outcome of Pregnancy

	Miscarriage	Delivered Full Term
Heavy alcohol use	14	4
No heavy alcohol use	36	46

TABLE 3–11 Incident Coronary Artery Disease by Treatment

	Number of Participants	Number with Coronary Artery Disease
Cholesterol medication	400	28
Placebo	400	42

TABLE 3–12 Total Follow-Up Time by Treatment

	Number with Coronary Artery Disease	Total Follow-Up (years)
Cholesterol medication	28	3451
Placebo	42	2984

5. In the study described in Problem 4, some patients were not followed for a total of 10 years. Some suffered events (i.e., developed coronary artery disease during the course of follow-up), whereas others dropped out of the study. Table 3–12 displays the total number of person-years of follow-up in each group.

a. Compute the incidence rate of coronary artery disease in patients receiving the new cholesterol medication.

b. Compute the incidence rate of coronary artery disease in patients receiving a placebo.

6. A small cohort study is conducted in 13 patients with an aggressive cellular disorder linked to cancer. The clinical courses of the patients are depicted graphically in Figure 3–2.

a. Compute the prevalence of cancer at 12 months.

b. Compute the cumulative incidence of cancer at 12 months.

c. Compute the cumulative incidence of cancer at 24 months.

d. Compute the incidence rate (per month) of cancer.

REFERENCES

1. Hennekens, C.H. and Buring, J.E. *Epidemiology in Medicine.* Philadelphia: Lippincott, Williams & Wilkins, 1987.

2. Allison, P. *Survival Analysis Using SAS: A Practical Guide.* Cary, NC: SAS Institute, 1995.

FIGURE 3-2 Clinical Course for Patients with Aggressive Cellular Disorder

CHAPTER 4

Summarizing Data Collected in the Sample

Before any biostatistical analyses are performed, we must define the population of interest explicitly. The composition of the population depends on the investigator's research question. It is important to define it explicitly as inferences based on the study sample will only be generalizable to the specified population. The *population* is the collection of all individuals about whom we wish to make generalizations. For example, if we wish to assess the prevalence of cardiovascular disease (CVD) among all adults 30 to 75 years of age living in the United States, then all adults in that age range living in the United States at the specified time of the study constitute the population of interest. If we wish to assess the prevalence of CVD among all adults 30 to 75 years of age living in the state of Massachusetts, then all adults in that age range living in Massachusetts at the specified time of the study constitute the population of interest. If we wish to assess the prevalence of CVD among all adults 30 to 75 years of age living in the city of Boston, then all adults in that age range living in Boston at the specified time of the study constitute the population of interest.

In most applications, the population is so large that it is impractical to study the entire population. Instead, we select a sample (a subset) from the population and make inferences about the population based on the results of an analysis on the sample. The *sample* is a subset of individuals from the population. Ideally, individuals are selected from the population into the sample at random. (We discuss this procedure and other concepts related to sampling in detail in Chapter 5.)

There are a number of techniques that can be used to select a sample. Regardless of the specific techniques used, the sample should be representative of the population (i.e., the characteristics of individuals in the sample should be similar to those in the population). By definition, the number of individuals in the sample is smaller than the number of individuals in the population. There are formulas to determine the appropriate number of individuals to include in the sample that depend on the characteristic being measured (i.e., exposure, risk factor, or outcome) and the desired level of precision in the estimate. We present details about sample size computations in Chapter 8.

Once a sample is selected, the characteristic of interest must be summarized in the sample using appropriate techniques. This is the first step in an analysis. Once the sample is appropriately summarized, statistical inference procedures are then used to generate inferences about the population based on the sample. We discuss statistical inference procedures in Chapter 6, Chapter 7, and Chapter 9.

In this chapter, we present techniques to summarize data collected in a sample. The appropriate numerical summaries and graphical displays depend on the type of characteristic under study. Characteristics—sometimes called variables, outcomes, or endpoints—are classified as one of the following types: dichotomous, ordinal, categorical, or continuous.

Dichotomous variables have only two possible responses. The response options are usually coded "yes" or "no." Exposure to a particular risk factor (e.g., smoking) is an example of a dichotomous variable. Prevalent disease status is another example of a dichotomous variable, where each individual in a sample would be classified as having or not having the disease of interest at a point in time.

Ordinal and categorical variables have more than two possible responses but the response options are ordered and

TABLE 4–1 Blood Pressure Categories

Classification of Blood Pressure	SBP and/or DBP
Normal	<120 and <80
Pre-Hypertension	120–139 or 80–89
Stage I Hypertension	140–159 or 90–99
Stage II Hypertension	>160 and >100

unordered, respectively. Symptom severity is an example of an *ordinal variable* with possible responses of minimal, moderate, and severe. The National Heart, Lung, and Blood Institute (NHLBI) issues guidelines to classify blood pressure as normal, pre-hypertension, Stage I hypertension or Stage II hypertension.[1] The classification scheme is shown in Table 4–1 and is based on specific levels of systolic blood pressure (SBP) and diastolic blood pressure (DBP). Participants are classified into the highest category, as defined by their SBP and DBP.

Categorical variables, sometimes called nominal variables, are similar to ordinal variables except that the responses are unordered. Race/ethnicity is an example of a categorical variable. It is often measured using the following response options: white, black, Hispanic, American Indian or Alaskan native, Asian or Pacific Islander, or other. Another example of a categorical variable is blood type, with response options A, B, AB, and O.

Continuous variables, sometimes called quantitative or measurement variables, in theory take on an unlimited number of responses between defined minimum and maximum values. Systolic blood pressure, diastolic blood pressure, total cholesterol level, CD4 cell count, platelet count, age, height, and weight are all examples of continuous variables. For example, systolic blood pressure is measured in millimeters of mercury (mmHg) and an individual in a study could have a systolic blood pressure of 120, 120.2, or 120.23, depending on the precision of the instrument used to measure systolic blood pressure.

Almost all numerical summary measures depend on the specific type of variable under consideration. One exception is the sample size, which is an important summary measure for any variable type (dichotomous, ordinal, categorical, or continuous). The sample size, denoted as n, reflects the number of independent or distinct units (participants) in the sample. For example, if a study is conducted to assess the total cholesterol in a population and a random sample of 100 individuals is selected for participation, then $n = 100$ (assuming all individuals selected agree to participate). In some applications, the unit of analysis is not an individual participant but might be a blood sample or specimen.

Suppose in the example study that each of the 100 participants provides blood samples for cholesterol testing at three distinct points in time (e.g., at the start of the study, 6 and 12 months later). The unit of analysis could be the blood sample, in which case the sample size would be $n = 300$. It is important to note that these 300 blood samples are not 300 independent or unrelated observations because multiple blood samples were taken from each participant. Multiple measurements taken on the same individual are referred to as clustered or repeated measures data. Statistical methods that account for the clustering of measurements taken on the same individual must be used in analyzing the 300 total cholesterol measurements taken on participants over time. Details of these techniques can be found in Sullivan.[2] The sample size in most of the analyses discussed in this textbook refers to the number of individuals participating in the study. In the examples that follow, we will indicate the sample size. It is always important to report the sample size when summarizing data.

Numerical summary measures computed on samples are called statistics. (Summary measures computed on populations are called parameters.) The sample size is an example of an important statistic that should always be reported when summarizing data. In the following sections, we present sample statistics as well as graphical displays for each type of variable.

4.1 DICHOTOMOUS VARIABLES

Dichotomous variables take on one of only two possible responses. Gender is an example of a dichotomous variable, with response options of "male" or "female," as are current smoking status and diabetes status, with response options of "yes" or "no."

4.1.1 Descriptive Statistics for Dichotomous Variables

Dichotomous variables are often used to classify participants as possessing or not possessing a particular characteristic, having or not having a particular attribute. For example, in a study of cardiovascular risk factors we might collect information on participants such as whether or not they have diabetes, whether or not they smoke, and whether or not they are on treatment for high blood pressure or high cholesterol. The response options for each of these variables are "yes" or "no."

When analyzing dichotomous variables, responses are often classified as success or failure, with success denoting the response of interest. The success response is not necessarily the positive or healthy response but instead the response of interest. In fact, in many medical applications the focus is often on the unhealthy or "at-risk" response.

Example 4.1. The seventh examination of the offspring in the Framingham Heart Study was conducted between 1998 and 2001. A total of $n = 3539$ participants (1625 men and 1914 women) attended the seventh examination and completed an extensive physical examination. At that examination, numerous variables were measured including demographic characteristics such as gender, educational level, income, and marital status, clinical characteristics such as height, weight, systolic and diastolic blood pressure, and total cholesterol, and behavioral characteristics such as smoking and exercise.

Dichotomous variables are often summarized in frequency distribution tables. Table 4–2 displays a frequency distribution table for the variable gender measured in the seventh examination of the Framingham Offspring Study. The first column of the frequency distribution table indicates the specific response options of the dichotomous variable (in this example, male and female). The second column contains the frequencies (counts or numbers) of individuals in each response category (the numbers of men and women, respectively). The third column contains the relative frequencies, which are computed by dividing the frequency in each response category by the sample size (1625 / 3539 = 0.459). The relative frequencies are often expressed as percents by multiplying by 100 and are most often used to summarize dichotomous variables. For example, in this sample 45.9% are men and 54.1% are women.

Another example of a frequency distribution table is presented in Table 4–3, showing the distribution of treatment with anti-hypertensive medication in persons attending the seventh examination of the Framingham Offspring Study. Notice that there are only $n = 3532$ valid responses, although the sample size is actually $n = 3539$. There are seven individuals with missing data on this particular question. Missing data occurs in studies for a variety of reasons. When there is very little missing data (e.g., less than 5%) and there is no apparent pattern to the missingness (e.g., there is no systematic reason for missing data), then statistical analyses based on the available data is generally appropriate. However, if there is extensive missing data or if there is a pattern to the missingness, then

TABLE 4–3 Frequency Distribution Table for Treatment with Anti-Hypertensive Medication

	Frequency	Relative Frequency (%)
No treatment	2313	65.5
Treatment	1219	34.5
Total	3532	100.0

caution must be exercised in performing statistical analyses. Techniques for handling missing data are beyond the scope of this book; more details can be found in Little and Rubin.[3] From Table 4.3, we can see that 34.5% of the participants are currently being treated for hypertension.

Sometimes it is of interest to compare two or more groups on the basis of a dichotomous outcome variable. For example, suppose we wish to compare the extent of treatment with anti-hypertensive medication in men and women. Table 4–4 summarizes treatment with anti-hypertensive medication in men and women who attended the seventh examination of the Framingham Offspring Study. The first column of the table indicates the gender of the participant. Gender is a dichotomous variable and in this example, it is used to distinguish the comparison groups (men and women). The outcome variable is also a dichotomous variable and represents treatment with anti-hypertensive medication or not. A total of $n = 611$ men and $n = 608$ women are on anti-hypertensive treatment. Because there are different numbers of men and women (1622 versus 1910) in the study sample, comparing frequencies (611 versus 608) is not the most appropriate comparison. The frequencies indicate that almost equal numbers of men and women are on treatment. A more appropriate comparison is based on relative frequencies, 37.7% versus 31.8%, which incorporate the different numbers of men and women in the sample. Notice that the sum of the right-most column is not 100%, as it was in previous examples. In this example, the bottom row contains data on the total sample and

TABLE 4–2 Frequency Distribution Table for Gender

	Frequency	Relative Frequency (%)
Male	1625	45.9
Female	1914	54.1
Total	3539	100.0

TABLE 4–4 Treatment with Anti-Hypertensive Medication in Men and Women Attending the Seventh Examination of the Framingham Heart Study

	n	Number On Treatment	Relative Frequency (%)
Male	1622	611	37.7
Female	1910	608	31.8
Total	3532	1219	34.5

34.5% of all participants are being treated with anti-hypertensive medication. In Chapter 6 and Chapter 7, we will discuss formal methods to compare relative frequencies between groups.

4.1.2   Bar Charts for Dichotomous Variables

Graphical displays are very useful for summarizing data. There are many options for graphical displays, and many widely available software programs offer a variety of displays. However, it is important to choose the graphical display that accurately conveys information in the sample. The appropriate graphical display depends on the type of variable being analyzed. Dichotomous variables are best summarized using *bar charts*. The response options (yes/no, present/absent) are shown on the horizontal axis, and either the frequencies or relative frequencies are plotted on the vertical axis, producing a frequency bar chart or relative frequency bar chart, respectively.

Figure 4–1 is a frequency bar chart depicting the distribution of men and women who attended the seventh examination of the Framingham Offspring Study. The horizontal axis displays the two response options (men and women), and the vertical axis displays the frequencies (the numbers of men and women who attended the seventh examination).

Figure 4–2 is a relative frequency bar chart of the distribution of treatment with anti-hypertensive medication measured in the seventh examination of the Framingham Offspring Study. Notice that the vertical axis in Figure 4–2 displays relative frequencies and not frequencies, as was the case in Figure 4–1. In Figure 4–2, it is not necessary to show both responses as the relative frequencies, expressed as percentages, sum to 100%. If 65.5% of the sample is not being treated, then 34.5% must be on treatment. These types of bar charts are very useful for comparing relative frequencies between groups.

Figure 4–3 is a relative frequency bar chart describing treatment with anti-hypertensive medication in men versus women who attended the seventh examination of the Framingham Offspring Study. Notice that the vertical axis displays relative frequencies and in this example, 37.7% of men were using anti-hypertensive medications as compared to 31.8% of women. Figure 4–4 is an alternative display of the same data. Notice the scaling of the vertical axis. How do the relative frequencies compare visually? Finally, consider a third display of the same data, shown in Figure 4–5. How do the relative frequencies compare?

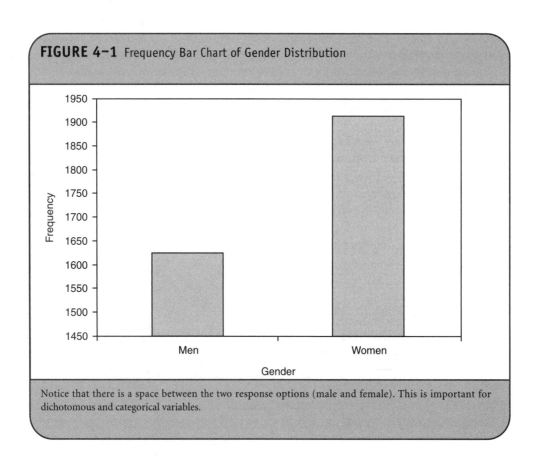

FIGURE 4–1 Frequency Bar Chart of Gender Distribution

Notice that there is a space between the two response options (male and female). This is important for dichotomous and categorical variables.

FIGURE 4-2 Relative Frequency Bar Chart of Distribution of Treatment with Anti-hypertensive Medication

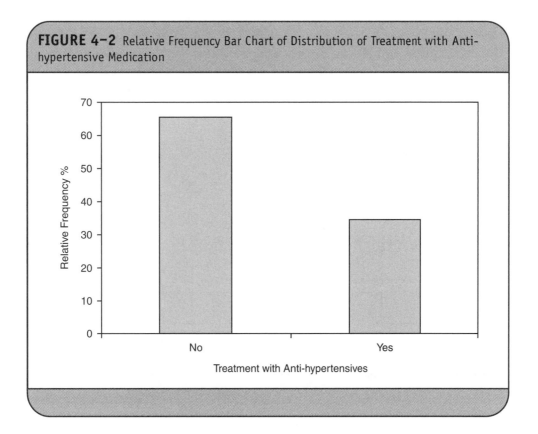

FIGURE 4-3 Relative Frequency Bar Chart of Distribution of Treatment with Anti-hypertensive Medication in Men and Women

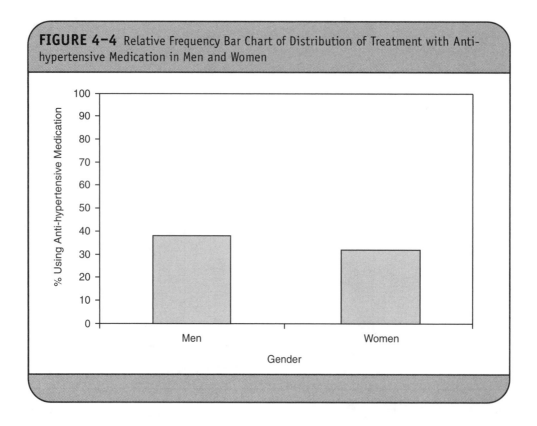

FIGURE 4–4 Relative Frequency Bar Chart of Distribution of Treatment with Anti-hypertensive Medication in Men and Women

The axes in any graphical display should be scaled to accommodate the range of the data. While relative frequencies can, in theory, range from 0% to 100%, it is not necessary to always scale the axes from 0% to 100%. It is also potentially misleading to restrict the scaling of the vertical axis, as was done in Figure 4–5, to exaggerate the difference in the use of anti-hypertensive medication between men and women, at least from a visual standpoint. In this example, the relative frequencies are 31.8% and 37.7%, and thus scaling from 0% to 40% is appropriate to accommodate the data. It is always important to label axes clearly so that readers can appropriately interpret the data.

4.2   ORDINAL AND CATEGORICAL VARIABLES

Ordinal and categorical variables have a fixed number of response options that are ordered and unordered, respectively. Ordinal and categorical variables typically have more than two distinct response options, whereas dichotomous variables have exactly two response options. Summary statistics for ordinal and categorical variables again focus primarily on relative frequencies (or percentages) of responses in each response category.

4.2.1   Descriptive Statistics for Ordinal and Categorical Variables

Consider again a study of cardiovascular risk factors such as the Framingham Heart Study. In the study, we might collect information on participants such as their blood pressure, total cholesterol, and body mass index (BMI). Often, clinicians classify patients into categories. Each of these variables—blood pressure, total cholesterol, and BMI—are continuous variables. In this section, we will organize continuous measurements into ordinal categories. For example, the NHLBI and the American Heart Association use the classification of blood pressure given in Table 4–1.[1,4,5] The American Heart Association uses the following classification for total cholesterol levels: desirable, less than 200 mg/dl; borderline high risk, 200–239 mg/dl; and high risk, 240 mg/dl or more.[4] Body mass index (BMI) is computed as the ratio of weight in kilograms to height in meters squared and the following categories are often used: underweight, less than 18.5; normal weight, 18.5–24.9; overweight, 25.0–29.9; and obese, 30.0 or greater. These are all examples of ordinal variables. In each case, it is healthier to be in a lower category.

Example 4.2. Using data from the seventh examination of the Offspring in the Framingham Heart Study ($n = 3539$), we can create the categories as defined previously for blood pressure, total cholesterol, and BMI. Frequency distribution tables, similar to those presented for dichotomous data, are also used to summarize categorical and ordinal variables. Table 4–5 is a frequency distribution table for the ordinal blood pressure variable. The mutually exclusive and exhaustive categories are shown in the first column of the table. The frequencies, or

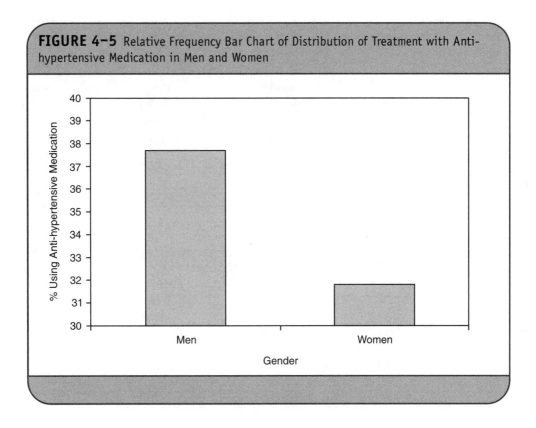

FIGURE 4–5 Relative Frequency Bar Chart of Distribution of Treatment with Anti-hypertensive Medication in Men and Women

numbers of participants in each response category, are shown in the middle column and the relative frequencies, as percents, are shown in the rightmost column.

Notice that there are only $n = 3533$ valid responses, whereas the sample size is $n = 3539$. There are six individuals with missing blood pressure data. More than a third of the sample (34.1%) has normal blood pressure, 41.1% are classified as pre-hypertensive, 18.5% have Stage I hypertension, and 6.3% have Stage II hypertension. With ordinal variables, two additional columns are often displayed in the frequency distribution table, called the cumulative frequency and cumulative relative frequency, respectively (see Table 4–6).

The cumulative frequencies in this example reflect the number of patients at the particular blood pressure level or below. For example, 2658 patients have normal blood pressure or pre-hypertension. There are 3311 patients with normal, pre-hypertension, or Stage I hypertension. The cumulative relative frequencies are very useful for summarizing ordinal variables and indicate the percent of patients at a particular level or below. In this example, 75.2% of the patients are not classified as hypertensive (i.e., they have normal blood pressure or pre-hypertension). Notice that for the last (highest) blood pressure category, the cumulative frequency is equal to the sample size ($n = 3533$) and the cumulative relative frequency is 100%, indicating that all of the patients are at the highest level or below.

Table 4–7 shows the frequency distribution table for total cholesterol. The total cholesterol categories are defined as follows and again are based on the measured cholesterol values. Persons are classified as having desirable total cholesterol if the measured total cholesterol is less than 200 mg/dl; borderline high total cholesterol, 200–239 mg/dl; and high total cholesterol, 240 mg/dl or more. At the seventh examination of the Framingham Offspring Study, 51.6% of the patients are classified as having desirable total cholesterol levels and another 34.3% have borderline high total cholesterol. Using the cumulative relative frequencies, we can summarize the data as

TABLE 4–5 Frequency Distribution Table for Blood Pressure Categories

	Frequency	Relative Frequency (%)
Normal	1206	34.1
Pre-hypertension	1452	41.1
Stage I hypertension	653	18.5
Stage II hypertension	222	6.3
Total	3533	100.0

TABLE 4–6 Frequency Distribution Table for Blood Pressure Categories with Cumulative Frequency and Cumulative Relative Frequency

	Frequency	Relative Frequency (%)	Cumulative Frequency	Cumulative Relative Frequency (%)
Normal	1206	34.1	1206	34.1
Pre-hypertension	1452	41.1	2658	75.2
Stage I Hypertension	653	18.5	3311	93.7
Stage II Hypertension	222	6.3	3533	100.0
Total	3533	100.0		

TABLE 4–7 Frequency Distribution Table for Total Cholesterol Categories

	Frequency	Relative Frequency (%)	Cumulative Frequency	Cumulative Relative Frequency (%)
Desirable	1712	51.6	1712	51.6
Borderline high	1139	34.3	2851	85.9
High	469	14.1	3320	100.0
Total	3320	100.0		

follows: 85.9% of patients have total cholesterol levels that are desirable or borderline high. The remaining 14.1% of patients are classified as having high cholesterol.

Table 4–8 is a frequency distribution table for the ordinal BMI variable. Both the weight and height are measured directly and the BMI is computed as described previously. In the seventh examination of the Framingham Offspring Study sample, 28.0% of the patients are classified as normal weight, 41.3% are classified as overweight, and 30.1% are classified as obese. Using the cumulative relative frequencies, almost 70% are underweight, normal weight, or overweight. This is equivalent to reporting that 70% of the sample is not obese.

Table 4–5 through Table 4–8 contain summary statistics for ordinal variables. The key summary statistics for ordinal variables are relative frequencies and cumulative relative frequencies. Table 4–9 through Table 4–11 contain summary statistics for categorical variables. Categorical variables are variables with two or more distinct responses but the responses are unordered. Some examples of categorical variables measured in the Framingham Heart Study include marital status, handedness, and smoking status. For categorical variables, frequency distribution tables with frequencies and relative frequencies provide appropriate summaries. Cumulative frequencies and cumulative relative frequencies are generally not useful for

TABLE 4–8 Frequency Distribution Table for Body Mass Index Categories

	Frequency	Relative Frequency (%)	Cumulative Frequency	Cumulative Relative Frequency (%)
Underweight	20	0.6	20	0.6
Normal weight	932	28.0	952	28.6
Overweight	1374	41.3	2326	69.9
Obese	1000	30.1	3326	100.0
Total	3326	100.0		

categorical variables, as it is usually not of interest to combine categories (as there is no inherent ordering).

Table 4–9 is a frequency distribution table for the categorical marital status variable. The mutually exclusive (non-overlapping) and exhaustive (covering all possible options) categories are shown in the first column of the table. The frequencies, or numbers of participants in each response category, are shown in the middle column, and the relative frequencies, as percents, are shown in the rightmost column. There are $n = 3530$ valid responses to the marital status question. A total of 9 participants did not provide marital status data. The majority of the sample is married (73.1%) and approximately 10% of the sample is divorced, another 10% is widowed, 6% is single, and 1% is separated. The relative frequencies are the most relevant statistics used to describe a categorical variable. Cumulative frequencies and cumulative relative frequencies are not generally informative descriptive statistics for categorical variables.

Because this is a categorical variable, there is no ordering to the responses and therefore the first column can be organized differently. For example, sometimes responses are presented from the most frequently to least frequently occurring in the sample, and sometimes responses are presented alphabetically. Any ordering is appropriate. In contrast, with ordinal variables there is an ordering to the responses and therefore response options can only be presented either from highest to lowest (healthiest to unhealthiest) or vice versa. The response options within an ordinal scale cannot be rearranged.

Table 4–10 is a frequency distribution table for a dichotomous categorical variable. Dichotomous variables are a special case of categorical variables with exactly two response options. Table 4–10 displays the distribution of the dominant hand of participants who attended the seventh examination of the Framingham Offspring Study. The response options are "right" or "left." There are $n = 3513$ valid responses to the dominant

hand assessment. A total of 26 participants did not provide data on their dominant hand. The majority of the Framingham sample is right-handed (89.5%). Table 4–11 is a frequency distribution table for a categorical variable reflecting smoking status. Smoking status here is measured as nonsmoker, former smoker, or current smoker. There are $n = 3536$ valid responses to the smoking status questions. Three participants did not provide adequate data to be classified. Almost half of the sample is former smokers (48.8%), over a third (37.6%) has never smoked, and approximately 14% are current smokers. The adverse health effects of smoking have been a major focus of public health messages in recent years, and the percentage of participants reporting as current smokers must be interpreted relative to the time of the study. Table 4–12 shows the proportions of participants reporting themselves as currently smoking at the time of each examination of the Framingham offspring. The dates of each exam are also provided.

In the next two sections, we present graphical displays for ordinal and categorical variables, respectively. Whereas the numerical summaries for ordinal and categorical variables are identical (at least in terms of the frequencies and relative frequencies), graphical displays for ordinal and categorical variables are different in a very important way.

4.2.2 Histograms for Ordinal Variables

Histograms are appropriate graphical displays for ordinal variables. A histogram is different from a bar chart in one important feature. The horizontal axis of a histogram shows

TABLE 4–10 Frequency Distribution Table for Dominant Hand

	Frequency	Relative Frequency (%)
Right	3143	89.5
Left	370	10.5
Total	3513	100.0

TABLE 4–9 Frequency Distribution Table for Marital Status

	Frequency	Relative Frequency (%)
Single	203	5.8
Married	2580	73.1
Widowed	334	9.5
Divorced	367	10.4
Separated	46	1.3
Total	3530	100.0

TABLE 4–11 Frequency Distribution Table for Smoking Status

	Frequency	Relative Frequency (%)
Nonsmoker	1330	37.6
Former	1724	48.8
Current	482	13.6
Total	3536	100.0

TABLE 4-12 Current Smoking in the Framingham Offspring Study by Date of Exam

Exam Cycle	Dates	Current Smokers (%)
1	Aug 1971–Sept 1975	59.7
2	Oct 1979–Oct 1983	28.5
3	Dec 1983–Sept 1987	23.9
4	Apr 1987–Sept 1991	21.7
5	Jan 1991–June 1995	17.4
6	Jan 1995–Sept 1998	13.8
7	Sept 1998–Oct 2001	13.6

the distinct ordered response options of the ordinal variable. The vertical axis can show either frequencies or relative frequencies, producing a frequency histogram or relative frequency histogram, respectively. The bars are centered over each response option and scaled according to frequencies or relative frequencies as desired. The difference between a histogram and a bar chart is that the bars in a histogram run together; there is no space between adjacent responses. This reinforces the idea that the response categories are ordered and based on an underlying continuum. This underlying continuum may or may not be measurable.

Figure 4–6 is a frequency histogram for the blood pressure data displayed in Table 4–5. The horizontal axis displays the ordered blood pressure categories and the vertical axis displays the frequencies or numbers of participants classified in each category. The histogram immediately conveys the message that the majority of participants are in the lower two categories of the distribution. A small number of participants are in the Stage II hypertension category. The histogram in Figure 4–7 is a relative frequency histogram for the same data. Notice that the figure is the same except for the vertical axis, which is scaled to accommodate relative frequencies instead of frequencies.

Usually, relative frequency histograms are preferred over frequency histograms, as the relative frequencies are most appropriate for summarizing the data. From Figure 4–7, we can see that approximately 34% of the participants have normal blood pressure, 41% have pre-hypertension, just under 20% have Stage I hypertension, and 6% have Stage II hypertension.

Figure 4–8 is a relative frequency histogram for the total cholesterol variable summarized in Table 4–7. The bars of the histogram run together to reflect the fact that there is an underlying continuum of total cholesterol measurements. From Figure 4–8, we see that over 50% of the participants have desirable total cholesterol levels and just under 15% have high total cholesterol levels. The horizontal axis could be scaled

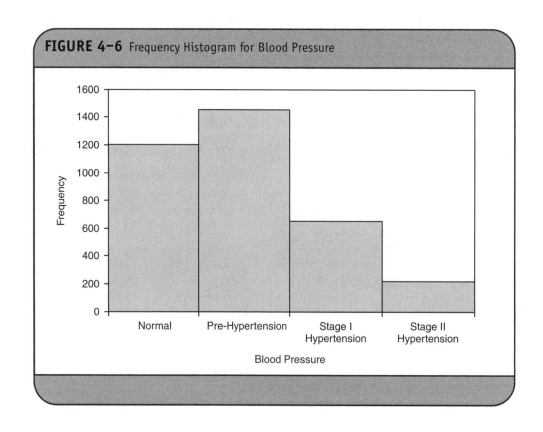

FIGURE 4-6 Frequency Histogram for Blood Pressure

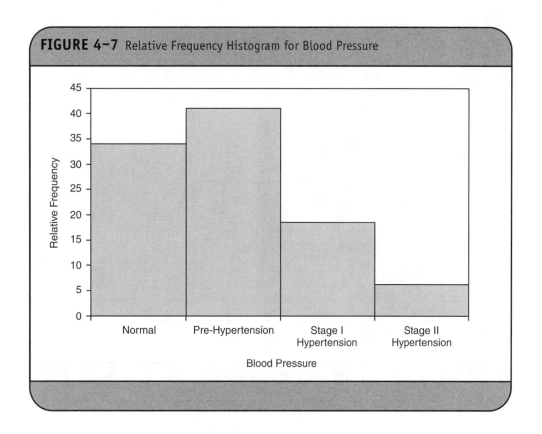

FIGURE 4-7 Relative Frequency Histogram for Blood Pressure

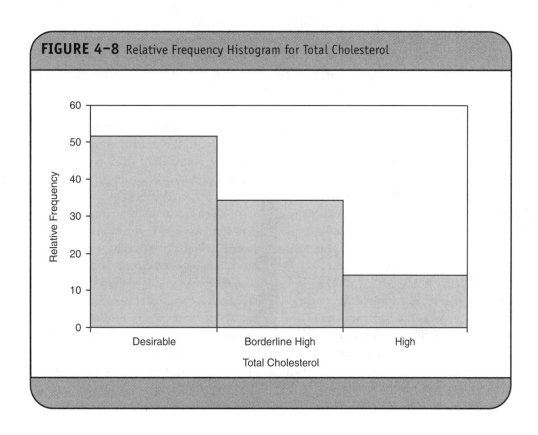

FIGURE 4-8 Relative Frequency Histogram for Total Cholesterol

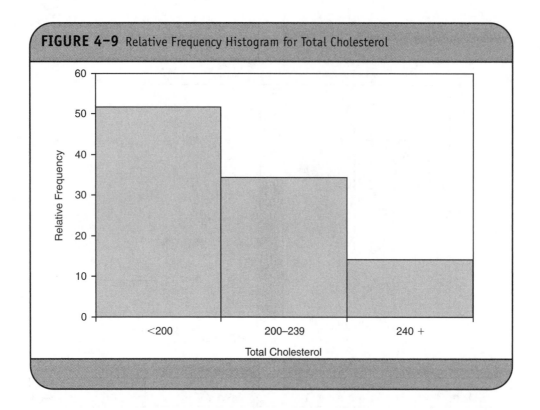

FIGURE 4-9 Relative Frequency Histogram for Total Cholesterol

differently. Figure 4–9 makes the continuum of total cholesterol underlying the categories used here to summarize the data more obvious. Another alterative is to mark the transition points. In Figure 4–9, the horizontal axis could be labeled 200 and 240 at the points of intersection of adjacent bars.

Figure 4–10 is a relative frequency histogram for the BMI data summarized in Table 4–8. The ordered BMI categories are shown in text along the horizontal axis and relative frequencies, as percents, are displayed along the vertical axis. From Figure 4–10, it is immediately evident that a small percentage of the participants are underweight and that the majority of the participants are overweight or obese, with the former more likely than the latter. The horizontal axis of Figure 4–10 could be scaled differently to show the numerical values of BMI that defined the ordinal categories or with labels to indicate the BMI values that separate adjacent bars (e.g., 18.5, 25.0, 30.0).

4.2.3   Bar Charts for Categorical Variables

Bar charts are appropriate graphical displays for categorical variables. Bar charts for categorical variables with more than two responses are constructed in the same fashion as bar charts for dichotomous variables. The horizontal axis of the bar chart again displays the distinct responses of the categorical variable. Because the responses are unordered, they can be

arranged in any order (e.g., from the most frequently to least frequently occurring in the sample, or alphabetically). The vertical axis can show either frequencies or relative frequencies, producing a frequency bar chart or relative frequency bar chart, respectively. The bars are centered over each response option and scaled according to frequencies or relative frequencies as desired.

Figure 4–11 is an example of a frequency bar chart displaying the distribution of marital status in the participants who attended the seventh examination of the Framingham Offspring Study. The distinct response options are shown on the horizontal axis, arranged as they were in Table 4–9. Frequencies, or numbers of respondents selecting each response, are shown on the vertical axis. It is immediately evident from the bar chart that the majority of respondents are married. Notice the spaces between the bars, indicating a clear separation between distinct response options. Because there is no inherent ordering to the response options, as is always the case with a categorical variable, the horizontal axis can be scaled differently. Figure 4–12 and Figure 4–13 show alternative arrangements of the response options. Each of the bar charts displays identical data. All three presentations are appro-priate as the categorical responses can be ordered in any way. Figure 4–12 arranges the responses from most

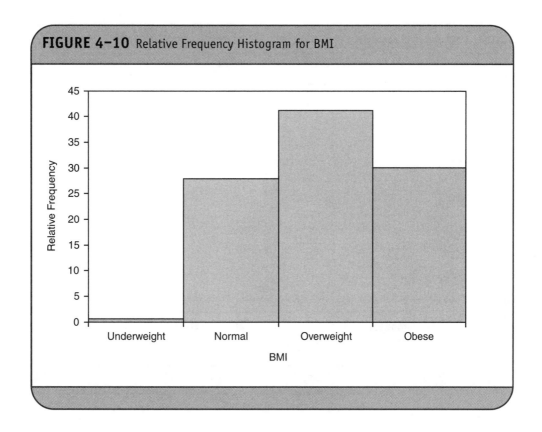

FIGURE 4-10 Relative Frequency Histogram for BMI

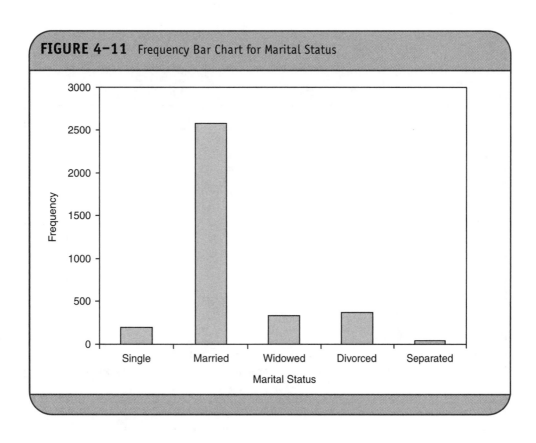

FIGURE 4-11 Frequency Bar Chart for Marital Status

FIGURE 4-12 Frequency Bar Chart for Marital Status

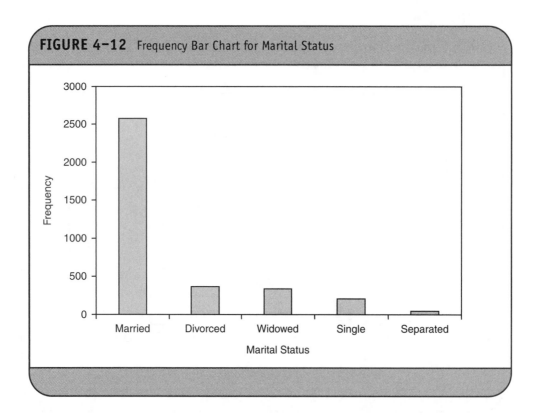

FIGURE 4-13 Frequency Bar Chart for Marital Status

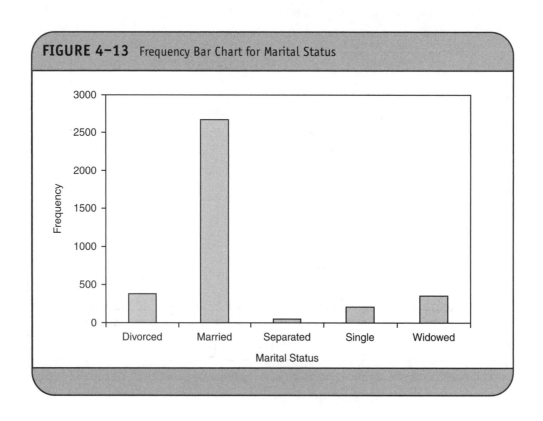

frequently to least frequently occurring, and Figure 4–13 arranges the responses alphabetically.

It is more typical to present relative frequency bar charts with relative frequencies displayed as proportions or percentages on the horizontal axis. Figure 4–14 is a relative frequency bar chart displaying the distribution of the dominant hand and is summarized in Table 4–10. Figure 4–14 clearly displays that the vast majority of participants in the seventh examination of the Framingham Heart Study are right-handed. Because the dominant hand is a dichotomous variable, we only need to display the relative frequency for one bar, as the second is determined from the first.

Figure 4–15 is a relative frequency bar chart displaying the distribution of smoking status measured at the seventh examination of the Framingham Offspring Study and summarized in Table 4–11. Figure 4–15 gives the clear impression that a small percentage of the participants are current smokers. Almost 50% are former smokers. Again, the response options in Figure 4–14 and Figure 4–15 may be rearranged, as there is no inherent ordering to these ordinal scales.

4.3   CONTINUOUS VARIABLES

Continuous variables, sometimes called measurement or quantitative variables, take on an unlimited number of distinct responses between a theoretical minimum value and maximum value. In a study of cardiovascular risk factors, we might measure participants' ages, heights, weights, systolic and diastolic blood pressures, total serum cholesterol levels, and so on. The measured values for each of these continuous variables depend on the scale of measurement. For example, in adult studies such as the Framingham Heart Study, age is usually measured in years. Studies of infants might measure age in days or even hours, whichever is more appropriate. Heights can be measured in inches or centimeters, weights can be measured in pounds or kilograms. Assuming weight is measured in pounds, measurements might be to the nearest pound, the nearest tenth of a pound, or the nearest hundredth (e.g., 145, 145.1, 145.13), depending on the precision of the scale.

4.3.1   Descriptive Statistics for Continuous Variables

To illustrate the computations of descriptive statistics in detail, we selected a small subset of the Framingham Heart Study data. After performing computations by hand on the small subset, we provide descriptive statistics for the full sample that were generated by computer.

Example 4.3. At the seventh examination of the Offspring in the Framingham Heart Study ($n = 3539$), numerous continuous variables were measured, including systolic and diastolic blood pressure, total serum cholesterol, height, and weight. Using the heights and weights measured on each participant, we computed the BMI. In this study, height was

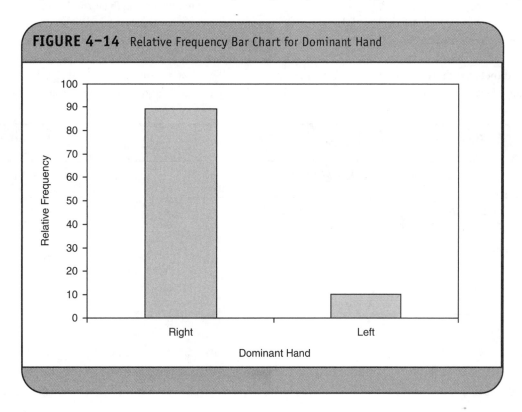

FIGURE 4–14 Relative Frequency Bar Chart for Dominant Hand

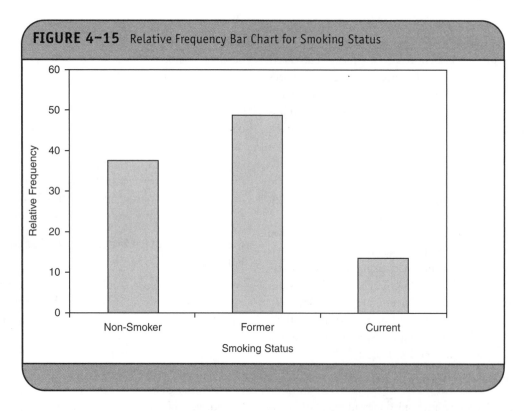

FIGURE 4-15 Relative Frequency Bar Chart for Smoking Status

measured in inches and weight in pounds. The following formula can be used to compute BMI using these metrics:

$$BMI = 703.03 \times \frac{Weight\ in\ pounds}{(Height\ in\ inches)^2}$$

To illustrate the computation of descriptive statistics for continuous variables, we randomly selected a subset of 10 participants who completed the seventh examination of the Framingham Offspring Study. The data values are shown in Table 4–13. The first

column contains a unique identification number for each participant, the second through sixth columns contain the actual measurements on participants, and the rightmost column contains the computed BMI using the formula shown. Descriptive statistics for each continuous variable are computed following. Formulas for the computations will be presented within examples and then summarized at the end of this chapter.

The first summary statistic for a continuous variable (as well as for dichotomous, categorical, and ordinal variables)

TABLE 4-13 Subsample of $n = 10$ Participants Attending the Seventh Examination of the Framingham Offspring Study

Participant ID	Systolic Blood Pressure	Diastolic Blood Pressure	Total Serum Cholesterol	Weight (lbs)	Height (in.)	BMI
1	141	76	199	138	63.00	24.4
2	119	64	150	183	69.75	26.4
3	122	62	227	153	65.75	24.9
4	127	81	227	178	70.00	25.5
5	125	70	163	161	70.50	22.8
6	123	72	210	206	70.00	29.6
7	105	81	205	235	72.00	31.9
8	113	63	275	151	60.75	28.8
9	106	67	208	213	69.00	31.5
10	131	77	159	142	61.00	26.8

is the sample size. The sample size here is $n = 10$. It is always important to report the sample size to convey the size of the study. Larger studies are generally viewed more favorably, as larger sample sizes generally produce more precise results. However, there is a point at which increasing the sample size will not materially increase the precision of the analysis. (Sample size computations will be discussed in detail in Chapter 8.)

Because this sample is small ($n = 10$), it is relatively easy to summarize the sample by inspecting the observed values. Suppose we first consider the diastolic blood pressures. To facilitate interpretation, we order the diastolic blood pressures from smallest to largest:

$$62 \quad 63 \quad 64 \quad 67 \quad 70$$
$$72 \quad 76 \quad 77 \quad 81 \quad 81$$

Diastolic blood pressures less than 80 are considered normal (see Table 4.1), thus the participants in this sample can be summarized as having fairly normal diastolic pressures. There are two participants with diastolic blood pressures of 81 but they hardly exceed the upper limit of the "normal" classification. The diastolic blood pressures in this sample are not all identical (with the exception of the two measured values of 81) but they are relatively similar. In general, the participants in this sample can be described as having healthy diastolic blood pressures from a clinical standpoint.

For larger samples, such as the full seventh examination of the Framingham Offspring Study with $n = 3539$, it is impossible to inspect individual values to generate a summary, so summary statistics are necessary. There are two general aspects of a useful summary for a continuous variable. The first is a description of the center or average of the data (i.e., what is a typical value) and the second addresses variability in the data.

Using the diastolic blood pressures, we now illustrate the computation of several statistics that describe the average value and then the variability of the data. In biostatistics, the term "average" is a very general term. There are several statistics that describe the average value of a continuous variable. The first is probably the most familiar—the sample mean. The sample mean is computed by summing all of the values and dividing by the sample size. For the sample of diastolic blood pressures, the sample mean is computed as follows:

$$\text{Sample Mean} = \frac{62+63+64+67+70+72+76+77+81+81}{10}$$

$$= \frac{713}{10} = 71.3$$

To simplify the formulas for sample statistics (and for population parameters), we usually denote the variable of interest as X. X is simply a placeholder for the variable being analyzed. Here $X =$ diastolic blood pressure. The sample mean is denoted $\overline{X}$ (read "X bar") and the formula for the sample mean is

$$\overline{X} = \frac{\Sigma X}{n}$$

where Σ indicates summation (i.e., the sum of the diastolic blood pressures in this sample). The mean diastolic blood pressure is $\overline{X} = 71.3$.

When reporting summary statistics for a continuous variable, the convention is to report one more decimal place than the number of decimal places measured. Systolic and diastolic blood pressures, total serum cholesterol, and weight were measured to the nearest integer, therefore the summary statistics are reported to the nearest tenths place. Height was measured to the nearest quarter inch (hundredths), therefore the summary statistics are reported to the nearest thousandths place. BMI was computed to the nearest tenth, so summary statistics are reported to the nearest hundredths place.

The sample mean is one measure of the average diastolic blood pressure. A second measure of the average value is the sample median. The sample median is the middle value in the ordered dataset, or the value that separates the top 50% of the values from the bottom 50%. When there is an odd number of observations in the sample, the median is the value that holds as many values above it as below it in the ordered dataset. When there is an even number of observations in the sample, the median is defined as the mean of the two middle values in the ordered dataset. In the sample of $n = 10$ diastolic blood pressures, the two middle values are 70 and 72, and thus the median is $(70 + 72)/2 = 71$. Half of the diastolic blood pressures are above 71 and half are below.

The mean and median provide different information about the average value of a continuous variable. Suppose the sample of 10 diastolic blood pressures looked like:

$$62 \quad 63 \quad 64 \quad 67 \quad 70$$
$$72 \quad 76 \quad 77 \quad 81 \quad 140$$

The sample mean for this sample is $\overline{X} = 772/10 = 77.2$. This does not represent a typical value, as the majority of diastolic blood pressures in this sample are below 77.2. The extreme value of 140 is affecting the computation of the mean. For this same sample, the median is 71. The median is unaffected by extreme or outlying values. For this reason, the median is preferred over the mean when there are extreme values (either very small or very large values relative to the others). When there are no extreme values, the mean is the preferred measure of a typical value, in part because each observation is considered in the computation of the mean. When there are no extreme values in a sample, the mean and median of the sample will be close in value.

Table 4–14 displays the sample means and medians for each of the continuous measures in the sample of $n = 10$. For each continuous variable measured in this subsample of participants, the means and medians are not identical but are relatively close in value, suggesting that the mean is the most appropriate summary of a typical value for each of these variables. (If the mean and median are very different, it suggests that there are outliers affecting the mean.)

A third measure of a typical value for a continuous variable is the mode. The mode is defined as the most frequent value. The mode of the diastolic blood pressures is 81, the mode of the total cholesterol levels is 227, and the mode of the heights is 70.00 because these values each appear twice, whereas the other values only appear once. For each of the other continuous variables, there are 10 distinct values and thus there is no mode (because no value appears more frequently than any other). Suppose the diastolic blood pressures looked like:

$$62 \quad 63 \quad 64 \quad 64 \quad 70$$
$$72 \quad 76 \quad 77 \quad 81 \quad 81$$

In this sample, there are two modes 64 and 81. The mode is a useful summary statistic for a continuous variable. It is not presented instead of either the mean or the median but rather in addition to the mean or median.

The second aspect of a continuous variable that must be summarized is the variability in the sample. A relatively crude yet important measure of variability in a sample is the sample range. The sample range is computed as:

Sample range = Maximum value – Minimum value

Table 4–15 displays the sample ranges for each of the continuous measures in the subsample of $n = 10$ observations.

The range of a variable depends on the scale of measurement. The blood pressures are measured in millimeters of mercury, total cholesterol is measured in milligrams per deciliter, weight in pounds, and so on. The range of total serum cholesterol is large with the minimum and maximum in the sample of size $n = 10$ differing by 125 units. In contrast, the heights of participants are more homogeneous with a range of 11.25 inches. The range is an important descriptive statistic for a continuous variable but it is based only on two values in the dataset. Like the mean, the sample range can be affected by extreme values and thus it must be interpreted with caution. The most widely used measure of variability for a continuous variable is called the standard deviation, which will be described later.

Assuming that there are no extreme or outlying values of the variable, the mean is the most appropriate summary of a typical value. To summarize variability in the data, we specifically estimate the variability in the sample around the sample mean. If all of the observed values in a sample are close to the sample mean, the standard deviation will be small (i.e., close to zero), and if the observed values vary widely around the sample mean, the standard deviation will be large. If all of the values in the sample are identical, the sample standard deviation will be zero.

In the sample of $n = 10$ diastolic blood pressures, we found $\overline{X} = 71.3$. Table 4–16 displays each of the observed values along with the respective deviations from the sample mean. The deviations from the mean reflect how far each individual's diastolic blood pressure is from the mean diastolic blood pressure. The first participant's diastolic blood pressure is 4.7 units above the mean, whereas the second participant's diastolic blood pressure is 7.3 units below the mean. What we need is a summary of these deviations from the mean, in particular a measure of how far (on average) each participant is from the mean diastolic blood pressure. If we

TABLE 4–14 Means and Medians of Variables in Subsample of Size $n = 10$

	Mean	Median
Diastolic blood pressure	71.3	71.0
Systolic blood pressure	121.2	122.5
Total serum cholesterol	202.3	206.5
Weight (lbs)	176.0	169.5
Height (in.)	67.175	69.375
Body mass index (BMI)	27.26	26.60

TABLE 4–15 Ranges of Variables in Subsample of Size $n = 10$

	Minimum	Maximum	Range
Diastolic blood pressure	62	81	19
Systolic blood pressure	105	141	36
Total serum cholesterol	150	275	125
Weight (lbs)	138	235	97
Height (in.)	60.75	72.00	11.25
Body mass index (BMI)	22.8	31.9	9.1

TABLE 4–16 Deviations from the Mean

Diastolic Blood Pressure (X)	Deviation from the Mean ($X-\overline{X}$)
76	4.7
64	-7.3
62	-9.3
81	9.7
70	-1.3
72	0.7
81	9.7
63	-8.3
67	-4.3
77	5.7
$\Sigma X = 713$	$\Sigma(X-\overline{X}) = 0$

TABLE 4–17 Squared Deviations from the Mean

Diastolic Blood Pressure (X)	Deviation from the Mean ($X-\overline{X}$)	Squared Deviation from the Mean ($X-\overline{X})^2$
76	4.7	22.09
64	-7.3	53.29
62	-9.3	86.49
81	9.7	94.09
70	-1.3	1.69
72	0.7	0.49
81	9.7	94.09
63	-8.3	68.89
67	-4.3	18.49
77	5.7	32.49
$\Sigma X = 713$	$\Sigma(X-\overline{X}) = 0$	$\Sigma(X-\overline{X})^2 = 472.10$

compute the mean of the deviations by summing the deviations and dividing by the sample size, we run into a problem: the sum of the deviations from the mean is zero. This will always be the case as it is a property of the sample mean—the sum of the deviations below the mean will always equal the sum of the deviations above the mean.

The goal is to capture the magnitude of these deviations in a summary measure. To address this problem of the deviations summing to zero, we could take absolute values or square each deviation from the mean. Both methods would address the problem. The more popular method to summarize the deviations from the mean involves squaring the deviations. (Absolute values are difficult in mathematical proofs, which are beyond the scope of this book.) Table 4–17 displays each of the observed values, the respective deviations from the sample mean, and the squared deviations from the mean.

The squared deviations are interpreted as follows. The first participant's squared deviation is 22.09, meaning that their diastolic blood pressure is 22.09 units squared from the mean diastolic blood pressure, and the second participant's diastolic blood pressure is 53.29 units squared from the mean diastolic blood pressure. A quantity that is often used to measure variability in a sample is called the sample variance, and it is essentially the mean of the squared deviations. The sample variance is denoted s^2 and is computed as:

$$s^2 = \frac{\Sigma(X-\overline{X})^2}{n-1}$$

The sample variance is not actually the mean of the squared deviations because we divide by $(n-1)$ instead of n. In statistical inference (which is described in detail in Chapter 6, Chapter 7, and Chapter 9), we make generalizations or estimates of

population parameters based on sample statistics. If we were to compute the sample variance by taking the mean of the squared deviations and dividing by n, we would consistently underestimate the true population variance. Dividing by $(n-1)$ produces a better estimate of the population variance. The sample variance is nonetheless usually interpreted as the average squared deviation from the mean. In this sample of $n = 10$ diastolic blood pressures, the sample variance is $s^2 = 472.10 / 9 = 52.46$. Thus, on average, diastolic blood pressures are 52.46 units squared from the mean diastolic blood pressure.

Because of the squaring, the variance is not particularly interpretable. The more common measure of variability in a sample is the sample standard deviation, defined as the square root of the sample variance:

$$s = \sqrt{s^2} = \sqrt{\frac{\Sigma(X-\overline{X})^2}{n-1}}$$

The sample standard deviation of the diastolic blood pressures is $s = \sqrt{52.46} = 7.2$. On average, diastolic blood pressures are 7.2 units from (above or below) the mean diastolic blood pressure.

When a dataset has outliers, or extreme values, we summarize a typical value using the median as opposed to the mean. When a dataset has outliers, variability is often summarized by a statistic called the interquartile range (IQR). The interquartile range is the difference between the first and third quartiles. The first quartile, denoted Q_1, is the value in the dataset that holds 25% of the values below it. The third quartile, denoted Q_3, is the value in the dataset that holds 25% of the values above it. The IQR is defined as

$$IQR = Q_3 - Q_1$$

For the sample of $n = 10$ diastolic blood pressures, the median is 71 (50% of the values are above 71 and 50% are below). The quartiles can be computed in the same way we computed the median but we consider each half of the dataset separately (see Figure 4–16).

There are five values below the median (lower half) and the middle value is 64, which is the first quartile. There are five values above the median (upper half) and the middle value is 77, which is the third quartile. The IQR is $77 - 64 = 13$; the IQR is the range of the middle 50% of the data. When the sample size is odd, the median and quartiles are determined in the same way. Suppose in the previous example that the lowest value (62) was excluded and the sample size was $n = 9$. The median and quartiles are indicated graphically in Figure 4–17. When the sample size is 9, the median is the middle number, 72. The quartiles are determined in the same way looking at the lower and upper halves, respectively. There are four values in the lower half, so the first quartile is the mean of the two middle values in the lower half, $(64 + 64) / 2 = 64$. The same approach is used in the upper half to determine the third quartile, $(77 + 81) / 2 = 79$.

When there are no outliers in a sample, the mean and standard deviation are used to summarize a typical value and the variability in the sample, respectively. When there are outliers in a sample, the median and IQR are used to summarize a typical value and the variability in the sample, respectively.

An important issue is determining whether a sample has outliers or not. There are several methods to determine outliers in a sample. A very popular method is based on the following:

Outliers are values below $Q_1 - 1.5 \times (Q_3 - Q_1)$

or above $Q_3 + 1.5 \times (Q_3 - Q_1)$,

or equivalently, values below $Q_1 - 1.5 \times IQR$

or above $Q_3 + 1.5 \times IQR$

These are referred to as Tukey fences.[6] For the diastolic blood pressures, the lower limit is $64 - 1.5 \times (77 - 64) = 44.5$ and the upper limit is $77 + 1.5 \times (77 - 64) = 96.5$. The diastolic blood pressures range from 62 to 81, therefore there are no outliers. The best summary of a typical diastolic blood pressure is the mean ($\bar{X} = 71.3$) and the best summary of variability is given by the standard deviation ($s = 7.2$).

Table 4–18 displays the means, standard deviations, medians, quartiles, and IQRs for each of the continuous variable displayed in Table 4–13 in the subsample of $n = 10$ participants who attended the seventh examination of the Framingham Offspring Study. Table 4–19 displays the observed minimum and maximum values along with the limits to determine outliers using the quartile rule for each of the variables in the subsample of $n = 10$ participants. Are there outliers in any of the variables? Which statistics are most appropriate to summarize the average or typical value and the dispersion? Because there are no suspected outliers in the subsample of $n = 10$ participants, the mean and standard deviation are the most appropriate statistics to summarize average values and dispersion, respectively, of each of these characteristics.

Table 4–20 displays the means, standard deviations, medians, quartiles, and IQRs for each of the continuous variables displayed in Table 4–13 in the full sample ($n = 3539$) of participants who attended the seventh examination of the Framingham Heart Study. Looking just at the means and medians, does it appear that any of the characteristics are subject to outliers in the full sample?

Table 4–21 displays the observed minimum and maximum values along with the limits to determine outliers using

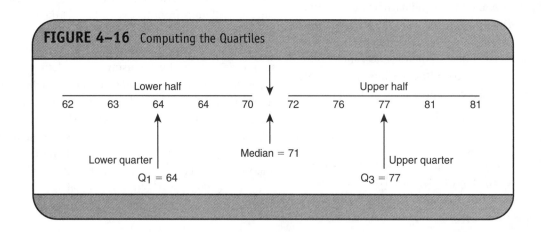

FIGURE 4–16 Computing the Quartiles

FIGURE 4–17 Median and Quartiles

TABLE 4–18 Summary Statistics on $n = 10$ Participants Attending the Seventh Examination of the Framingham Offspring Study

	Mean ($\bar{X}$)	Standard Deviation (s)	Median	Q_1	Q_3	IQR
Systolic blood pressure	121.2	11.1	122.5	113.0	127.0	14.0
Diastolic blood pressure	71.3	7.2	71.0	64.0	77.0	13.0
Total serum cholesterol	202.3	37.7	206.5	163.0	227.0	64.0
Weight (lbs)	176.0	33.0	169.5	151.0	206.0	55.0
Height (in.)	67.175	4.205	69.375	63.0	70.0	7.0
Body mass index (BMI)	27.26	3.10	26.60	24.9	29.6	4.7

the quartile rule for each of the variables in the full sample ($n = 3539$) of participants who attended the seventh examination of the Framingham Offspring Study. Are there outliers in any of the variables? Which statistics are most appropriate to summarize the average or typical values and the dispersion for each variable?

In the full sample, each of the characteristics has outliers on the upper end of the distribution, as the maximum values exceed the upper limits in each case. There are also outliers on the low end for diastolic blood pressure and total cholesterol, as the minimums are below the lower limits. For some of these characteristics, the difference between the upper limit and the

TABLE 4–19 Limits for Assessing Outliers in Characteristics Measured in $n = 10$ Participants Attending the Seventh Examination of the Framingham Offspring Study

	Minimum	Maximum	Lower Limit[a]	Upper Limit[b]
Systolic blood pressure	105	141	92	148
Diastolic blood pressure	62	81	44.5	96.5
Total serum cholesterol	150	275	67	323
Weight (lbs)	138	235	68.5	288.5
Height (in.)	60.75	72.00	52.5	80.5
Body mass index (BMI)	22.8	31.9	17.85	36.65

[a] Determined by $Q_1 - 1.5(Q_3 - Q_1)$.
[b] Determined by $Q_3 + 1.5(Q_3 - Q_1)$.

TABLE 4–20 Summary Statistics on Sample of Participants Attending the Seventh Examination of the Framingham Offspring Study $n = 3{,}539$)

	Mean ($\overline{X}$)	Standrd Deviation (s)	Median	Q_1	Q_3	IQR
Systolic blood pressure	127.3	19.0	125.0	114.0	138.0	24.0
Diastolic blood pressure	74.0	9.9	74.0	67.0	80.0	13.0
Total serum cholesterol	200.3	36.8	198.0	175.0	223.0	48.0
Weight (lbs)	174.4	38.7	170.0	146.0	198.0	52.0
Height (in.)	65.957	3.749	65.750	63.000	68.750	5.75
Body mass index (BMI)	28.15	5.32	27.40	24.5	30.8	6.3

TABLE 4–21 Limits for Assessing Outliers in Characteristics Measured in Participants Attending the Seventh Examination of the Framingham Offspring Study

	Minimum	Maximum	Lower Limit[a]	Upper Limit[b]
Systolic blood pressure	81.0	216.0	78	174
Diastolic blood pressure	41.0	114.0	47.5	99.5
Total serum cholesterol	83.0	357.0	103	295
Weight (lbs)	90.0	375.0	68.0	276.0
Height (in.)	55.00	78.75	54.4	77.4
Body mass index (BMI)	15.8	64.0	15.05	40.25

[a] Determined by $Q_1 - 1.5(Q_3 - Q_1)$.
[b] Determined by $Q_3 + 1.5(Q_3 - Q_1)$.

maximum (or the lower limit and the minimum) is small (e.g., height, systolic and diastolic blood pressures), whereas for others (e.g., total cholesterol, weight, and BMI) the difference is much larger. This method for determining outliers is a popular one but not generally applied as a hard and fast rule. In this application, it would be reasonable to present means and standard deviations for height, systolic and diastolic blood pressures, and medians and IQRs for total cholesterol, weight, and BMI. Another method for assessing whether a distribution is subject to outliers or extreme values is through graphical displays.

4.3.2 Box-Whisker Plots for Continuous Variables

Box-whisker plots are very useful plots for displaying the distribution of a continuous variable. In Example 4.3, we considered a subsample of $n = 10$ participants who attended the seventh examination of the Framingham Offspring Study. We computed the following summary statistics on diastolic blood pressures: These statistics are sometimes referred to as quantiles, or

percentiles, of the distribution. A specific quantile or percentile is a value in the dataset that holds a specific percentage of the values at or below it. For example, the first quartile is the 25th percentile, meaning that it holds 25% of the values at or below it. The median is the 50th percentile, the third quartile is the 75th percentile, and the maximum is the 100th percentile (i.e., 100% of the values are at or below it).

Minimum:	62
Q_1:	64
Median:	71
Q_3:	77
Maximum:	81

A *box-whisker* plot is a graphical display of these percentiles. Figure 4.18 is a box-whisker plot of the diastolic blood pressures measured in the subsample of $n = 10$ participants described in Example 4.3. The horizontal lines represent (from the top) the maximum, the third quartile, the median (also

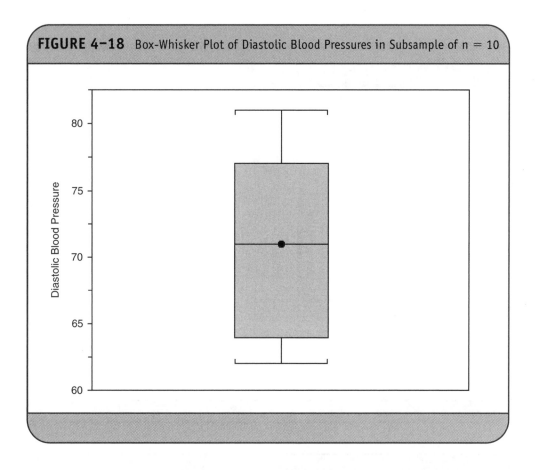

FIGURE 4-18 Box-Whisker Plot of Diastolic Blood Pressures in Subsample of n = 10

indicated by the dot), the first quartile, and the minimum. The shaded box represents the middle 50% of the distribution (between the first and third quartiles). A box-whisker plot is meant to convey the distribution of a variable at a quick glance.

Figure 4–19 is a box-whisker plot of the diastolic blood pressures measured in the full sample of participants who attended the seventh examination of the Framingham Offspring Study. In the full sample, we determined that there were outliers both at the low and the high end (see Table 4–21). In Figure 4–19, the outliers are displayed as horizontal lines at the top and bottom of the distribution. At the low end of the distribution, there are five values that are considered outliers (i.e., values below 47.5, which was the lower limit for determining outliers). At the high end of the distribution, there are 12 values that are considered outliers (i.e., values above 99.5, which was the upper limit for determining outliers). The "whiskers" of the plot (the notched horizontal lines) are the limits we determined for detecting outliers (47.5 and 99.5).

Figure 4–20 is a box-whisker plot of the total serum cholesterol levels measured in the full sample of participants who attended the seventh examination of the Framingham Offspring Study. In the full sample, we determined that there were outliers both at the low and the high end (see Table 4–21).

Again in Figure 4–20, the outliers are displayed as horizontal lines at the top and bottom of the distribution. The outliers of total cholesterol are more numerous than those we observed for diastolic blood pressure, particularly on the high end of the distribution.

Box-whisker plots are very useful for comparing distributions. Figure 4–21 shows side-by-side box-whisker plots of the distributions of weights (in pounds) for men and women who attended the seventh examination of the Framingham Offspring Study. The figure clearly shows a shift in the distributions, with men having much higher weights. In fact, the 25th percentile of the weights in men is approximately 180 lbs, equal to the 75th percentile in women. Specifically, 25% of the men weigh 180 lbs or less as compared to 75% of the women. There are a substantial number of outliers at the high end of the distribution among both men and women. There are two outlying low values among men.

Because men are generally taller than women (see Figure 4–22), it is not surprising that men have greater weights than women. A more appropriate comparison is of BMI (see Figure 4–23). The distributions of BMI are similar for men and women. There are again a substantial number of outliers in the distributions in both men and women. However, when

FIGURE 4-19 Box-Whisker Plot of Diastolic Blood Pressures in Participants Attending the Seventh Examination of the Framingham Offspring Study

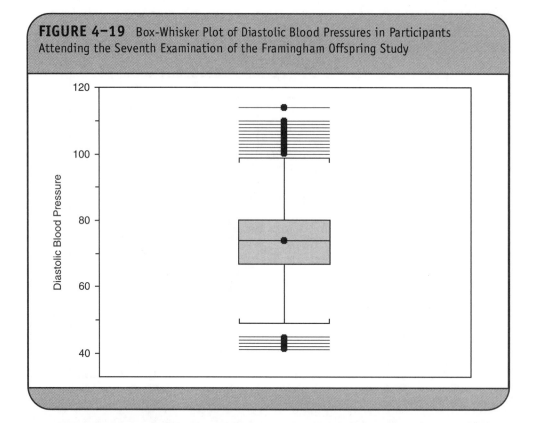

FIGURE 4-20 Box-Whisker Plot of Total Serum Cholesterol Levels in Participants Attending the Seventh Examination of the Framingham Offspring Study

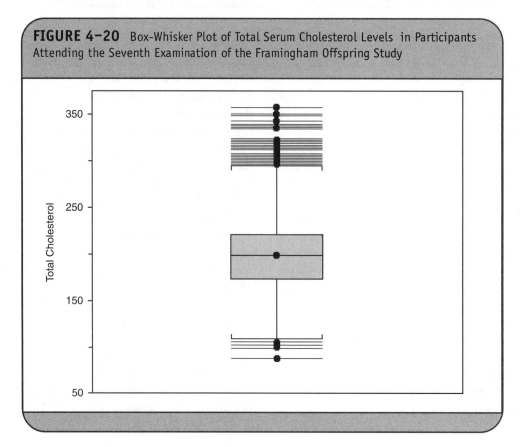

FIGURE 4-21 Side-by-side Box-Whisker Plots of Weights in Men and Women Attending the Seventh Examination of the Framingham Offspring Study

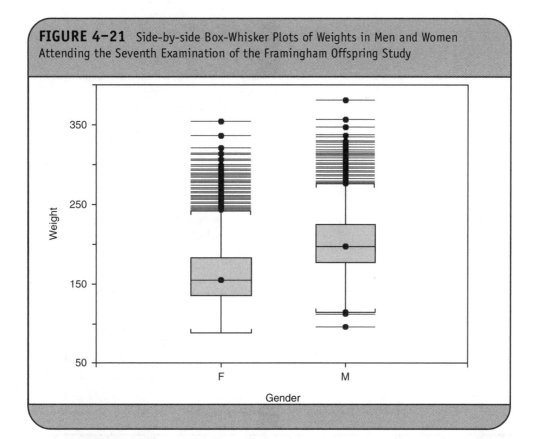

FIGURE 4-22 Side-by-side Box-Whisker Plots of Heights in Men and Women Attending the Seventh Examination of the Framingham Offspring Study

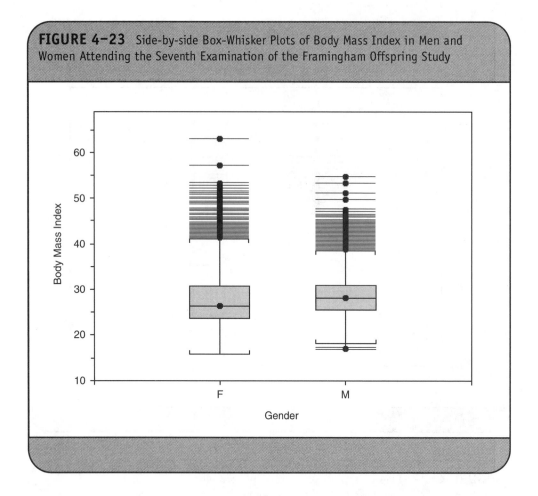

FIGURE 4–23 Side-by-side Box-Whisker Plots of Body Mass Index in Men and Women Attending the Seventh Examination of the Framingham Offspring Study

taking height into account (by comparing BMI instead of comparing weights alone), we see that the most extreme outliers are among the women. What statistics would be most appropriate to summarize typical BMI for men and women?

In the box-whisker plots, outliers are values that either exceed $Q_3 + 1.5 \times IQR$ or fall below $Q_1 - 1.5 \times IQR$. Some statistical computing packages use the following to determine outliers: values which either exceed $Q_3 + 3 \times IQR$ or fall below $Q_1 \times 3 \times IQR$, which would result in fewer observations being classified as outliers.[7,8] The rule using $1.5 \times IQR$ is the more commonly applied rule to determine outliers.

4.4 SUMMARY

The first important aspect of any statistical analys is an appropriate summary of the key variables. This involves first identifying the type of variable being analyzed. This step is extremely important, as the appropriate numerical and graphical summaries depend on the type of variable being analyzed. Variables are dichotomous, ordinal, categorical, or continuous. The best numerical summaries for dichotomous, ordinal, and categorical variables are relative frequencies. The best numerical summaries for continuous variables include the mean and standard deviation or the median and interquartile range, depending on whether or not there are outliers in the distribution. The mean and standard deviation, or the median and interquartile range, summarize location and dispersion, respectively. The best graphical summary for dichotomous and categorical variables is a bar chart, and the best graphical summary for an ordinal variable is a histogram. Both bar charts and histograms can be designed to display frequencies or relative frequencies, with the latter being the more popular display. Box-whisker plots provide a very useful and informative summary for continuous variables. Box-whisker plots are also useful for comparing the distributions of a continuous variable among mutually exclusive (i.e., non-overlapping) comparison groups. Figure 4–24 summarizes key statistics and graphical displays organized by variable type.

FIGURE 4–24 Key Statistics and Graphical Displays

Variable Type	Statistic/Graphical Display	Definition
Dichotomous, Ordinal, or Categorical	Relative Frequency	Frequency/n
Dichotomous or Categorical	Frequency or Relative Frequency Bar Chart	
Ordinal	Frequency or Relative Frequency Histogram	
Continuous	Mean	$\overline{X} = \dfrac{\Sigma X}{n}$
	Standard Deviation	$s = \sqrt{\dfrac{\Sigma(X-\overline{X})^2}{n-1}}$
	Median	Middle value in ordered dataset
	First Quartile	Q_1 = Value holding 25% below it
	Third Quartile	Q_3 = Value holding 25% above it
	Interquartile Range	$Q_3 - Q_1$
	Criteria for Outliers	Values below $Q_1 - 1.5(Q_3 - Q_1)$ or above $Q_3 + 1.5(Q_3 - Q_1)$
	Box-Whisker Plot	

4.5 PRACTICE PROBLEMS

1. A study is run to estimate the mean total cholesterol level in children 2 to 6 years of age. A sample of 9 participants is selected and their total cholesterol levels are measured as follows.

   185   225   240   196   175
   180   194   147   223

   a. Compute the sample mean.
   b. Compute the sample standard deviation.
   c. Compute the median.
   d. Compute the first and third quartiles.
   e. Which measure, the mean or median, is a better measure of a typical value? Justify.
   f. Which measure, the standard deviation or the interquartile range, is a better measure of dispersion? Justify.

2. Generate a box-whisker plot for the data in Problem 1.

3. The box plot of Figure 4–25 shows the distributions of total cholesterol levels in boys and girls 10 to 15 years of age.
   a. What is the median total cholesterol level in boys?
   b. Are there any outliers in total cholesterol in boys? Justify briefly.
   c. What proportion of the boys has total cholesterol less than 205?

   d. What proportion of the girls has total cholesterol less than 205?

4. The following data were collected as part of a study of coffee consumption among graduate students. The following reflects cups per day consumed:

   3   4   6   8   2   1   0   2

   a. Compute the sample mean.
   b. Compute the sample standard deviation.
   c. Compute the median.
   d. Compute the first and third quartiles.
   e. Which measure, the mean or median, is a better measure of a typical value? Justify.
   f. Which measure, the standard deviation or the interquartile range, is a better measure of dispersion? Justify.

5. In a study of a new anti-hypertensive medication, systolic blood pressures are measured at baseline. The data are as follows:

   120   112   138   145   135
   150   145   163   148   128
   143   156   160   142   150

   a. Compute the sample mean.
   b. Compute the sample median.

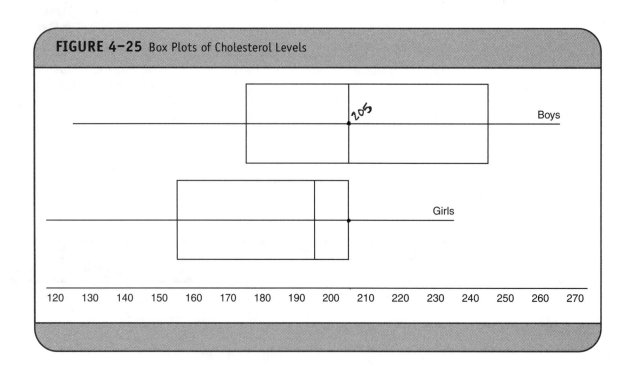

FIGURE 4–25 Box Plots of Cholesterol Levels

| 120 | 130 | 140 | 150 | 160 | 170 | 180 | 190 | 200 | 210 | 220 | 230 | 240 | 250 | 260 | 270 |

c. Compute the sample standard deviation.

d. Compute the sample range.

e. Are there any outliers?

6. Organize the systolic blood pressures of Problem 5 into categories and develop a frequency distribution table.

7. Generate a relative frequency histogram using the data in Problem 6.

8. Figure 4–26 shows birth weights (in grams) of infants who were delivered full-term, classified by their mother's weight gain during pregnancy:

   a. What is the median birth weight for mothers who gained 50 to 74 pounds?

   b. What is the interquartile range for mothers who gained 75 pounds or more?

   c. Are there any outliers in birth weights among mothers who gained less than 50 pounds?

   d. What are the best measures of a typical birth weight and the variability in birth weights among women who gained less than 50 pounds?

9. The following are baby height measurements (in centimeters) for a sample of women participating in a study of pregnancy outcomes:

28	30	41	48	29
48	62	49	51	39

   a. Compute the sample mean.

   b. Compute the sample standard deviation.

   c. Compute the median.

   d. Compute the first and third quartiles.

   e. Which measure, the mean or median, is a better measure of a typical value? Justify.

   f. Which measure, the standard deviation or the interquartile range, is a better measure of dispersion? Justify.

10. Construct a frequency distribution table using the data in Problem 9 and the following categories: less than 35, 35–44, 45–54, 55 or more.

11. Generate a relative frequency histogram using the data in Problem 10.

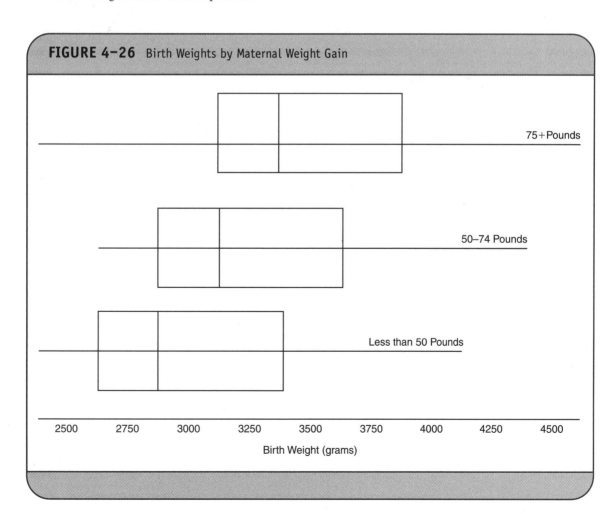

FIGURE 4-26 Birth Weights by Maternal Weight Gain

REFERENCES

1. National Heart, Lung, and Blood Institute. Available at *http://www.nhlbi.nih.gov*.

2. Sullivan, L.M. "Repeated measures." *Circulation* (in press).

3. Little, R.J. and Rubin, D.B. *Statistical Analysis with Missing Data.* New York: John Wiley & Sons, 1987.

4. American Heart Association. Available at *http://www.americanheart.org*.

5. The Expert Panel. "Expert panel on detection, evaluation, and treatment of high blood cholesterol in adults: summary of the second report of the NCEP expert panel (Adult Treatment Panel II)." *Journal of the American Medical Association*, 1993; 269: 3015–3023.

6. Hoaglin, D.C. "John W. Tukey and data analysis." *Statistical Science*, 2003; 18(3): 311–318.

7. SAS version 9.1 © 2002–2003 by SAS Institute, Cary, NC.

8. S-PLUS version 7.0 © 1999–2006 by Insightful Corp., Seattle, WA.

CHAPTER 5

The Role of Probability

Probabilities are numbers that reflect the likelihood that a particular event will occur. We hear about probabilities in many everyday situations, ranging from weather forecasts (probability of rain or snow) to the lottery (probability of hitting the big jackpot). In biostatistical applications, it is probability theory that underlies statistical inference. *Statistical inference* involves making generalizations or inferences about unknown population parameters based on sample statistics. A *population parameter* is any summary measure computed on a population (e.g., the population mean, which is denoted μ; the population variance, which is denoted σ^2; or the population standard deviation, which is denoted σ). In Chapter 4, we presented a number of different statistics to summarize sample data. In Chapter 6, Chapter 7, and Chapter 9, we will discuss statistical inference in detail. Specifically, we will present formulas and procedures to make inferences about a population based on a single sample. There are many details to consider but, in general, we select a sample from the population of interest, measure the characteristic under study, summarize this characteristic in our sample, and then make inferences about the population based on what we observe in the sample.

This process can be very powerful. In many statistical applications, we make inferences about a large number of individuals in a population based on a study of only a small fraction of the population (i.e., the sample). This is the power of biostatistics. If a study were to be replicated or repeated on another sample from the population, it is possible that we might observe slightly different results. This could be due to the fact that the second study involves a slightly different sample, again the sample being only a subset of the population. A third replication might produce yet different results. From any given population, there are often many different samples that can be selected. The results based on each sample can vary, and this variability is called *sampling variability*.

In practice, we select only one sample. Understanding how that study sample was produced is important for statistical inference. In our discussion of probability, we focus on probability as it applies to selecting individuals from a population into a sample. We will also focus on quantifying sampling variation. Whenever we make statistical inferences, we must recognize that we are making these inferences based on incomplete information—specifically, we are making inferences about a population based only on a single sample.

5.1 SAMPLING

Probability is important in selecting individuals from a population into a sample, and again in statistical inference when we make generalizations about the population based on that sample. When we select a sample from a population, we want that sample to be representative of the population. Specifically, we want the sample to be similar to the population in terms of key characteristics. For example, suppose we are interested in studying obesity in residents of the state of California. The Centers for Disease Control and Prevention (CDC) reports data on demographic information on the residents of each state, and some of these demographic characteristics are summarized for the state of California in Table 5–1.[1]

In California, the residents are almost equally split by gender, their median age is 33.3 years, and over 72.7% are

TABLE 5-1 Demographic Characteristics for California

Men (%)	49.8
Median age (years)	33.3
18 years of age and older (%)	72.7
White (%)	63.4
African-American (%)	7.4
High school graduate or higher (%)	76.8
Bachelors degree or higher (%)	26.6

18 years of age and older. The state has 63.4% Caucasians, 7.4% African Americans, and the remainder are other races. Almost 77% of the residents have a high school diploma, and over 26% have a bachelors degree or higher. For example, if we were to select a sample of the residents of California for a study, we would not want the sample to be 75% men with a median age of 50. That would not be representative of the population. Table 5–2 contains the same demographic information for California, Massachusetts, Florida, and Alabama.[1]

Notice the differences in demographic characteristics among these states. Previous studies have shown that obesity is related to gender, race, and educational level; therefore, when we select a sample to study obesity, we must be careful to accurately reflect these characteristics.[2–4] Studies have shown that prevalent obesity is inversely related to educational level (i.e., persons with higher levels of education are less likely to be obese). If we select a sample to assess obesity, we would want to take care not to over-represent (or under-represent) persons with lower educational levels as this could inflate (or diminish) our estimate of obesity in that state.

Sampling individuals from a population into a sample is a critically important step in any biostatistical analysis. There are two popular types of sampling, probability sampling and non-probability sampling. In *probability sampling*, each

member of the population has a known probability of being selected. In *non-probability sampling*, each member of the population is selected without the use of probability. Popular methods of each type of sampling are described here. More details can be found in Cochran and Kish.[5,6]

5.1.1 Probabilty Sampling: Simple Random Sampling

In *simple random sampling*, we start with what is called the *sampling frame*, a complete list or enumeration of the entire population. Each member of the population is assigned a unique identification number, and then a set of numbers are selected at random to determine the individuals to be included in the sample. Many introductory statistical textbooks contain tables of random numbers that can be used, and there are also statistical computing packages that can be used to generate random numbers.[7,8] Simple random sampling is a technique against which many other sampling techniques are compared. It is most useful when the population is relatively small because it requires a complete enumeration of the population as a starting point. In this sampling scheme, each individual in the population has the same chance of being selected.

5.1.2 Probability Sampling: Systematic Sampling

In *systematic sampling*, we again start with the complete sampling frame and members of the population are assigned unique identification numbers. However, in systematic sampling every third or every fifth person is selected. The spacing or interval between selections is determined by the ratio of the population to the sample size (N / n). For example, if the population size is $N = 1000$ and a sample size of $n = 100$ is desired, then the sampling interval is $1000 / 100 = 10$; so every tenth person is selected into the sample. The first person is selected at random from among the first ten in the list, with this first selection made at random using a random

TABLE 5-2 Demographic Characteristics for California, Massachusetts, Florida, and Alabama

	California	Massachusetts	Florida	Alabama
Men (%)	49.8	48.2	48.8	48.3
Median age (years)	33.3	36.5	38.7	35.8
18 years of age and older (%)	72.7	76.4	77.2	74.7
White (%)	63.4	86.2	79.7	72.0
African-American (%)	7.4	6.3	15.5	26.3
High school graduate or higher (%)	76.8	84.8	79.9	75.3
Bachelors degree or higher (%)	26.6	33.2	22.3	19.0

numbers table or a computer-generated random number. If the desired sample size is $n = 175$, then the sampling fraction is $1000 / 175 = 5.7$. Clearly, we cannot take every 5.7th person, so we round this down to 5 and take every fifth person. Once the first person is selected at random, every fifth person is selected from that point on through the end of the list.

There is a possibility that a systematic sample might not be representative of a population. This can occur if there is a systematic arrangement of individuals in the population. Suppose that the population were married couples and that the sampling frame was set up to list each husband and then his wife. Selecting every tenth person (or any even-numbered multiple) would result in selecting all men or women depending on the starting point. This is a very extreme example but as a general principle, all potential sources of systematic bias should be considered in the sampling process.

5.1.3 Probabilty Sampling: Stratified Sampling

In *stratified sampling*, we split the population into non-overlapping groups or strata (e.g., men and women; people under 30 years of age and people 30 years of age and older) and then sample within each strata. Sampling within each strata can be by simple random sampling or systematic sampling. The idea behind stratified sampling is to ensure adequate representation of individuals within each strata. For example, if a population contains 70% men and 30% women and we want to ensure the same representation in the sample, we can stratify and sample the requisite numbers of men and women to ensure the same representation. For example, if the desired sample size is $n = 200$, then $n = 140$ men and $n = 60$ women could be sampled either by simple random sampling or by systematic sampling.

Non-probability samples are often used in practice because in many applications, it is not possible to generate a sampling frame. In non-probability samples, the probability that any individual is selected into the sample is unknown. Whereas it is informative to know the likelihood that any individual is selected from the population into the sample (which is only possible with a complete sampling frame), it is not possible here. However, what is most important is selecting a sample that is representative of the population. Some examples of non-probability samples are described here.

5.1.4 Non-Probability Sampling: Convenience Sampling

In *convenience sampling*, we select individuals into our sample by any convenient contact. For example, we might approach patients seeking medical care at a particular hospital in a waiting or reception area. Convenience samples are useful for collecting preliminary or pilot data. They should not be used for statistical inference as they are generally not constructed to be representative of any specific population.

5.1.5 Non-Probability Sampling: Quota Sampling

In *quota sampling*, we determine a specific number of individuals to select into our sample in each of several specific groups. The idea is similar to stratified sampling in that we develop non-overlapping groups and sample a predetermined number of individuals within each group. For example, suppose we wish to ensure that the distribution of participant's ages in the sample is similar to that in the population. Suppose our desired sample size is $n = 300$ and we know from census data that in the population, approximately 30% are under age 20, 40% are between 20 and 49, and 30% are 50 years of age and older. We would then sample $n = 90$ persons under age 20, $n = 120$ between the ages of 20 and 49, and $n = 90$ who are 50 years of age and older. Sampling proceeds until these totals, or quotas, are reached. Quota sampling is different from stratified sampling because in a stratified sample, individuals within each stratum are selected at random. Here we enroll participants until the quota is reached.

5.2 BASIC CONCEPTS

We now discuss how probabilities are determined and we consider sampling by simple random sampling. A *probability* is a number that reflects the likelihood that a particular event, such as sampling a particular individual from a population into a sample, will occur. Probabilities range from 0 to 1. Sometimes probabilities are converted to percentages, in which case the range is 0% to 100%. A probability of 0 indicates that there is no chance that a particular event will occur, whereas a probability of 1 indicates that an event is certain to occur. In most applications, we are dealing with probabilities between 0 and 1, not inclusive.

Example 5.1. Suppose we wish to conduct a study of obesity in children 5 to 10 years of age who are seeking medical care at a particular pediatric practice. The population includes all children who were seen in the practice in the past 12 months and is summarized in Table 5–3.

TABLE 5–3 Children Seen Over the Past 12 Months							
	Age (years)						Total
	5	6	7	8	9	10	
Boys	432	379	501	410	420	418	2560
Girls	408	513	412	436	461	500	2730
Total	840	892	913	846	881	918	5290

If we select a child at random (by simple random sampling), then each child has the same probability of being selected. In statistics, the phrase "at random" is synonomous with "equally likely." In this application, each child has the same probability of being selected and that probability is determined by $1 / N$, where N is the population size. Thus, the probability that any child is selected is $1 / 5290 = 0.0002$. In most sampling situations, we are generally not concerned with sampling a specific individual but instead concern ourselves with the probability of sampling certain "types" of individuals. For example, what is the probability of selecting a boy or a child 7 years of age? The following formula can be used to compute probabilities of selecting individuals with specific attributes or characteristics.

P(characteristic) =

$$\frac{\text{Number of persons with characteristic}}{\text{Total number of persons in the population}(N)}.$$

If we select a child at random, the probability that we select a boy is computed as follows: P(boy) = $2560 / 5290 = 0.484$. This probability can be interpreted in two ways. The probability that we select a boy at random from the population is 0.484, or 48.4%. A second interpretation is that the proportion of boys in the population is 48.4%. The probability that we select a child who is 7 years of age is P(7 years of age) = $913 / 5290 = 0.173$.

This formula can also be used to compute probabilities of characteristics defined more narrowly or more broadly. For example, what is the probability of selecting a boy who is 10 years of age? P(boy who is 10 years of age) = $418 / 5290 = 0.079$. What is the probability of selecting a child (boy or girl) who is at least 8 years of age? P(at least 8 years of age) = $(846 + 881 + 918) / 5290 = 2645 / 5290 = 0.500$.

To use this formula to compute probabilities, we must enumerate the population as in Example 5.1. Once the population is enumerated, we can compute probabilities relatively easily by counting the numbers of individuals who possess the characteristic of interest and dividing by the population size.

5.3 CONDITIONAL PROBABILITY

Each of the probabilities computed in the previous section are unconditional probabilities. In each case, the denominator is the total population size $N = 5290$, reflecting the fact that everyone in the entire population is eligible to be selected. Sometimes it is of interest to focus on a particular subset of the population (e.g., a subpopulation). For example, suppose we are interested just in the girls and ask the question, what is the

probability of selecting a 9-year-old from the subpopulation of girls? There are a total of $N_G = 2730$ girls (here N_G refers to the population size of girls) and the probability of selecting a 9-year-old from the subpopulation of girls is written as follows: P(9-year-old | girls), where "|" refers to the fact that we are conditioning on or referring to a specific subgroup, and that subgroup specified to the right of "|".

The conditional probability is computed using the same approach we used to compute unconditional probabilities. P(9-year-old | girls) = $461 / 2730 = 0.169$. This means that 16.9% of the girls are 9 years of age. Note that this is not the same as the probability of selecting a 9-year-old girl, which is P(girl who is 9 years of age) = $461 / 5290 = 0.087$. What is the probability of selecting a boy from among the 6-year-olds? P(boy | 6 years of age) = $379 / 892 = 0.425$. Thus, 42.5% of the 6-year-olds are boys (and 57.5% of the 6-year-olds are girls). Some popular applications of conditional probability in medicine are described here.

5.3.1 Evaluating Screening Tests

Screening tests are often used in clinical practice to assess the likelihood that a person has a particular medical condition. Many screening tests are based on laboratory tests that detect particular markers that are related to a specific disease. For example, a popular screening test for prostate cancer is called the prostate-specific antigen (PSA) test and is recommended for men over 50 years of age. The test measures PSA, which is a protein produced by the prostate gland. The PSA screening test measures the amount of PSA in the blood. Low levels of PSA are normal but elevated levels have been shown to be associated with prostate cancer. The PSA test alone does not provide a diagnosis of prostate cancer. A more invasive test, such as a biopsy—in which tissue is extracted and examined under a microscope—is needed to make a diagnosis. Data such as that shown in Example 5.2 are often compiled to evaluate the usefulness of a screening test.

Example 5.2. Suppose that we wish to investigate whether the PSA test is a useful screening test for prostate cancer. To be useful clinically, we would want the test to distinguish between men with and without prostate cancer. Suppose that a population of $N = 120$ men over 50 years of age who are considered high-risk for prostate cancer have both the PSA screening test and a biopsy. The PSA results are reported as low, slightly to moderately elevated, or highly elevated. The classifications are based on the following levels of measured protein, respectively: $0-2.5$, $2.6-19.9$, and 20 or more nanograms per milliliter (ng/ml).[9] The biopsy provides the diagnosis of prostate cancer. The results of the study are shown in Table 5–4.

TABLE 5–4 Evaluation of PSA Test

| PSA Level | Biopsy Results | | Total |
	Prostate Cancer	No Prostate Cancer	
Low	3	61	64
Slightly–moderately elevated	13	28	41
Highly elevated	12	3	15
Total	28	92	120

The probability that a man has prostate cancer given that he has a low level of PSA is P(prostate cancer | low PSA) = 3 / 64 = 0.047. The probability that a man has prostate cancer given that he has a slightly to moderately elevated level of PSA is P(prostate cancer | slightly to moderately elevated PSA) = 13 / 41 = 0.317. The probability that a man has prostate cancer given that he has a highly elevated level of PSA is P(prostate cancer | highly elevated PSA) = 12 / 15 = 0.80. The probability or likelihood that a man has prostate cancer is highly dependent on his PSA level. Based on these data, is the PSA test a clinically important screening test?

Some screening tests are based on a set of self-administered questions that address a specific state, such as depression, anxiety, or stress. Patients who screen positive (e.g., score high or low on a set of questions) might be referred to undergo subsequent screening or more involved testing to make a diagnosis.

Example 5.3. In pregnancy, women often undergo screening to assess whether their fetus is likely to have Down Syndrome. The screening test evaluates levels of specific hormones in the blood. The screening tests are reported as positive or negative, indicating that a woman is more or less likely to be carrying an affected fetus. Suppose that a population of $N = 4810$ pregnant women undergo the screening test and are scored as either positive or negative depending on the levels of hormones in the blood. In addition, suppose that each woman in the study has an amniocentesis. Amniocentesis is an invasive procedure that provides a more definitive assessment as to whether a fetus is affected with Down Syndrome. Amniocentesis is called a diagnostic test, or the gold standard (i.e., the true state). The results of the screening tests and the amniocentesis (diagnostic test) are summarized in Table 5–5.

Using the data from Table 5–5, the probability that a woman with a positive test has an affected fetus is P(affected fetus | screen positive) = 9 / 360 = 0.025, and the probability that a woman with a negative test has an affected fetus is P(affected fetus | negative screen positive) = 1 / 4450 = 0.0002. Is the screening test a useful test?

TABLE 5–5 Evaluation of Prenatal Screening Test

	Affected Fetus	Unaffected Fetus	Total
Positive	9	351	360
Negative	1	4449	4450
Total	10	4800	4810

5.3.2 Sensitivity and Specificity

Screening tests are not used to make medical diagnoses but instead to identify individuals most likely to have a certain condition. Ideally, screening tests are not excessively costly and pose little risk to the patients undergoing the test. There are a number of widely used screening tests available today, including the PSA test for prostate cancer, mammograms for breast cancer, and serum and ultrasound assessments for prenatal diagnosis.

When a screening test is proposed, there are two measures that are often used to evaluate its performance, the sensitivity and specificity of the test. Suppose that the results of the screening test are dichotomous—specifically, each person is classified as either positive or negative for having the condition of interest. *Sensitivity* is also called the true positive fraction and is defined as the probability that a diseased person screens positive. *Specificity* is also called the true negative fraction and is defined as the probability that a disease-free person screens negative. To evaluate the screening test, each participant undergoes the test and is classified as positive or negative based on criteria that are specific to the test (e.g., high levels of a marker in a serum test, or the presence of a mass on a mammogram). Each participant also undergoes a diagnostic test, which provides a definitive diagnosis (e.g., an amniocentesis, or a biopsy). A total of N patients complete both the screening test and the diagnostic test. The data are often organized as shown in Table 5–6. The results of the screening test are shown

TABLE 5–6 Data Layout for Evaluating Screening Tests

	Diseased	Disease Free	Total
Screen positive	a	b	$a+b$
Screen negative	c	d	$c+d$
Total	$a+c$	$b+d$	N

in the rows of the table, and the results of the diagnostic test are shown in the columns.

The definitions of sensitivity and specificity are given as:

$$\text{Sensitivity} = \text{True Positive Fraction} =$$
$$\text{P(screen positive | disease)} = a / (a + c).$$

$$\text{Specificity} = \text{True Negative Fraction} =$$
$$\text{P(screen negative | disease free)} = d / (b + d).$$

$$\text{False Positive Fraction} =$$
$$\text{P(screen positive | disease free)} = b / (b + d).$$

$$\text{False Negative Fraction} =$$
$$\text{P(screen negative | disease)} = c / (a + c).$$

The false positive fraction is 1-specificity and the false negative fraction is 1-sensitivity. Therefore, knowing sensitivity and specificity captures the information in the false positive and false negative fractions. These are simply alternate ways of expressing the same information. Often, sensitivity and the false positive fraction are reported for a test.

Example 5.4. Consider again the study presented in Example 5.3 in which a population of $N = 4810$ pregnant women have a screening test and an amniocentesis to assess the likelihood of carrying a fetus with Down Syndrome. The results are summarized in Table 5–5.

The performance characteristics of the test are:

$$\text{Sensitivity} = \text{P(screen positive | affected fetus)} =$$
$$9 / 10 = 0.900.$$

$$\text{Specificity} = \text{P(screen negative | unaffected fetus)} =$$
$$4449 / 4800 = 0.927.$$

$$\text{False Positive Fraction} =$$
$$\text{P(screen positive | unaffected fetus)} = 351 / 4800 = 0.073.$$

$$\text{False Negative Fraction} =$$
$$\text{P(screen negative | affected fetus)} = 1 / 10 = 0.100.$$

These results are interpreted as follows. If a woman is carrying an affected fetus, there is a 90.0% probability that the screening test will be positive. If the woman is carrying an unaffected fetus (defined here as a fetus free of Down Syndrome, because this test does not assess other abnormalities), there is a 92.7% probability that the screening test will be negative. If a woman is carrying an unaffected fetus, there is a 7.3% probability that the screening test will be positive, and if a woman is carrying an affected fetus, there is a 10.0% probability that the test will be negative. The false positive and false negative fractions quantify errors in the test. The errors are often of greatest concern. For example, if a woman is carrying an unaffected fetus, there is a 7.3% probability that the test will incorrectly come back positive. This is potentially a serious problem, as a positive test result would likely produce great anxiety for the woman and her family. A false negative result is also problematic. If a woman is carrying an affected fetus, there is a 10.0% probability that the test will come back negative. The woman and her family might feel a false sense of assurance that the fetus is not affected when, in fact, the screening test missed the abnormality.

The sensitivity and false positive fractions often are reported for screening tests. However, for some tests the specificity and false negative fractions might be the most important. The most important characteristics of any screening test depend on the implications of an error. In all cases, it is important to understand the performance characteristics of any screening test to appropriately interpret results and their implications.

5.3.3 Positive and Negative Predictive Value

Patients undergoing medical testing often ask the following questions: What is the probability that I have the disease if my screening test comes back positive? What is the probability that I do not have the disease if my test comes back negative? These questions again can be answered with conditional probabilities. These quantities are called the *positive* and *negative predictive values* of a test and are defined in the following sections. Consider again the data layout of Table 5–6 summarizing the results of screening and diagnostic tests applied to a population of N individuals. The definitions of positive and negative predictive values are given as: Positive predictive value = P(disease | screen positive) = $a / (a + b)$. Negative predictive value = P(disease free | screen negative) = $d / (c + d)$. Notice the difference in the definitions of the positive and negative predictive values as compared to the sensitivity and specificity provided previously.

Example 5.5. Consider again the study presented in Example 5.3 and Example 5.4, in which a population of $N = 4810$ pregnant women have a screening test and an amniocentesis to assess the likelihood of carrying a fetus with Down Syndrome. The results are summarized in Table 5–5. The positive predictive value P(affected fetus | screen positive) = 9/360 = 0.025 and negative predictive value P(unaffected | screen negative) = 4449/4450 = 0.999. These results are interpreted as follows. If a woman screens positive, there is a 2.5% probability that she is carrying an affected fetus. If a woman screens negative, there is a 99.9% probability that she is carrying an unaffected fetus.

Patients often want to know the probability of having the disease if they screen positive (positive predictive value). As with this example, the positive predictive value can be very low (2.5%) because it depends on the prevalence of the disease in the population. Thankfully, the prevalence of Down Syndrome in the population is low. Using the data in Example 5.5, the prevalence of Down Syndrome in the population of $N = 4810$ women is 10 / 4810 = 0.002 (i.e., Down Syndrome affects 2 fetuses per 1000). Whereas this screening test has good performance characteristics (sensitivity of 90.0% and specificity of 92.7%) because the prevalence of the condition is so low, even a test with a high probability of detecting an affected fetus does not translate into a high positive predictive value. Because positive and negative predictive values depend on the prevalence of the disease, they cannot be estimated in case control designs (see Section 2.2.4 for more details).

5.4   INDEPENDENCE

In probability, two events are said to be *independent* if the probability of one is not affected by the occurrence or non-occurrence of the other. The definition alone is difficult to digest.

Example 5.6. In Example 5.2, we analyzed data from a population of $N = 120$ men who had both a PSA test and a biopsy for prostate cancer. Suppose we have a different test for prostate cancer. This prostate test produces a numerical risk that classifies a man as at low, moderate, or high risk for prostate cancer. A sample of 100 men underwent the new test and also had a biopsy. The data are summarized in Table 5–7.

The probability that a man has prostate cancer given he has a low risk is P(prostate cancer | low risk) = 10 / 60 = 0.167. The probability that a man has prostate cancer given he has a moderate risk is P(prostate cancer | moderate risk) = 6 / 36 = 0.167. The probability that a man has prostate cancer given he has a high risk is P(prostate cancer | high risk) = 4 / 24 = 0.167. The probability or likelihood that a man has prostate cancer here is unrelated or independent of his risk based on the prostate test. Knowing a man's prostate test result does not affect the likelihood that he has prostate cancer in this example. Thus, the likelihood that a man has prostate cancer is independent of his prostate test result.

Independence can be demonstrated in several ways. Consider two events—call them A and B (A could be a low-risk based on the prostate test and B a diagnosis of prostate cancer). Two events are independent if

$$P(A \mid B) = P(A) \text{ or if } P(B \mid A) = P(B).$$

For example, define A = *Low Risk* and B = *Prostate Cancer*. To check independence, we must compare a conditional and an unconditional probability: P(A | B) = P(low risk | prostate cancer) = 10 / 20 = 0.50, and P(A) = P(low risk) = 60 / 120 = 0.50. The equality of the conditional and unconditional probabilities here indicates independence. Independence can also be checked using P(B | A) = P(prostate cancer | low risk) = 10 / 60 = 0.167, and P(B) = P(prostate cancer) = 20 / 120 = 0.167. Both versions of the definition of independence will give the same result.

Example 5.7. Table 5–8 contains information on a population of $N = 6732$ individuals who are classified as having or

TABLE 5-7 Prostate Test and Biopsy Results

Prostate Test Risk	Biopsy Results		Total
	Prostate Cancer	No Prostate Cancer	
Low	10	50	60
Moderate	6	30	36
High	4	20	24
Total	20	100	120

TABLE 5-8 Family History and Prevalent CVD

	Prevalent CVD	Free of CVD	Total
Family history of CVD	491	368	859
No family history of CVD	152	5721	5873
Total	643	6089	6732

not having prevalent cardiovascular disease (CVD). Each individual is also classified in terms of having a family history of cardiovascular disease. In this analysis, family history is defined as a first degree relative (parent or sibling) with diagnosed CVD before age 60.

Are family history and prevalent CVD independent? Another way to ask the question is as follows: Is there a relationship between family history and prevalent CVD? This is a question of independence of events. Let A = *Prevalent CVD* and B = *Family History of CVD*. (Note that it does not matter how we define A and B; the result will be identical.) We now must check whether $P(A | B) = P(A)$ or if $P(B | A) = P(B)$. Again, it makes no difference which definition is used, the results will be identical. We will compute $P(A | B) = $ P(prevalent CVD | family history of CVD) = 491 / 859 = 0.572 and compare it to $P(A) = $ P(prevalent CVD) = 643 / 6732 = 0.096. These probabilities are not equal, therefore family history and prevalent CVD are not independent. In the population, the probability of prevalent CVD is 9.6%, or 9.6% of the population has prevalent CVD. Individuals with a family history of CVD are much more likely to have prevalent CVD. The probability of prevalent CVD given a family history is 57.2%, as compared to 2.6% among patients with no family history.

5.5   BAYES' THEOREM

Bayes' Theorem is a probability rule that can be used to compute a conditional probability based on specific available information. There are several versions of the theorem, ranging from simple to more involved. The following is the simple statement of the rule:

$$P(A | B) = \frac{P(B | A)\, P(A)}{P(B)}$$

Example 5.8. Suppose a patient exhibits symptoms raising concern with his physician that he may have a particular disease. Suppose the disease is relatively rare with a prevalence

of 0.2% (meaning it affects 2 out of every 1000 persons). The physician recommends testing, starting with a screening test. The screening test is noninvasive, based on a blood sample and costs $250. Before agreeing to the screening test, the patient wants to know what will be learned from the test—specifically, he wants to know his chances of having the disease if the test comes back positive. The physician reports that the screening test is widely used and has a reported sensitivity of 85%. In addition, the test comes back positive 8% of the time and negative 92% of the time.

The patient wants to know P(disease | screen positive). Using Bayes' Theorem, we can compute this as follows:

P(disease | screen positive) = P(screen positive | disease) P(disease)/P(screen positive).

We know that P(disease) = 0.002, P(screen positive | disease) = 0.85 and P(screen positive) = 0.08. We can now substitute the values into the above equation to compute the desired probability:

P(disease | screen positive) = (0.85)(0.002) / (0.08) = 0.021.

If the patient undergoes the test and it comes back positive, there is a 2.1% chance that he has the disease. Without the test, there is a 0.2% chance that he has the disease (the prevalence in the general population). Should the patient have the screening test?

Another important question that the patient might ask is, What is the chance of a false positive result? Specifically, what is P(screen positive | no disease)? We can compute this conditional probability with the available information using Bayes' Theorem:

P(screen positive | no disease) =

$$\frac{P(\text{no disease} | \text{screen positive})P(\text{screen positive})}{P(\text{no disease})},$$

P(screen positive | no disease) =

(1 − 0.021)(0.08) / (1 − 0.002) = 0.078.

Note that if P(disease) = 0.002, then P(no disease) = 1 − 0.002. The events *Disease* and *No Disease* are called complementary events. The *No Disease* group includes all members of the population not in the *Disease* group. The probabilities of complementary events must sum to 1, i.e., P(disease) + P(no disease) = 1. Similarly, P(no disease | screen positive) +

P(disease | screen positive) = 1. Using Bayes' Theorem, there is a 7.8% probability that the screening test will be positive in patients free of disease, which is the false positive fraction of the test.

5.6 PROBABILITY MODELS

To compute the probabilities in the previous sections, we counted the number of participants that had the characteristic of interest and divided by the population size. For conditional probabilities, the population size (denominator) was modified to reflect the subpopulation of interest. In each of the examples in the previous sections, we had a tabulation of the population (the sampling frame) that allowed us to compute the desired probabilities. There are instances where a complete enumeration or tabulation is not available. In some of these instances, probability models or mathematical equations can be used to generate probabilities.

There are many probability models and the model appropriate for a specific application depends on the specific attributes of the application. If an application satisfies specific attributes of a probability model, the model can be used to generate probabilities. In the following two sections, we describe two very popular probability models. These probability models will be extremely important in statistical inference, which is discussed in detail in Chapter 6, Chapter 7, and Chapter 9.

5.6.1 A Probability Model for a Discrete Outcome: The Binomial Distribution

The binomial distribution model is an important probability distribution model that is appropriate when a particular experiment or process has two possible outcomes. The name itself, *binomial*, reflects the dichotomy of responses. There are many different probability models and if a particular process results in more than two distinct outcomes, a multinomial probability model might be appropriate. Here we focus on the situation in which the outcome is dichotomous. For example, adults with allergies might report relief with medication or not, children with a bacterial infection might respond to antibiotic therapy or not, adults who suffer a myocardial infarction might survive or not, or a medical device such as a coronary stent might be successfully implanted or not. These are just a few examples of applications or processes where the outcome of interest has two possible values.

The two outcomes are often labeled "success" and "failure," with "success" denoting the outcome of interest. In some medical and public health applications, we are interested in

quantifying the extent of disease (the unhealthy response). Clearly, the unhealthy response is not a "success"; this nomenclature is simply used for the application of the binomial distribution model. In any application of the binomial distribution, we must clearly specify which outcome is the success and which is the failure.

The binomial distribution model allows us to compute the probability of observing a specified number of successes when the process is repeated a specific number of times (e.g., in a set of patients) and the outcome for a given patient is either a success or a failure. We must first introduce some notation that is necessary for the binomial distribution model. First, we let n denote the number of times the application or process is repeated and x denote the number of successes, out of n, of interest. We let p denote the probability of success for any individual. The binomial distribution model is defined as

$$P(x \text{ successes}) = \frac{n!}{x!(n-x)!} p^x (1-p)^{n-x},$$

where ! denotes factorial, defined as $k! = k(k-1)(k-2)...1$. For example, $4! = 4(3)(2)1 = 24$, $2! = 2(1) = 2$ and $1! = 1$. There is one special case where $0! = 1$.

Appropriate use of the binomial distribution model depends on satisfying the following three assumptions about the application or process under investigation: each replication of the process results in one of two possible outcomes (success or failure); the probability of success is the same for each replication; and the replications are independent, meaning here that a success in one patient does not influence the probability of success in another.

Example 5.9. Consider the example where adults with allergies report relief from allergic symptoms with a specific medication. Suppose we know that the medication is effective in 80% of patients with allergies who take it as prescribed. If we provide the medication to 10 patients with allergies, what is the probability that it is effective in exactly 7 patients?

Do we satisfy the three assumptions of the binomial distribution model? Each replication of this application involves providing medication to a patient and assessing whether he or she reports relief of symptoms. The outcome is relief from symptoms ("yes" or "no") and here we will call a reported relief from symptoms a success. The probability of success for each person is 0.8. The final assumption is that the replications are independent. In this setting, this essentially means that the probability of success for any given patient does not depend on the success or failure of any other patient (For more details, see D'Agostino, Sullivan and Beiser.[10]) This is a reasonable assumption in this case. We now need to set the notation: $n = 10$, $x = 7$, and $p = 0.80$. The desired probability is

$$P(7 \text{ successes}) = \frac{10!}{7!(10-7)!} \, 0.80^7 (1-0.80)^{10-7}.$$

The first (factorial) portion of the formula is computed as follows:

$$\frac{10!}{7!(10-7)!} = \frac{10(9)(8)(7)(6)(5)(4)(3)(2)1}{\{7(6)(5)(4)(3)(2)(1)\}\{(3)(2)(1)\}} =$$

$$\frac{10(9)(8)}{3(2)} = 120.$$

Substituting,

$$P(7 \text{ successes}) = (120)(0.2097)(0.008) = 0.2013.$$

There is a 20.13% probability that exactly 7 of 10 patients will report relief from symptoms when the probability that anyone reports relief is 80%.

What is the probability that none report relief? We can again use the binomial distribution model with $n = 10$, $x = 0$, and $p = 0.80$:

$$P(0 \text{ successes}) = \frac{10!}{0!(10-0)!} \, 0.80^0 (1-0.80)^{10-0}.$$

The first (factorial) portion of the formula is computed as follows:

$$\frac{10!}{0!(10-0)!} = \frac{10!}{\{1\}\{10!\}} = 1.$$

Substituting,

$$P(0 \text{ successes}) = (1)(1)(0.0000001024) = 0.0000001024.$$

There is practically no chance that none of the 10 will report relief from symptoms when the probability of reporting relief for any individual patient is 80%.

What is the most likely number of patients who will report relief when the medication is given to 10 patients? If 80% report relief and we consider 10 patients, we would expect that 8 report relief. What is the probability that 8 of 10 report relief?

$$P(8 \text{ successes}) = \frac{10!}{8!(10-8)!} \, 0.80^8 (1-0.80)^{10-8}.$$

The first (factorial) portion of the formula is computed as follows:

$$\frac{10!}{8!(10-8)!} = \frac{10(9)(8)(7)(6)(5)(4)(3)(2)1}{\{8(7)(6)(5)(4)(3)(2)(1)\}\{(2)(1)\}} =$$

$$\frac{10(9)}{2} = 45.$$

Substituting,

$$P(8 \text{ successes}) = (45)(0.1678)(0.04) = 0.3020.$$

There is a 30.20% probability that exactly 8 of 10 patients will report relief from symptoms when the probability that anyone reports relief is 80%. The probability that exactly 8 report relief will be the highest probability of all possible outcomes (0 through 10).

Many statistical textbooks provide tables of binomial probabilities for specific combinations of n, x, and p.[10] These tables can be used to determine the probability of observing x successes out of n replications when the probability of success is p. The tables can be of limited use as they often contain only some combinations of n, x, and p. The binomial formula can always be used as long as assumptions are appropriately satisfied.

Example 5.10. The likelihood that a patient with a heart attack dies of the attack is 0.04 (i.e., 4 of 100 die of the attack). Suppose we have 5 patients who suffer a heart attack. What is the probability that all will survive?

Here we are provided with the probability that an attack is fatal. For this example, we will call a success a fatal attack, and thus $p = 0.04$. We have $n = 5$ patients and want to know the probability that all survive or, in other words, that none are fatal (0 successes). We again need to assess the assumptions. Each attack is fatal or non-fatal, the probability of a fatal attack is 4% for all patients, and the outcome of individual patients are independent. It should be noted that the assumption that the probability of success applies to all patients must be evaluated carefully. The probability that a patient dies from a heart attack depends on many factors including age, the severity of the attack, and other co-morbid conditions.

To apply the 4% probability, we must be convinced that all patients are at the same risk of a fatal attack. The assumption of the independence of events must also be evaluated carefully. As long as the patients are unrelated, the assumption is usually appropriate. Prognosis of disease could be related or correlated in members of the same family or in individuals who are co-habitating. In this example, suppose that the 5 patients being analyzed are unrelated, of similar age, and free of co-morbid conditions:

$$P(0 \text{ successes}) = \frac{5!}{0!(5-0)!} \, 0.04^0 (1-0.04)^{5-0}.$$

The first (factorial) portion of the formula is computed as follows:

$$\frac{5!}{0!(5-0)!} = \frac{5!}{\{1\}\{5\}} = 1.$$

Substituting,

$$P(0 \text{ successes}) = (1)(1)(0.8154) = 0.8154.$$

There is an 81.54% probability that all patients will survive the attack when the probability that any one dies is 4%. In this example, the possible outcomes are 0, 1, 2, 3, 4, or 5 successes (fatalities). Because the probability of fatality is so low, the most likely response is 0 (all patients survive).

The binomial formula generates the probability of observing exactly x successes out of n. If we want to compute the probability of a range of outcomes, we need to apply the formula more than once. Suppose in this example we wanted to compute the probability that no more than 1 person dies of the attack. Specifically, we want P(no more than 1 success) = P(0 or 1 successes) = P(0 successes) + P(1 success). To compute this probability, we apply the binomial formula twice. We already computed P(0 successes), we now compute P(1 success):

$$P(1 \text{ successes}) = \frac{5!}{1!(5-1)!} \, 0.04^1 (1-0.04)^{5-1}.$$

The first (factorial) portion of the formula is computed as follows:

$$\frac{5!}{1!(5-1)!} = \frac{5(4)(3)(2)1}{\{1\}\{4(3)(2)(1)\}} = 5.$$

Substituting,

$$P(1 \text{ success}) = (5)(0.04)(0.8493) = 0.1697.$$

P(no more than 1 success) = P(0 or 1 successes) =
P(0 successes) + P(1 success) = 0.8154 + 0.1697 = 0.9851.

The probability that no more than 1 of 5 (or equivalently, that at most 1 of 5) die from the attack is 98.51%.

What is the probability that 2 or more of 5 die from the attack? Here we want to compute P(2 or more successes). The possible outcomes are 0, 1, 2, 3, 4, or 5, and the sum of the probabilities of each of these outcomes is 1 (i.e., we are certain to observe either 0, 1, 2, 3, 4, or 5 successes). We just computed P(0 or 1 successes) = 0.9851, so P(2, 3, 4, or 5 successes) = 1 − P(0 or 1 successes) = 0.0149. There is a 1.49% probability that 2 or more of 5 will die from the attack.

The mean of a binomial population is defined as $\mu = np$, and the standard deviation is $\sigma = \sqrt{n(p)(1-p)}$. In Example 5.9, we considered a binomial population with $n = 10$ and $p = 0.80$. The mean, or expected, number of successes is $\mu = np = 10(0.80) = 8$, and the standard deviation is $\sigma = \sqrt{n(p)(1-p)} = \sqrt{10(0.8)(0.2)} = 1.3$.

5.6.2 A Probability Model for a Continuous Outcome: The Normal Distribution

The normal distribution model is an important probability distribution model that is appropriate when a particular experiment or process results in a continuous outcome. There are many different probability models for continuous outcomes and the appropriate model depends on the distribution of the outcome of interest. The normal probability model applies when the distribution of the continuous outcome follows what is called the Gaussian distribution, or is well described by a bell-shaped curve (Figure 5–1).

The horizontal or x-axis is used to display the scale of the characteristic being analyzed (e.g., height, weight, systolic blood pressure). The height of the curve reflects the probability of observing each value. Notice that the curve is highest in the middle, suggesting that the middle values have higher probabilities or are more likely to occur. The curve tails off above and below the middle, suggesting that values at either extreme are much less likely to occur. Similar to the binomial distribution model, there are some assumptions for appropriate use of the normal distribution model. The normal distribution model is appropriate for a continuous outcome if the following conditions are true. First, in a normal distribution the mean is equal to the median and also equal to the mode, which is defined as the most frequently observed value. As we discussed in Chapter 4, it is not always the case that the mean and median are equal. For example, if a particular characteristic is subject to outliers, then the mean will not be equal to the median and therefore the characteristic will not follow a normal distribution. An example might be the length of stay in the hospital (measured in days) following a specific procedure. Length of stay often follows a skewed distribution, as illustrated in Figure 5–2.

Many characteristics are approximately normally distributed, such as height and weight for specific age and gender groups, as are many laboratory and clinical measures such as cholesterol level and systolic blood pressure. The first property of the normal distribution implies the following: $P(x > \mu) = P(x < \mu) = 0.5$, where x denotes the continuous variable of interest and μ is the population mean. The probability that a value exceeds the mean is 50% and equivalent to the probability that a value is below the mean, which is the definition of the median. In a normal distribution, the mean, median, and mode (the most frequent value) are equal. A

FIGURE 5–1 Normal Distribution

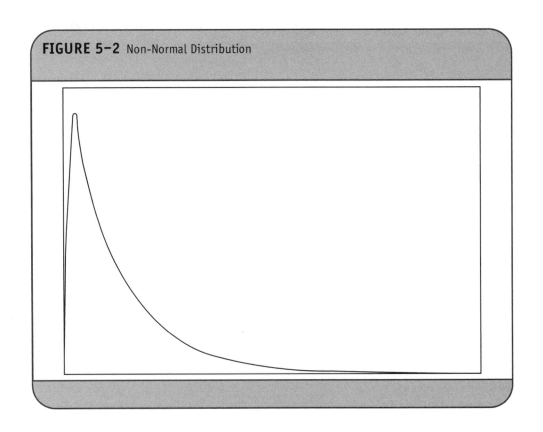

FIGURE 5–2 Non-Normal Distribution

continuous variable that follows a normal distribution is one for which the following three statements are also true.

i. Approximately 68% of the values fall between the mean and one standard deviation (in either direction), i.e., $P(\mu-\sigma < x < \mu+\sigma) = 0.68$, where **m** is the population mean and **s** is the population standard deviation.

ii. Approximately 95% of the values fall between the mean and two standard deviations (in either direction), i.e., $P(\mu-2\sigma < x < \mu+2\sigma) = 0.95$.

iii. Approximately 99.9% of the values fall between the mean and three standard deviations (in either direction), i.e., $P(\mu-3\sigma < x < \mu+3\sigma) = 0.999$.

Part (iii) of the preceding indicates that for a continuous variable following a normal distribution, almost all of the observations fall between $\mu-3$**s** and $\mu+3\sigma$, thus the minimum value is approximately $\mu-3\sigma$ and the maximum is approximately $\mu+3\sigma$. In the following examples, we will illustrate how these probabilities 68%, 95%, and 99.9% were derived.

Another attribute of a normal distribution is that it is symmetric about the mean. The curve to the right of the mean is a mirror image of that to the left. A continuous variable with a distribution like that displayed in Figure 5–1—whose mean, median, and mode are equal—is symmetric and satisfies the preceding conditions (i) through (iii) and follows a normal distribution. Similar to the binomial case, there is a normal

distribution model that can be used to compute probabilities. The normal probability model is shown below and computing probabilities with the normal distribution model requires calculus,

$$P(x) = \frac{1}{\sigma\sqrt{2p}}\, e^{-(x-\mu)^2/(2\sigma^2)},$$

where **m** is the population mean and **s** is the population standard deviation. There is an alternative to using calculus to compute probabilities for normal variables, and it involves the use of probability tables. This is the approach we will use.

Example 5.11. Body mass index (BMI) for specific gender and age groups is approximately normally distributed. The mean BMI for men aged 60 is 29 with a standard deviation of 6, and for women aged 60 the mean BMI is 28 with a standard deviation of 7. Suppose we consider the distribution of BMI among men aged 60. Knowing that the distribution is normal and having the mean and standard deviation allow us to completely generate the distribution. The distribution of BMI among men aged 60 is shown in Figure 5–3.

Notice that the mean (**m** = 29) is in the center of the distribution, the horizontal axis is scaled in units of the standard deviation (**s** = 6), and the distribution essentially ranges from $\mu-3\sigma$ to $\mu+3\sigma$. This is not to say that there are not BMI values below 11 or above 47; there are such values

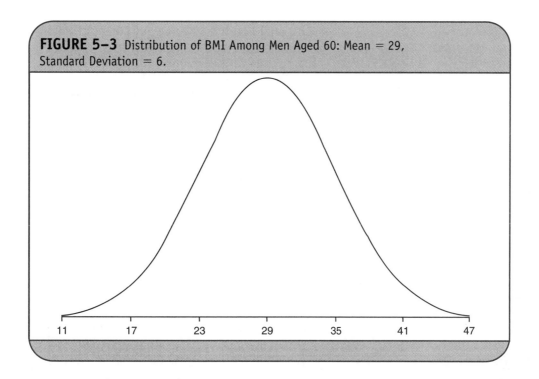

FIGURE 5–3 Distribution of BMI Among Men Aged 60: Mean = 29, Standard Deviation = 6.

but they occur very infrequently. To compute probabilities about normal distributions, we compute areas under the curve. For example, suppose a man aged 60 is selected at random—what is the probability his BMI is less than 29? The probability is displayed graphically and represented by the area under the curve to the left of the value 29 in Figure 5–4.

The probability that a male has a BMI less than 29 is equivalent to the area under the curve to the left of the line drawn at 29. For any probability distribution, the total area under the curve is 1. For the normal distribution, we know that the mean is equal to median and thus half (50%) of the area under the curve is above the mean and half is below, so $P(BMI < 29) = 0.50$.

We might want to compute the probability that a male has a BMI of 29 or less, $P(x \leq 29)$. This can be thought of as $P(x \leq 29) = P(x < 29) + P(x = 29)$. We know that $P(x < 29) = 0.50$. With the normal distribution, $P(x = 29)$ is defined as 0. In fact, the probability of being exactly equal to any value is always defined as 0. That is not to say that there are no men with a BMI of 29. There is no area in a single line, and thus $P(X = 29)$ is defined as 0. Thus, $P(x \leq 29) = P(x < 29)$. This concept will be illustrated further.

Suppose we want to know the probability that a male has a BMI less than 35. The probability is displayed graphically and represented by the area under the curve to the left of the value 35 in Figure 5–5. The probability that a male has a BMI less than 35 is equivalent to the area under the curve

to the left of the line drawn at 35. For the normal distribution, we know that approximately 68% of the area under the curve lies between the mean plus or minus one standard deviation. For men aged 60, 68% of the area under the curve lies between 23 and 35. We also know that the normal distribution is symmetric about the mean, therefore $P(29 < x < 35) = P(23 < x < 29) = 0.34$. Thus, $P(x < 35) = 0.5 + 0.34 = 0.84$.

What is the probability that a male aged 60 has a BMI less than 41? Using similar logic and the fact that approximately 95% of the area under the curve lies between the mean plus or minus two standard deviations—i.e., $P(29 < x < 41) = P(17 < x < 29) = 0.475$—we can compute $P(x < 41) = 0.5 + 0.475 = 0.975$.

Suppose we now want to compute the probability that a male aged 60 has a BMI less than 30 (the threshold for classifying someone as obese). The area of interest, reflecting the probability, is displayed graphically in Figure 5–6. Because 30 is not the mean nor a multiple of standard deviations above or below the mean, we cannot use the properties of a normal distribution to determine $P(x < 30)$. The $P(x < 30)$ is certainly between 0.5 and 0.84, based on the previous computations, but we can determine a more exact value. To do so, we need a table of probabilities for the normal distribution.

Because every application we face could potentially involve a normal distribution with a different mean and standard

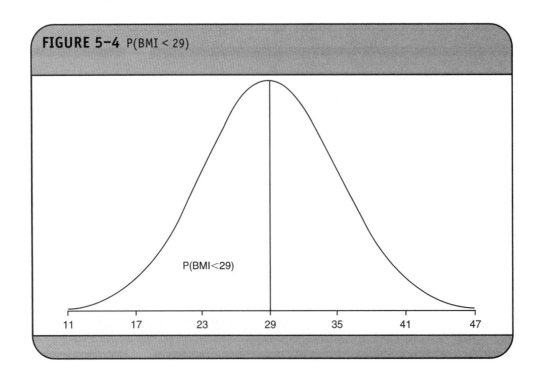

FIGURE 5-4 P(BMI < 29)

P(BMI<29)

11   17   23   29   35   41   47

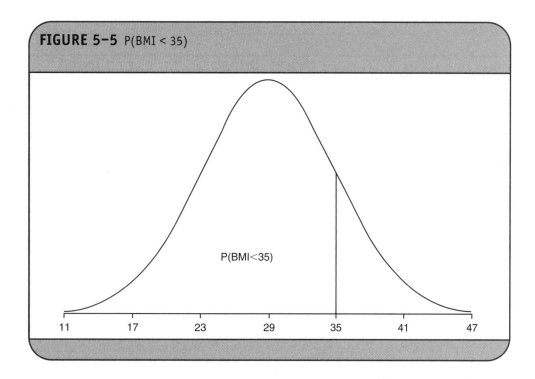

FIGURE 5–5 P(BMI < 35)

P(BMI<35)

11   17   23   29   35   41   47

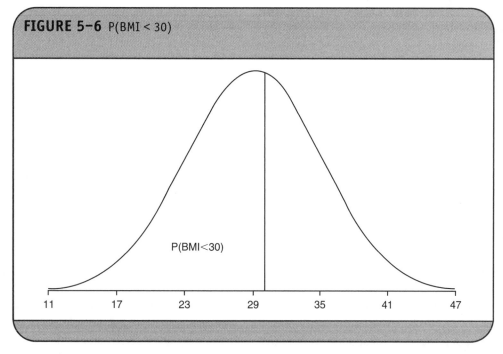

FIGURE 5–6 P(BMI < 30)

P(BMI<30)

11   17   23   29   35   41   47

deviation, we will use a table of probabilities for the standard normal distribution. The standard normal distribution is a normal distribution with a mean of 0 and standard deviation of 1. We will always use z to refer to a standard normal variable. Up to this point, we have been using x to denote the variable of interest (e.g., x = BMI, x = height, x = weight). z will be reserved to refer to the standard normal distribution. The standard normal distribution is displayed in Figure 5–7.

The mean of the standard normal distribution is 0, thus the distribution is centered at 0. Multiples of the standard deviation above and below the mean are by units of the standard deviation ($\sigma = 1$). The range of the standard normal

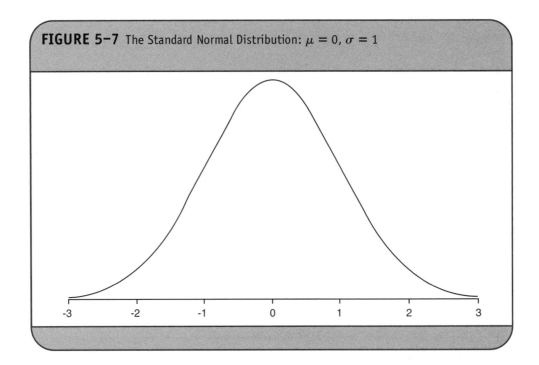

FIGURE 5-7 The Standard Normal Distribution: $\mu = 0$, $\sigma = 1$

distribution is approximately −3 to 3. Table 1 in the Appendix contains probabilities for the standard normal distribution.

The body of Table 1 contains probabilities for the standard normal distribution. These correspond to areas under the standard normal curve. Specifically, Table 1 is organized to provide the area under the curve to the left of or less than the specified z value. Table 1 can accommodate two decimal places of z. The units place and the first decimal place are shown in the left column and the second decimal place is displayed across the top row. For example, suppose we want to compute $P(z < 0)$. Because Table 1 contains z to two decimal places, this is equivalent to $P(z < 0.00)$. We locate 0.0 in the left column (units and tenths place) and 0.00 across the top row (hundredths place). $P(z < 0.00) = 0.5000$. Similarly, $P(z < 0.52) = 0.6985$.

The question of interest is $P(x < 30)$. We now have Table 1, which contains all of the probabilities for the standard normal distribution. BMI follows a normal distribution with a mean of 29 and a standard deviation of 6. We can use the standard normal distribution to solve this problem.

Figure 5–8 shows the distributions of BMI for men aged 60 and the standard normal distribution side-by-side. The areas under the curve are identical; only the scaling of the x-axis is different. BMI ranges from 11 to 47 while the standard normal variable, z, ranges from −3 to 3. We want to compute $P(x < 30)$. We determine the z value that

corresponds to $x = 30$ and then use Table 1 to find the probability or area under the curve. The following formula converts an x value into a z score, also called a standardized score:

$$Z = \frac{x - \mu}{\sigma},$$

where μ is the mean and σ is the standard deviation of the variable x. We want to compute $P(x < 30)$. Using the preceding formula, we convert ($x = 30$) to its corresponding z score (this is called standardizing):

$$Z = \frac{30 - 29}{6} = \frac{1}{6} = 0.17.$$

Thus, $P(x < 30) = P(z < 0.17)$. We can solve the latter using Table 1: $P(x < 30) = P(z < 0.17) = 0.5675$. Notice in Figure 5–9 that the area below 30 and the area below 0.17 in the x and z distributions, respectively, are identical.

Using Table 1, $P(z < 0.17) = 0.5675$. Thus, the probability that a male aged 60 has a BMI less than 30 is 56.75%.

Suppose we now want to compute the probability that a male aged 60 has a BMI of 30 or less. Specifically, we want $P(x \leq 30)$. $P(x \leq 30) = P(x < 30) + P(x = 30)$. The second term reflects the probability of observing a male age 60 with a BMI of exactly 30. We are computing probabilities for the normal distribution as areas under the curve. There is no area

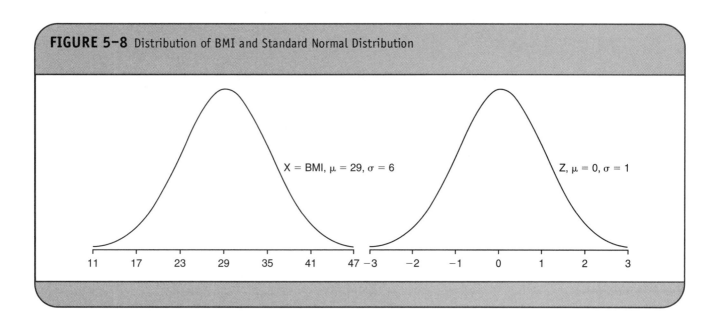

FIGURE 5-8 Distribution of BMI and Standard Normal Distribution

in a single line and thus P(x = 30) is defined as 0. For the normal distribution, and for other probability distributions for continuous variables, this will be the case. Therefore, P(x < 30) = P(x ≤ 30) = 0.5675. Note that for the binomial distribution and for other probability distributions for discrete variables, the probability of taking on a specific value is not defined as 0 (see Section 5.6.1).

Consider again Example 5.11. What is the probability that a male aged 60 has a BMI exceeding 35? Specifically, what is P(x > 35)? Again we standardize:

$$P(x > 35) = P\left(z > \frac{35-29}{6} = \frac{6}{6} = 1\right).$$

We now need to compute P(z > 1). If we look up z = 1.00 on Table 1, we find that P(z < 1.00) = 0.8413. Table 1 always gives the probability that z is less than the specified value. We want P(z > 1) (see Figure 5–10). Table 1 give P(z < 1) = 0.8413, thus P(z > 1) = 1 − 0.8413 = 0.1587. Almost 16% of men aged 60 have BMI over 35.

What is the probability that a male aged 60 has a BMI between 30 and 35? Note that this is the same as asking what proportion of men aged 60 have a BMI between 30 and 35. Specifically, we want P(30 < x < 35). To solve this, we standardize and use Table 1. From the preceding examples, P(30 < x < 35) = P(0.17 < z < 1). This can be computed as P(0.17 < z < 1) = 0.8413 − 0.5675 = 0.2738. This probability can be thought of as P(0.17 < z < 1) = P(z < 1) − P(z < 0.17).

Now consider BMI in women. What is the probability that a female aged 60 has a BMI less than 30? We use the same approach, but recall that for women aged 60, the mean is 28 and the standard deviation is 7,

$$P(x < 30) = P\left(z < \frac{30-28}{7} = \frac{2}{7} = 0.29\right).$$

Using Table 1, P(z < 0.29) = 0.6141. Therefore, 61.41% of women aged 60 have a BMI less than 30, and 38.59% of women have a BMI of 30 or more.

What is the probability that a female aged 60 has a BMI exceeding 40? Specifically, what is P(x > 40)? Again, we standardize:

$$P(x > 40) = P\left(z > \frac{40-28}{7} = \frac{12}{7} = 1.71\right).$$

We need now to compute P(z > 1.71). If we look up z =1.71 on Table 1, we find that P(z < 1.71) = 0.9564. P(z < 1.71) = 1 − 0.9564 = 0.0436. Less than 5% of the women aged 60 have a BMI exceeding 40.

Table 1 is very useful for computing probabilities about normal distributions. To do this, we first standardize or convert a problem about a normal distribution (x) into a problem about the standard normal distribution (z). Once we have the problem in terms of z, we use Table 1 in the Appendix to compute the desired probability.

The standard normal distribution can also be useful for computing percentiles. A *percentile* is a value in the distribution that holds a specified percentage of the population below

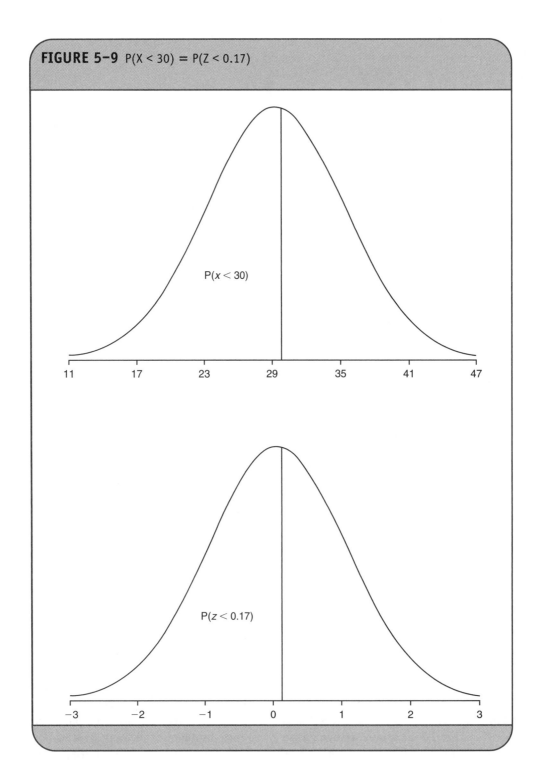

FIGURE 5–9 $P(X < 30) = P(Z < 0.17)$

it. The pth percentile is the value that holds p% of the values below it. For example, the median is the 50th percentile, the first quartile is the 25th percentile, and the third quartile is the 75th percentile. In some instances, it may be of interest to compute other percentiles, for example, the 5th or 95th. The following formula is used to compute percentiles of a normal distribution.

$$x = \mu + z\sigma,$$

where μ is the mean, σ is the standard deviation of the variable x, and z is the value from the standard normal distribution for the desired percentile.

Example 5.12. Consider again Example 5–11, where we analyzed BMI in men and women aged 60. The mean BMI for

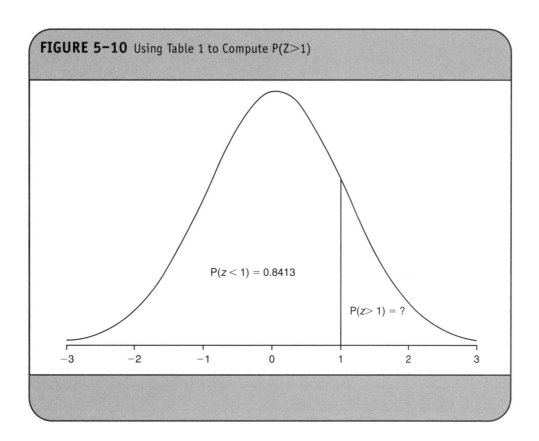

FIGURE 5–10 Using Table 1 to Compute P(Z>1)

P(z < 1) = 0.8413

P(z> 1) = ?

men aged 60 is 29 with a standard deviation of 6, and for women aged 60 the mean BMI is 28 with a standard deviation of 7. What is the 90th percentile of BMI for men?

Figure 5–11 shows the distribution of BMI in men aged 60. The 90th percentile is the BMI that holds 90% of the BMI values below it. It therefore must be a value in the high (right) end of the distribution if 90% of the values are below it, and therefore only 10% are above it. The vertical line in Figure 5–11 is an estimate of the value of the 90th percentile.

To compute the 90th percentile, we use the formula $x = \mu + z\sigma$. The mean and standard deviation are 29 and 6, respectively; what is needed is the z value reflecting the 90th percentile of the standard normal distribution. To compute this value, we use Table 1—however, we use Table 1 almost in "reverse." When computing percentiles, we know the area under the curve (or probability) and want to compute the z score. In Example 5.11, we computed z scores and used Table 1 to determine areas under the curve, or probabilities. Here we know that the area under the curve below the desired z value is 0.90 (or 90%). What z score holds 0.90 below it? The interior of Table 1 contains areas under the curve below z. If the area under the curve below z is 0.90, we find 0.90 in the body (center) of Table 1. The value 0.90 is not there exactly; however, the values 0.8997 and 0.9015 are contained in Table 1. These correspond

to z values of 1.28 and 1.29, respectively (i.e., 89.97% of the area under the standard normal curve is below 1.28). The exact z value holding 90% of the values below it is 1.282. This value was determined by a statistical computing package (e.g., Excel) with more precision than that shown in Table 1. Using $z = 1.282$, we can now compute the 90th percentile of BMI for men: $x = 29 + 1.282(6) = 36.69$. Ninety percent of the BMIs in men aged 60 are below 36.69, and 10% of the BMIs in men aged 60 are above 36.69. What is the 90th percentile of BMI among women aged 60? $x = 28 + 1.282(7) = 36.97$. Ninety percent of the BMIs in women aged 60 are below 36.97, and 10% of the BMIs in women aged 60 are above 36.97.

Table 1A in the Appendix was developed using Table 1 and contains the z values for popular percentiles. It can be used to compute percentiles for normal distributions. A popular application of percentiles is in anthropometrics, which is the study of human measurements. These measures, such as weight and height, are used to study patterns in body size. For example, pediatricians often measure a child's weight, length, or height, and head circumference. The observed values are often converted into percentiles to assess where a particular child falls relative to his or her peers (i.e., children of the same gender and age). For example, if a child's weight for their age is extremely low, it might be an indication of malnutrition. Growth charts for boys and

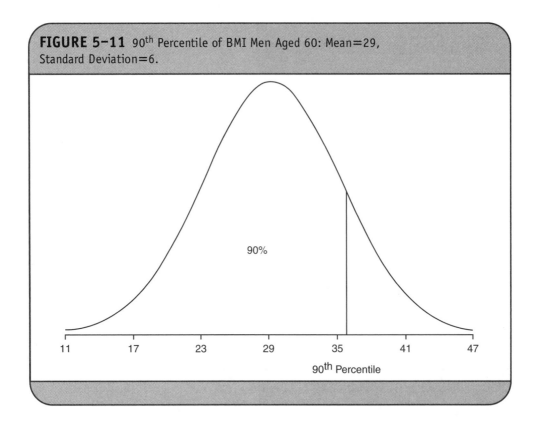

FIGURE 5-11 90th Percentile of BMI Men Aged 60: Mean=29, Standard Deviation=6.

girls including length-for-age, weight-for-age, BMI-for-age, head circumference-for-age, and other anthropometric charts are available for infants from birth to 36 months and children 2 to 20 years old on the Centers for Disease Control (CDC) website at *http://www.cdc.gov/nchs/about/major/nhanes/growthcharts*.

Example 5.13. For infant girls, the mean length at 10 months is 72 cm with a standard deviation of 3 cm. Suppose a girl of 10 months has a measured length of 67 cm. How does her length compare to other girls of 10 months?

We can compute her percentile by determining the proportion of girls with lengths below 67. Specifically,

$$P(x < 67) = P\left(z < \frac{67 - 72}{3} = \frac{-5}{3} = -1.67\right).$$

Using Table 1, $P(z < -1.67) = 0.0475$. This girl is in the 4.75th percentile. Fewer than 5% of girls of 10 months are below 67 cm. This may be an instance where some intervention is needed.

5.6.3 Sampling Distributions

In Chapter 6, Chapter 7, and Chapter 9, we will focus on statistical inference, where we will make inferences or generalizations about population parameters based on observed sample statistics. In Chapter 4, we presented techniques and a number of statistics to summarize sample data. Suppose we want to generate an estimate of a continu-ous variable in a population (e.g., weight, HDL cholesterol level). It is very typical to estimate the mean of a continuous variable in a population. The mean of a representative sample would be a very good estimate of the unknown population mean. If a second sample were selected, that sample might produce a slightly different estimate (i.e., the mean of the second sample might be slightly different than the mean of the first). Whenever we perform statistical inference, we must recognize that we are essentially working with incomplete information—specifically, only a fraction of the population. When we make estimates about population parameters based on sample statistics, it will be extremely important to quantify the precision in our estimates. This is done using probability and, in particular, the probability models we have just discussed.

Example 5.14. Consider the following small population consisting of $N = 6$ patients who recently underwent total hip replacement. We are interested in a patient's self-reported pain-free function, rated on a scale of 0 to 100, with higher scores representing better function (e.g., 0 = severely limited and painful functioning to 100 = completely pain-free function-ing), measured 3 months post-procedure. The data are shown below and ordered from smallest to largest:

25   50   80   85   90   100

The population mean is $\mu = \frac{\Sigma X}{N} = 71.7$ and the standard deviation is $\sigma = \sqrt{\frac{\Sigma(X-\mu)^2}{N}} = 28.4$. A box-whisker plot of the population data is shown in Figure 5–12.

The distribution of function scores is slightly skewed, with the majority of patients reporting high scores. Suppose we did not have the population data and instead were interested in estimating the mean functioning score based on a sample. Suppose we planned to take a sample of size $n = 4$. Table 5–9 shows all possible samples of size $n = 4$ from the population of $N = 6$ when sampling without replacement. (*Sampling without replacement* means that we select an individual and with that person aside, we select a second from those remaining, and so on. In contrast, when *sampling with replacement*, we make a selection, record that selection, and place that person back before making a second selection. When sampling with replacement, the same individual can be selected into the sample multiple times.) The right column shows the sample mean based on the four observations contained in that sample.

The probability of selecting any particular preceding sample is 1 / 15 = 0.07. Suppose by chance we selected Sample 1.

The mean of Sample 1 is 60.0. If we based our estimate of the unknown population mean on Sample 1, and particularly on the sample mean of Sample 1, we would underestimate the true population mean. If we selected Sample 15, we would overestimate the population mean because the mean of Sample 15 is 88.8.

The collection of all possible sample means (in this example, there are 15 distinct samples that are produced by sampling four individuals at random without replacement) is called the sampling distribution of the sample means. We can consider it a population because it includes all possible values produced in this case by a specific sampling scheme. If we compute the mean and standard deviation of this population of sample means, we get the following: $\mu_{\overline{x}} = 71.7$ and a standard deviation of $\sigma_{\overline{x}} = 8.5$. The subscripts here are to distinguish these parameters from those based on the population data (x). To be consistent, the parameters based on the population data could include a subscript x.

Notice that the mean of the sample means is 71.7, which is precisely the value of the population mean. This will always be the case. Specifically, the mean of the sampling distribution of the sample means will always be equivalent

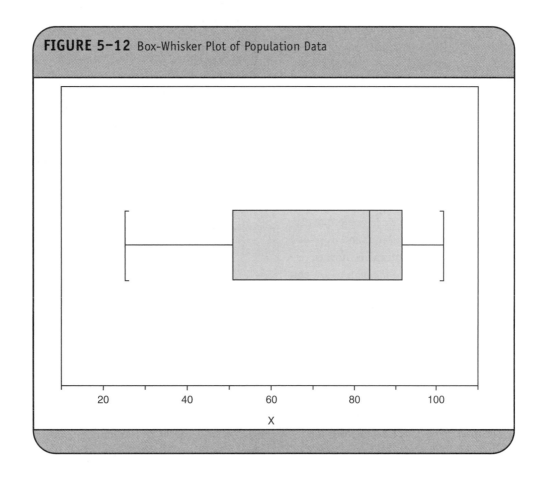

FIGURE 5–12 Box-Whisker Plot of Population Data

TABLE 5–9 All Samples of Size $n = 4$

Sample	Observations in the Sample				Sample Mean ($\overline{X}$)
1	25	50	80	85	60.0
2	25	50	80	90	61.3
3	25	50	80	100	63.8
4	25	50	85	90	62.5
5	25	50	85	100	65.0
6	25	50	90	100	66.3
7	25	80	85	90	70.0
8	25	80	85	100	72.5
9	25	80	90	100	73.8
10	25	85	90	100	75.0
11	50	80	85	90	76.3
12	50	80	85	100	78.8
13	50	80	90	100	80.0
14	50	85	90	100	81.3
15	80	85	90	100	88.8

to the population mean. This is important as it indicates that, on average, the sample mean is equal to the population mean. This is the definition of an unbiased estimator. Unbiasedness is a desirable property in an estimator. Notice also that the variability in the sample means is much smaller than the variability in the population; this will also always be the case. A box-whisker plot of the population of sample means is shown in Figure 5–13.

Notice that the distribution of the sample means is more symmetric and has a much more restricted range than the distribution of the population data shown in Figure 5–12. The importance of these observations is stated formally in the Central Limit Theorem.

Central Limit Theorem. Suppose we have a population with known mean and standard deviation, μ and σ, respectively. The distribution of the population can be normal or it can be non-normal (e.g., skewed toward the high or low end, or flat). If we take simple random samples of size n from the population with replacement, then for large samples (usually defined as samples with $n > 30$), the sampling distribution of the sample means is approximately normally distributed with a mean of $\mu_{\overline{x}} = \mu$ and a standard deviation $\sigma_{\overline{x}} = \frac{\sigma}{\sqrt{n}}$.

The importance of this theorem for applications is as follows. The theorem states that, regardless of the distribution of the population (normal or not), as long as the sample is sufficiently large (usually $n > 30$), then the distribution of the sample means is approximately normal. In Section 5.6.2, we learned that it is relatively straightforward to compute probabilities about a normal distribution. Therefore, when we make inferences about a population mean based on the sample mean, we can use the normal probability model to quantify uncertainty. This will become explicit in Chapter 6, Chapter 7, and Chapter 9.

Before illustrating the use of the Central Limit Theorem, we will first illustrate the result. For the result of the Central Limit Theorem to hold, the sample must be sufficiently large ($n > 30$). There are two exceptions to this: If the population is normal, then the result holds for samples of any size (i.e., the sampling distribution of the sample means will be approximately normal even for samples of size less than 30). If the population is binomial, then the result holds for samples that meet the following criteria: $\min[np, n(1 - p)] > 5$, where n is the sample size and p is the probability of success in the population. We will next illustrate the results of the Central Limit Theorem for a non-normal, a normal, and a binomial population.

Example 5.15. Suppose we measure a characteristic in a population and that this characteristic follows a normal distribution with a mean of 75 and standard deviation of 8. The distribution of the measure in the population is shown in Figure 5–14.

If we take simple random samples with replacement of size $n = 10$ from the population and for each sample we compute the sample mean, the Central Limit Theorem states that the distribution of sample means should be approximately normal. Note that the sample size $n = 10$ does not meet the criterion of $n > 30$, but in this case, our original population is normal and therefore the result holds. The distribution of sample means based on samples of size $n = 10$ is shown in Figure 5–15. The mean of the sample means is 75 and the standard deviation of the sample means is 2.5 (i.e., $\mu_{\overline{x}} = \mu = 75$ and a standard deviation of $\sigma_{\overline{x}} = \frac{\sigma}{\sqrt{n}} = \frac{8}{\sqrt{10}} = 2.5$).

If we take simple random samples with replacement of size $n = 5$, we get a similar distribution. The distribution of sample means based on samples of size $n = 5$ is shown in Figure 5–16. The mean of the sample means is again 75 and the standard deviation of the sample means is 3.6 (i.e., $\mu_{\overline{x}} = \mu = 75$ and a standard deviation of $\sigma_{\overline{x}} = \frac{\sigma}{\sqrt{n}} = \frac{8}{\sqrt{5}} = 3.6$).

Example 5.16. Suppose we measure a characteristic in a population and that this characteristic is dichotomous with 30% of the population classified as a success (i.e., $p = 0.30$). Recall that the binomial distribution is appropriate for a dichotomous outcome. The characteristic might

FIGURE 5–13 Box-Whisker Plot of Population of Sample Means

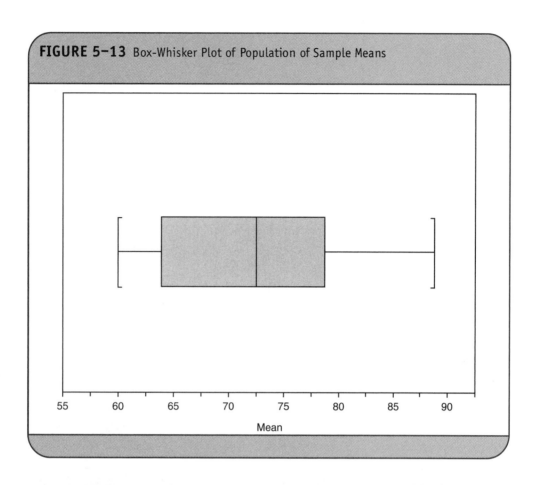

Mean

FIGURE 5–14 Normal Population

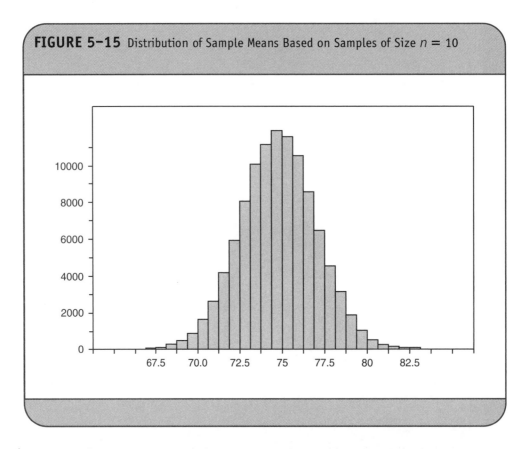

FIGURE 5–15 Distribution of Sample Means Based on Samples of Size $n = 10$

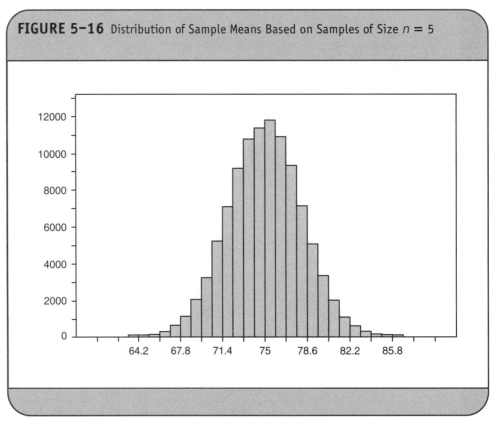

FIGURE 5–16 Distribution of Sample Means Based on Samples of Size $n = 5$

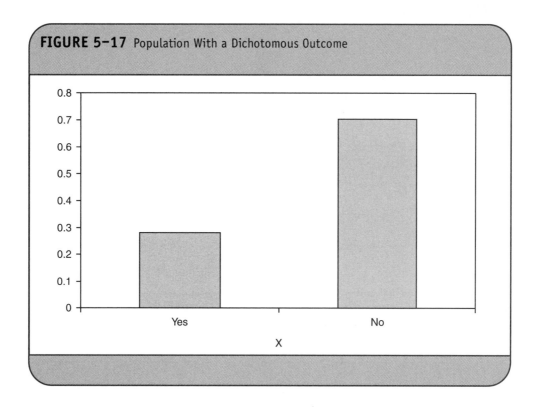

FIGURE 5–17 Population With a Dichotomous Outcome

represent disease status, the presence or absence of a genetic abnormality, or the success of a medical procedure. The distribution of the outcome in the population is shown in Figure 5–17.

This population is clearly not normal. The results of the Central Limit Theorem are said to apply to binomial populations as long as the minimum of np and $n(1 - p)$ is at least 5, where n refers to the sample size. If we take simple random samples with replacement of size $n = 20$ from this binomial population and for each sample we compute the sample mean, the Central Limit Theorem states that the distribution of sample means should be approximately normal because $\min[np, n(1 - p)] = \min[20(0.3), 20(0.7)] = \min(6, 14) = 6$. The distribution of sample means based on samples of size $n = 20$ is shown in Figure 5–18. The mean of the sample means is 6 and the standard deviation of the sample means is 0.4 (i.e., $\mu_{\bar{x}} = \mu = 6$ and a standard deviation of $\sigma_{\bar{x}} = \frac{\sigma}{\sqrt{n}} = \frac{2}{\sqrt{20}} = 0.4$).

Suppose we take simple random samples with replacement of size $n = 10$. In this scenario, we do not meet the sample size requirement for the results of the Central Limit Theorem to hold—i.e., $\min[np, n(1 - p)] = \min[10(0.3), 10(0.7)] = \min(3, 7) = 3$. The distribution of sample means based on samples of size $n = 10$ is shown in Figure 5–19. The distribution of sample means based on samples of size $n = 10$ is not quite normally distributed. The

sample size must be larger for the distribution to approach normality.

Example 5.17. Suppose we measure a characteristic in a population and that this characteristic follows a Poisson distribution with $\mu = 3$ and $\sigma = 1.7$. The Poisson is another probability model for a discrete variable and its distribution is shown in Figure 5–20. This population is not normal. The results of the Central Limit Theorem are said to apply when $n > 30$. The distribution of sample means based on samples of size $n = 30$ is shown in Figure 5–21.

The mean of the sample means is 3 and the standard deviation of the sample means is 0.3 (i.e., $\mu_{\bar{x}} = \mu = 3$ and a standard deviation of $\sigma_{\bar{x}} = \frac{\sigma}{\sqrt{n}} = \frac{1.7}{\sqrt{30}} = 0.3$).

Samples of smaller size from this population do not meet the requirements of the Central Limit Theorem, and thus the result would not hold. For example, suppose we take simple random samples with replacement of size $n = 10$. The distribution of sample means based on samples of size $n = 10$ is shown in Figure 5–22 and is not quite normally distributed. Samples of size 30 or greater will be approximately normally distributed. The distribution of sample means based on samples of size $n = 50$ is shown in Figure 5–23 and is normally distributed.

The mean of the sample means will always be equal to the population mean ($\mu_{\bar{x}} = \mu$). The standard deviation of the

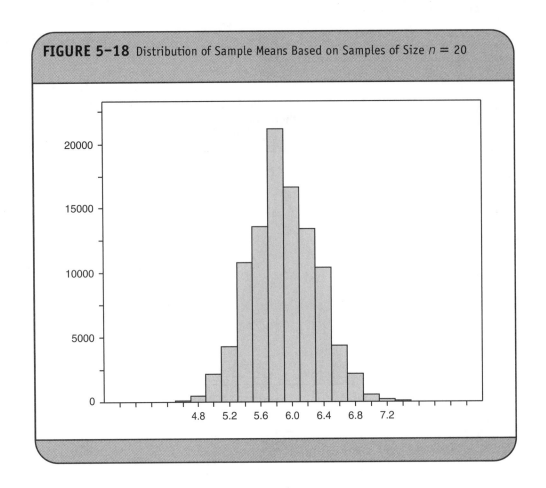

FIGURE 5–18 Distribution of Sample Means Based on Samples of Size $n = 20$

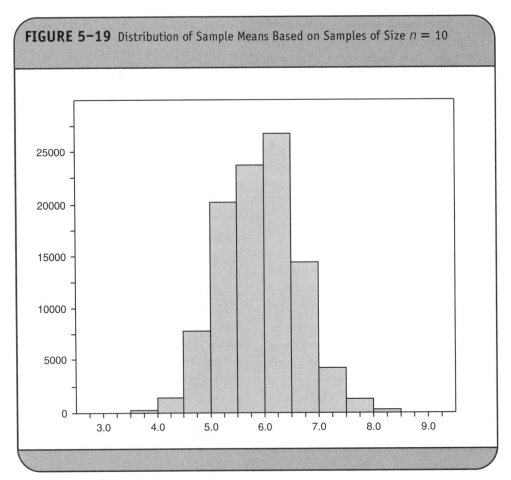

FIGURE 5–19 Distribution of Sample Means Based on Samples of Size $n = 10$

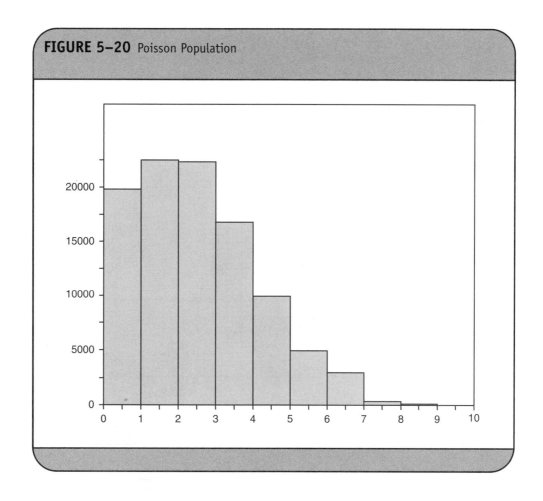

FIGURE 5–20 Poisson Population

sample means, defined as $\sigma_{\overline{x}}$, equals $\frac{\sigma}{\sqrt{n}}$ (i.e., $\sigma_{\overline{x}} = \frac{\sigma}{\sqrt{n}}$) and is also called the *standard error*. The standard error decreases as the sample size increases. Specifically, the variability in the sample means is smaller for larger sample sizes. This is intuitively sensible as extreme values will have less impact in samples of larger size. Notice in the previous examples how the standard errors decrease as the sample sizes increase.

Example 5.18. High density lipoprotein (HDL) cholesterol—the "good" cholesterol—has a mean of 54 and a standard deviation of 17 in patients over age 50. Suppose a physician has 40 patients over age 50 and wants to determine the probability that their mean HDL cholesterol is 60 or more. Specifically, we want to know $P(\overline{X} > 60)$.

Probability questions about a sample mean can be addressed with the Central Limit Theorem as long as the sample size is sufficiently large. In this example, we have $n = 40$. We can therefore assume that the sample mean is approximately normally distributed and can compute the desired probability by standardizing and using Table 1.

Standardizing involves subtracting the mean and dividing by the standard deviation. The mean of $\overline{X}$ is $\mu_{\overline{x}} = \mu$ and the

standard deviation of $\overline{X}$ is $s_{\overline{x}} = \frac{s}{\sqrt{n}}$. Therefore, the formula to standardize a sample mean is

$$Z = \frac{\overline{X} - \mu_{\overline{x}}}{\sigma_{\overline{x}}} = \frac{\overline{X} - \mu}{\sigma/\sqrt{n}}.$$

We want to compute

$$P(\overline{X} > 60) = P\left(z > \frac{60 - 54}{17/\sqrt{40}} = \frac{6}{2.7} = 2.22\right).$$

$P(z > 2.22)$ can be solved with Table 1 with $P(z > 2.22) = 1 - 0.9868 = 0.0132$. The probability that the mean HDL in these 40 patients will exceed 60 is 1.32%.

What is the probability that the mean HDL cholesterol among these 40 patients is less than 50? We now want

$$P(\overline{X} < 50) = P\left(z < \frac{50 - 54}{17/\sqrt{40}} = \frac{-4}{2.7} = -1.48\right).$$

$P(z < -1.48)$ can be solved with Table 1, $P(z < -1.48) = 0.0694$. The probability that the mean HDL among these 40 patients will be less than 50 is 6.94%.

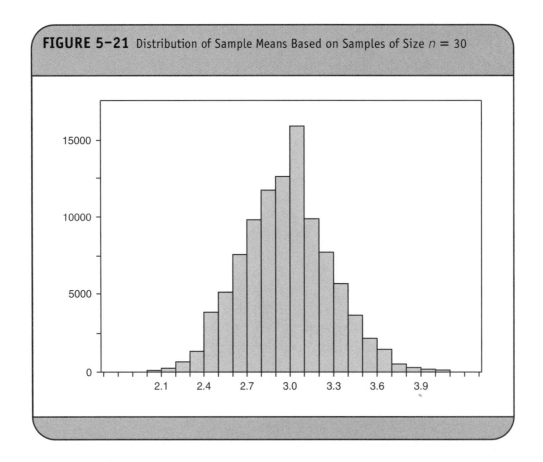

FIGURE 5–21 Distribution of Sample Means Based on Samples of Size $n = 30$

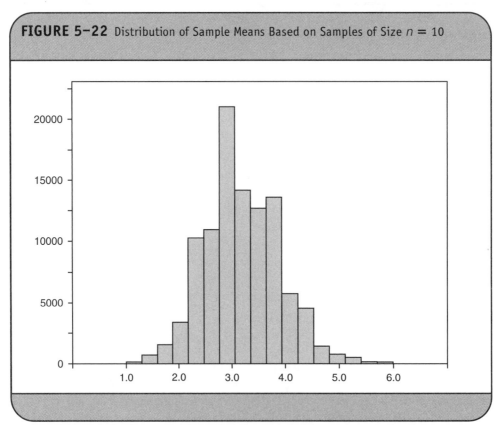

FIGURE 5–22 Distribution of Sample Means Based on Samples of Size $n = 10$

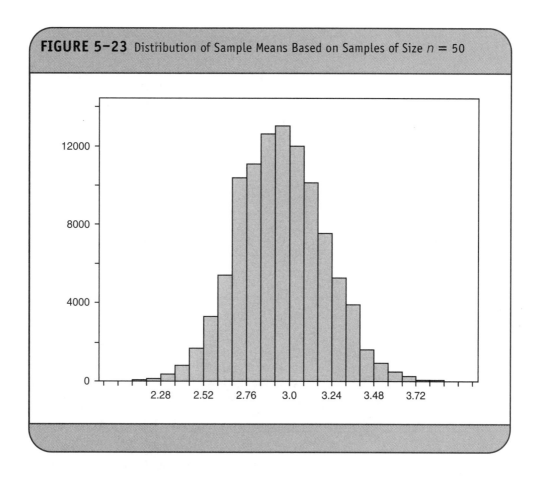

FIGURE 5–23 Distribution of Sample Means Based on Samples of Size $n = 50$

Example 5.19. Suppose we want to estimate the mean lowdensity lipoprotein (LDL)—the "bad" cholesterol—in the population of adults 65 years of age and older. Suppose that we know from studies of adults under age 65 that the standard deviation is 13 and we assume that the variability in LDL in adults 65 years of age and older is the same. We will select a sample of $n = 100$ participants 65 years of age and older and will use the mean of the sample as an estimate of the population mean. We want our estimate to be precise—specifically, we want it to be within 3 units of the true mean LDL value. What is the probability that our estimate (i.e., the sample mean) will be within 3 units of the true mean?

We can represent this question as $P(\mu - 3 < \overline{X} < \mu + 3)$. Because this is a probability about a sample mean, we appeal to the Central Limit Theorem. With a sample of size $n = 100$, we satisfy the sample size criterion and can use the Central Limit Theorem to solve the problem (i.e., convert to z and use Table 1). In the previous example, we asked questions around specific values of the sample mean (e.g., 50, 60) and converted those to z scores and worked with Table 1. Here the values of interest are $\mu - 3$ and $\mu + 3$. We will use these values below:

$$P(\mu - 3 < \overline{X} < \mu + 3) =$$

$$P\left(\frac{(\mu - 3) - \mu}{13/\sqrt{100}} < z < \frac{(\mu + 3) - \mu}{13/\sqrt{100}} \right) =$$

$$P\left(\frac{-3}{1.3} < z < \frac{3}{1.3} \right) = P(-2.31 < z < 2.31).$$

This we can solve with Table 1, $P(-2.31 < z < 2.31) = 0.9896 - 0.0104 = 0.9792$. There is a 97.92% probability that the sample mean, based on a sample of size $n = 100$, will be within 3 units of the true population mean. This is a very powerful statement. Looking only at 100 individuals aged 65 and older, we can obtain a very precise estimate of the population mean.

5.7   SUMMARY

In Chapter 6, Chapter 7, and Chapter 9, we will discuss statistical inference in detail. We will present formulas and procedures to make inferences about populations based on a single sample. The relationship between the sample statistic and the population parameter is based on the sampling distribution of that statistic and probability theory. Here we discussed probability as it applies to selecting individuals from a population into a sample. There are some basic concepts of probability that can be applied when the entire population can be enumerated.

When the population enumeration is not available, probability models can be used to determine probabilities as long as specific attributes are satisfied. The binomial and normal distribution models are popular models for discrete and continuous outcomes, respectively. A key concept here is the Central Limit Theorem, which brings together the concepts of probability and inference. We will rely heavily on the Central Limit Theorem in the next chapters, where we discuss statistical inference in detail. Table 5–10 summarizes key formulas and concepts in probability.

5.8   PRACTICE PROBLEMS

1. A recent study reported that the prevalence of hyperlipidemia (defined as total cholesterol over 200) is 30% in children 2 to 6 years of age. If 12 children are analyzed:
   a. What is the probability that at least 3 are hyperlipidemic?
   b. What is the probability that exactly 3 are hyperlipidemic?
   c. How many would be expected to meet the criteria for hyperlipidemia?

2. Hyperlipidemia in children has been hypothesized to be related to high cholesterol in their parents. The data in Table 5–11 were collected on parents and children.
   a. What is the probability that one or both parents are hyperlipidemic?
   b. What is the probability that a child and both parents are hyperlipidemic?
   c. What is the probability that a child is hyperlipidemic if neither parent is hyperlipidemic?
   d. What is the probability that a child is hyperlipidemic if both parents are hyperlipidemic?

3. Total cholesterol in children aged 10 to 15 is assumed to follow a normal distribution with a mean of 191 and a standard deviation of 22.4.
   a. What proportion of children 10 to 15 years of age have total cholesterol between 180 and 190?
   b. What proportion of children 10 to 15 years of age would be classified as hyperlipidemic? (Assume

TABLE 5–10 Summary of Key Formulas

$N =$ population size

Concept	Formula
Basic probability	$\text{P(Characteristic)} = \dfrac{\text{Number of persons with characteristic}}{N}$
Conditional probability rule	$\text{P}(A \mid B) = \dfrac{\text{P(A and B)}}{\text{P(B)}}$
Sensitivity	P(Screen positive | Disease)
Specificity	P(Screen negative | Disease free)
False positive fraction	P(Screen positive | Disease free)
False negative fraction	P(Screen negative | Disease)
Positive predictive value	P(Disease | Screen positive)
Negative predictive value	P(Disease free | Screen negative)
Independent events	$\text{P}(A \mid B) = \text{P}(A) \text{ or } \text{P}(B \mid A) = \text{P}(B)$
Bayes Theorem	$\text{P}(A \mid B) = \dfrac{\text{P}(B \mid A)\text{P}(A)}{\text{P}(B)}$
Binomial distribution	$\text{P}(x \text{ successes}) = \dfrac{n!}{x!(n-x)!}\, p^x (1-p)^{n-x}$
Standard normal distribution	$z = \dfrac{X - \mu}{\sigma}$ (Table 1)
Percentiles of the normal distribution	$X = \mu + z$
Result of Central Limit Theorem	$z = \dfrac{\bar{X} - \mu}{\sigma / \sqrt{n}}$ (Table 1)

TABLE 5–11 Hyperlipidemia in Parents and Children

Child	Both Parents Hyperlipidemic	One Parent Hyperlipidemic	Neither Parent Hyperlipidemic
Not hyperlipidemic	13	34	83
Hyperlipidemic	45	42	6

TABLE 5–12 Coffee Consumption in Graduate Students

	Do not drink coffee	Drink Decaffeinated Only	Drink Caffeinated Coffee
Male	145	94	365
Female	80	121	430

that hyperlipidemia is defined as a total cholesterol level over 200.)

   c. If a sample of 20 children are selected, what is the probability that the mean cholesterol level in the sample will exceed 200?

4. A national survey of graduate students is conducted to assess their consumption of coffee. Table 5–12 summarizes the data.

   a. What proportion of students drink decaffeinated coffee only?

   b. What proportion of coffee drinkers (caffeinated and decaffeinated) are female?

   c. What proportion of the females do not drink coffee?

5. Among coffee drinkers, men drink a mean of 3.2 cups per day with a standard deviation of 0.8 cups. Assume the number of cups per day follows a normal distribution.

   a. What proportion drink 2 cups per day or more?

   b. What proportion drink no more than 4 cups per day?

   c. If the top 5% of coffee drinkers are considered "heavy" coffee drinkers, what is the minimum number of cups consumed by a heavy coffee drinker?

   d. If a sample of 20 men is selected, what is the probability that the mean number of cups per day is greater than 3?

6. A study is conducted to assess the impact of caffeine consumption, smoking, alcohol consumption, and physical activity on cardiovascular disease. Suppose that 40% of participants consume caffeine and smoke. If 8 participants are evaluated, what is the probability that:

   a. Exactly half of them consume caffeine and smoke?

   b. More than 6 consume caffeine and smoke?

   c. Exactly 4 do not consume caffeine or smoke?

7. As part of the study described in Problem 6, investigators wanted to assess the accuracy of self-reported smoking status. Participants are asked whether they currently smoke or not. In addition, laboratory tests are performed on hair samples to determine the presence or absence of nicotine. The laboratory assessment is considered the gold standard, or the truth about nicotine consumption. The data are shown in Table 5–13.

   a. What is the sensitivity of the self-reported smoking status?

   b. What is the specificity of the self-reported smoking status?

8. A recent study of cardiovascular risk factors reported that 30% of adults met criteria for hypertension. If 15 adults are assessed, what is the probability that:

   a. Exactly 5 meet the criteria for hypertension?

   b. None meet the criteria for hypertension?

   c. How many would you expect to meet the criteria for hypertension?

TABLE 5–13 Self-Reported Smoking Status

	Nicotine Absent	Nicotine Present
Self-reported nonsmoker	82	14
Self-reported smoker	12	52

9. Table 5–14 displays blood pressure status by gender.
   a. What proportion of the participants have optimal blood pressure?
   b. What proportion of men have optimal blood pressure?
   c. What proportion of participants with hypertension are men?
   d. Are hypertensive status and male gender independent?

10. Diastolic blood pressures are assumed to follow a normal distribution with a mean of 85 and a standard deviation of 12.
    a. What proportion of people have diastolic blood pressures less than 90?
    b. What proportion have diastolic blood pressures between 80 and 90?
    c. If someone has a diastolic blood pressure of 100, what percentile does this represent?

11. Consider the data described in Problem 10. If 15 participants are sampled, what is the probability that their mean diastolic blood pressure exceeds 90?

12. A large national study finds that 10% of pregnant women deliver prematurely. A local obstetrician is seeing 16 pregnant women in his next clinic session.
    a. What is the probability that none will deliver prematurely?
    b. What is the probability that fewer than 3 will deliver prematurely?
    c. What is the probability that none will deliver prematurely if, in fact, the true proportion who deliver prematurely is 5.5%?
    d. If the true proportion is 10% and this obstetrician has 146 pregnant women under his care, how many would be expected to deliver prematurely?

13. Table 5–15 cross-classifies pregnant women in a study by their body mass index (BMI) at 16 weeks gestation and whether they had a pre-term delivery.
    a. What is the probability that a woman delivers pre-term?
    b. What is the probability a woman has a BMI less than 30 and delivers pre-term?
    c. What proportion of women with a BMI greater than 35 deliver pre-term?
    d. Are BMI and pre-term delivery independent? Justify.

14. In the study described in Problem 13, suppose the mean BMI at 16 weeks gestation is 28.5 with a standard deviation of 3.6, and that BMI is assumed to follow a normal distribution. Find the following:
    a. The proportion of women with a BMI greater than 30.
    b. The proportion of women with a BMI greater than 40.
    c. The BMI that separates the top 10% from the rest.

15. Suppose we want to estimate the mean BMI for women in pregnancy at 20 weeks gestation. If we have a sample of 100 women and measure their BMI at 20 weeks gestation, what is the probability that the sample mean is within 1 unit of the true BMI if the standard deviation in the BMI is taken to be 3.6?

TABLE 5–14 Blood Pressure by Gender

	Optimal	Normal	Hypertension	Total
Male	22	73	55	150
Female	43	132	65	240
Total	65	205	120	390

TABLE 5–15 Body Mass Index and Preterm Delivery

	BMI < 30	BMI 30–34.9	BMI 35+
Pre-term	320	80	120
Full term	4700	480	300

REFERENCES

1. National Center for Health Statistics. *Health, United States, 2003, with Chartbook on Trends in the Health of Americans*. Hyattsville, MD: US Government Printing Office, 2003.

2. Hedley, A.A., Ogden, C.L., Johnson, C.L., Carroll, M.D., Curtin, L.R., and Flegal, K.M. "Prevalence of overweight and obesity among U.S. children, adolescents, and adults, 1999–2002." *Journal of the American Medical Association* 2004; 291: 2847–2850.

3. Cope, M.B. and Allison, D.B. "Obesity: Person and population." *Obesity* 2006; 14: S156–S159.

4. Kim, J., Peterson, K.E., Scanlon, K.S., Fitzmaurice, G.M., Must, A., Oken, E., Rifas-Shiman, S.L., Rich-Edwards, J.W., and Gillman, M.W. "Trends in overweight from 1980 through 2001 among preschool-aged children enrolled in a health maintenance organization." *Obesity* 2006; 14: 1107–1112.

5. Cochran, W.G. *Sampling Techniques* (3rd ed.). New York: John Wiley & Sons, 1977.

6. Kish, L. *Survey Sampling (Wiley Classics Library)*. New York: John Wiley & Sons, 1995.

7. Rosner, B. *Fundamentals of Biostatistics*. Belmont, CA: Duxbury-Brooks/Cole, 2006.

8. SAS Version 9.1 © 2002–2003 by SAS Institute Inc., Cary, NC.

9. Thompson, I.M., Pauler, D.K., Goodman P.J., et al. "Prevalence of prostate cancer among men with a prostate-specific antigen level ≤ 4.0 ng per milliliter." *The New England Journal of Medicine* 2004; 350(22): 2239–2246.

10. D'Agostino, R.B., Sullivan, L.M. and Beiser, A. *Introductory Applied Biostatistics*. Belmont, CA: Duxbury–Brooks/Cole, 2004.

CHAPTER 6

Confidence Interval Estimates

We will now begin statistical inference. In Chapter 4, we presented descriptive statistics used to summarize sample data. In Chapter 5, we presented key concepts in probability and the Central Limit Theorem. In statistical inference, we use all of these concepts to make inferences about unknown population parameters based on sample statistics. There are two broad areas of statistical inference, estimation, and hypothesis testing. In estimation, sample statistics are used to generate estimates about unknown population parameters. In hypothesis testing, a specific statement or hypothesis is generated about a population parameter and sample statistics are used to assess the likelihood that the hypothesis is true. We will discuss estimation here and hypothesis testing in Chapter 7.

Estimation is the process of determining a likely value for a population parameter (e.g., the true population mean or population proportion) based on a random sample. In practice, we select a sample from the target population and use sample statistics (e.g., the sample mean or the sample proportion) as estimates of the unknown parameter. The sample should be representative of the population, with participants selected at random from the population. Because different samples can produce different results, it is necessary to quantify the precision—or lack thereof—that might exist among estimates from different samples.

The techniques for estimation as well as for other procedures in statistical inference depend on the appropriate classification of the key study variable (which we also call the outcome or endpoint) as continuous or dichotomous. (There are other types of variables which are discussed in Chapter 7; here we will focus on continuous and dichotomous outcomes.) Another key issue is the number of comparison groups in the investigation. For example, in the two-comparison group case it is also important to determine whether the samples from the groups are independent (i.e., physically separate, such as men versus women) or dependent (also called matched or paired). These issues dictate the appropriate estimation technique. Table 6–1 outlines these issues and identifies the estimation techniques that we will discuss here. Each will be discussed in detail.

TABLE 6–1 Estimation Techniques

Number of Samples	Outcome Variable	Parameter to be Estimated
One sample	Continuous	Mean
Two independent samples		Difference in means
Two dependent, matched samples		Mean difference
One sample	Dichotomous	Proportion (e.g., prevalence, cumulative incidence)
Two independent samples		Difference or ratio of proportions (e.g., attributable risk, relative risk, odds ratio)

6.1   INTRODUCTION TO ESTIMATION

There are two types of estimates that can be produced for any population parameter, point estimates and confidence interval estimates. A *point estimate* for a population parameter is a single-valued estimate of that parameter. A *confidence interval* (CI) estimate is a range of values for a population parameter with a level of confidence attached (e.g., 95% confidence that the interval contains the unknown parameter). The level of confidence is similar to a probability. The CI starts with the point estimate and builds in what is called a margin of error. The margin of error incorporates the confidence level (e.g., 90% or 95%, which is chosen by the investigator) and the sampling variability or the standard error of the point estimate.

A CI is a range of values that are likely to cover the true population parameter, and the general form is: *point estimate* ± *margin of error*. The point estimate is determined first. The point estimates for the population mean and proportion are the sample mean and sample proportion, respectively. These are our best single-valued estimates of the unknown population parameters. Recall from Chapter 5 that the sample mean is an unbiased estimator of the population mean. The same holds true for the sample proportion with regard to estimating the population proportion. Thus the starting point, or point estimate, for the CI for the population mean is the sample mean, and the point estimate for the population proportion is the sample proportion.

Next, a level of confidence is selected that reflects the likelihood that the CI contains the true, unknown parameter. Usually, confidence levels of 90%, 95%, and 99% are chosen, although theoretically any confidence level between 0% and 100% can be selected.

Suppose we want to generate a CI estimate for an unknown population mean. Again, the form of the CI is: *point estimate* ± *margin of error*, or $\overline{X}$ ± *margin of error*. Suppose we select a 95% confidence level. This means that there is a 95% probability that the CI will contain the true population mean. Thus,

$$\mathrm{P}(\overline{X} - margin\ of\ error < \mu < \overline{X} + margin\ of\ error) = 0.95.$$

In Chapter 5, we presented the Central Limit Theorem, which stated that for large samples, the distribution of the sample means is approximately normally distributed with a mean $\mu_{\overline{X}} = \mu$ and a standard deviation $\sigma_{\overline{X}} = \frac{\sigma}{\sqrt{n}}$. We will use the Central Limit Theorem to develop the margin of error.

For the standard normal distribution, the following is a true statement: $\mathrm{P}(-1.96 < z < 1.96) = 0.95$, i.e., there is a 95% probability that a standard normal variable will fall between -1.96 and 1.96. The Central Limit Theorem states that for large samples, $z = \frac{\overline{X} - \mu}{\sigma/\sqrt{n}}$. If we make this substitution, the following

statement is true: $\mathrm{P}(-1.96 < \frac{\overline{X} - \mu}{\sigma/\sqrt{n}} < 1.96) = 0.95$. Using algebra, we can rework this inequality such that the mean (μ) is the middle term. The steps are outlined below:

$$\mathrm{P}(-1.96 < \frac{\overline{X} - \mu}{\sigma/\sqrt{n}} < 1.96) = 0.95.$$

$$\mathrm{P}(-1.96\frac{\sigma}{\sqrt{n}} < \overline{X} - \mu < 1.96\frac{\sigma}{\sqrt{n}}) = 0.95.$$

$$\mathrm{P}(-\overline{X} - 1.96\frac{\sigma}{\sqrt{n}} < -\mu < -\overline{X} + 1.96\frac{\sigma}{\sqrt{n}}) = 0.95.$$

$$\mathrm{P}(\overline{X} - 1.96\frac{\sigma}{\sqrt{n}} < \mu < \overline{X} + 1.96\frac{\sigma}{\sqrt{n}}) = 0.95.$$

The 95% CI for the population mean is the interval in the last probability statement and is given by: $\overline{X} \pm 1.96\,\sigma/\sqrt{n}$. The margin of error is $1.96\,\sigma/\sqrt{n}$, where 1.96 reflects the fact that a 95% confidence level was selected and $\sigma/\sqrt{n}$ is the standard error (or the standard deviation of the point estimate, $\overline{X}$). The general form of a CI can be rewritten as follows:

point estimate ± *z* SE (*point estimate*),

where *z* is the value from the standard normal distribution reflecting the selected confidence level (e.g., for a 95% confidence level, $z = 1.96$). Table 1B in the Appendix contains the *z* values for popular confidence levels such as 90%, 95%, and 99%. In Table 1B, we find for 90%, $z = 1.645$; for 95%, $z = 1.96$; and for 99%, $z = 2.576$. Higher confidence levels have larger *z* values, which translate to larger margins of error and wider CIs. For example, to be 99% confident that a CI contains the true unknown parameter, we need a wider interval. In many applications, a confidence level of 95% is used. This is a generally accepted value but not a prescribed value.

In practice, we often do not know the value of the population standard deviation (σ). If the sample size is large ($n > 30$), then the sample standard deviation can be used to estimate the population standard deviation. Note that the prior derivation is based on the Central Limit Theorem, which requires a large sample size. There are instances in which the sample size is not sufficiently large (e.g., $n < 30$), and therefore the general result of the Central Limit Theorem does not apply. In this case, we cannot use the standard normal distribution (*z*) in the confidence interval. Instead we use another probability distribution, called the *t* distribution, which is appropriate for small samples.

The *t* distribution is another probability model for a continuous variable. The *t* distribution is similar to the standard normal distribution but takes a slightly different shape depending on the exact sample size. Specifically, the *t* values for CIs are larger for smaller samples resulting in larger margins of error (i.e., there is more imprecision with small samples). *t* values for

TABLE 6–2 *T* Values for Confidence Intervals

	Confidence Level				
df	80%	90%	95%	98%	99%
4	1.533	2.132	2.776	3.747	4.604
5	1.476	2.015	2.571	3.365	4.032
6	1.440	1.943	2.447	3.143	3.707
7	1.415	1.895	2.365	2.998	3.499
8	1.397	1.860	2.306	2.896	3.355
9	1.383	1.833	2.262	2.821	3.250

CIs are contained in Table 2 in the Appendix. *t* values are indexed by degrees of freedom (*df*) in Table 2, which are defined as $(n-1)$. Table 6–2 is an excerpt of Table 2 showing the *t* values for small samples ranging in size from 5 to 10 (thus, the degrees of freedom range from 4 to 9, as $df = n-1$).

Specific guidelines for using the standard normal (*z*) or *t* distributions are provided in subsequent sections as we discuss the CI formulas for specific applications. It is important to note that appropriate use of the *t* distribution assumes that the outcome of interest is approximately normally distributed.

Before providing specific formulas, we first discuss the interpretation of CIs in general. Suppose we want to estimate a population mean using a 95% confidence level. If we take 100 different samples (in practice, we take only one) and for each sample we compute a 95% CI, in theory, 95 out of the 100 CIs will contain the true mean value (μ). This leaves 5 of 100 CIs that will not include the true mean value. In practice, we select one random sample and generate one CI. This interval may or may not contain the true mean; the observed interval may overestimate μ or underestimate μ. The 95% CI is the likely range of the true, unknown parameter. It is important to note that a CI does not reflect the variability in the unknown parameter but instead provides a range of values that are likely to include the unknown parameter.

6.2 CONFIDENCE INTERVALS FOR ONE SAMPLE, CONTINUOUS OUTCOME

We wish to estimate the mean of a continuous outcome variable in a single population. For example, we wish to estimate the mean systolic blood pressure, body mass index (BMI), total cholesterol level, or white blood cell count in a single target population. We select a sample and compute descriptive statistics on the sample data using the techniques described in Chapter 4. Specifically, we compute the sample size (*n*), the sample mean ($\overline{X}$), and the sample standard deviation (*s*). The formulas for CIs for the population mean depend on the sample size and are given in Table 6–3.

Example 6.1. In Chapter 4, we presented data on $n = 3539$ participants who attended the seventh examination of the Offspring in the Framingham Heart Study. Descriptive statistics on variables measured in the sample are shown in Table 6–4 (these and other statistics were presented in Table 4–20). The numbers of participants (*n*) who provided information on each characteristic are shown in the second column of Table 6–4.

We wish to generate a 95% CI for systolic blood pressure using data collected in the Framingham Offspring Study. Because the sample size is large, we use the following expression,

$$\overline{X} \pm z \frac{s}{\sqrt{n}}.$$

The *z* value for 95% confidence is $z = 1.96$. Substituting the sample statistics and the *z* value for 95% confidence, we have

$$127.3 \pm 1.96 \frac{19.0}{\sqrt{3534}}.$$

Working through the computations, we have

$$127.3 \pm 0.63.$$

Adding and subtracting the margin of error, we get (126.7, 127.9). A point estimate for the true mean systolic blood

TABLE 6–3 Confidence Intervals for μ

$n \geq 30$	$\overline{X} \pm z \dfrac{s}{\sqrt{n}}$	(Find *z* in Table 1B)
$n < 30$	$\overline{X} \pm t \dfrac{s}{\sqrt{n}}$	(Find *t* in Table 2, df $= n-1$)

TABLE 6–4 Summary Statistics on Participants Attending the Seventh Examination of the Framingham Offspring Study ($n = 3{,}539$)

	n	Mean ($\overline{X}$)	Standard Deviation (*s*)
Systolic blood pressure	3534	127.3	19.0
Diastolic blood pressure	3532	74.0	9.9
Total serum cholesterol	3310	200.3	36.8
Weight (lbs)	3506	174.4	38.7
Height (in.)	3326	65.957	3.749
Body mass index (BMI)	3326	28.15	5.32

pressure in the population is 127.3, and we are 95% confident that the true mean is between 126.7 and 127.9. The margin of error is very small here because of the large sample size.

A 90% CI for BMI is given below. Notice that $z = 1.645$ to reflect the 90% confidence level:

$$28.15 \pm 1.645 \frac{5.32}{\sqrt{3326}},$$

$$28.15 \pm 0.152,$$

$$(28.00, 28.30).$$

We are 90% confident that the true BMI in the population is between 28.00 and 28.30. Again, the CI is very precise or narrow due to the very large sample size.

Example 6.2. In Chapter 4, we also presented data on a subsample of $n = 10$ participants who attended the seventh examination of the Framingham Offspring Study. Descriptive statistics on variables measured in the subsample are shown in Table 6–5 (these and other statistics were presented in Table 4–18).

Suppose we compute a 95% CI for the true systolic blood pressure using data in the subsample. Because the sample size is small, we must now use the CI formula that involves t rather than z,

$$\bar{X} \pm t \frac{s}{\sqrt{n}}.$$

We first need to determine the appropriate t value from Table 2. To do this, we need df $= n - 1 = 10 - 1 = 9$. The t value for 95% confidence with df $= 9$ is $t = 2.262$. Substituting the sample statistics and the t value for 95% confidence, we have

$$121.2 \pm 2.262 \frac{11.1}{\sqrt{10}}.$$

TABLE 6–5 Summary Statistics on $n = 10$ Participants Attending the Seventh Examination of the Framingham Offspring Study

	n	Mean ($\bar{X}$)	Standard Deviation (s)
Systolic blood pressure	10	121.2	11.1
Diastolic blood pressure	10	71.3	7.2
Total serum cholesterol	10	202.3	37.7
Weight (lbs)	10	176.0	33.0
Height (in.)	10	67.175	4.205
Body mass index (BMI)	10	27.26	3.10

Working through the computations, we have

$$121.2 \pm 7.94.$$

Adding and subtracting the margin of error, we get (113.3, 129.1). Based on this sample of size $n = 10$, our best estimate of the true mean systolic blood pressure in the population is 121.2. Based on this sample, we are 95% confident that the true systolic blood pressure in the population is between 113.3 and 129.1. Notice that the margin of error is larger here primarily due to the small sample size.

Using the subsample, we will now compute a 90% CI for BMI. Because the sample size is small, we again need to determine an appropriate value from the t distribution. For 90% confidence and df $= 9$, $t = 1.833$.

$$27.26 \pm 1.833 \frac{3.10}{\sqrt{10}},$$

$$27.26 \pm 1.80,$$

$$(25.46, 29.06).$$

We are 90% confident that the true BMI in the population is between 25.46 and 29.06. Again, because of the small sample size, the CI is less precise.

6.3   CONFIDENCE INTERVALS FOR ONE SAMPLE, DICHOTOMOUS OUTCOME

There are many applications where the outcome of interest is dichotomous. The parameter of interest is the unknown population proportion, denoted p. For example, suppose we wish to estimate the proportion of people with diabetes in a population, or the proportion of people with hypertension or obesity. The latter are defined by specific levels of blood pressure and BMI, respectively. Again, we select a sample and compute descriptive statistics on the sample data using the techniques described in Chapter 4. When the outcome of interest is dichotomous, we record on each member of the sample whether they have the characteristic of interest or not. The sample size is denoted by n and we let x denote the number of successes in the sample. Recall that for dichotomous outcomes, we define one of the outcomes a success and the other a failure. The specific response that is considered a success is defined by the investigator. For example, if we wish to estimate the proportion of people with diabetes in a population, we consider a diagnosis of diabetes as a success (the outcome of interest) and lack of diagnosis a failure. In this example, x represents the number of people with a diagnosis of diabetes in the sample. The sample proportion is denoted $\hat{p}$, and is computed

TABLE 6–6 Confidence Intervals for p

$$\min[n\,\hat{p}, n(1-\hat{p})]>5 \qquad \hat{p}\pm z\sqrt{\frac{\hat{p}(1-\hat{p})}{n}} \quad \text{Find } z \text{ in Table 1B}$$

$$\hat{p}\pm z\sqrt{\frac{\hat{p}(1-\hat{p})}{n}},$$

$$0.345\pm 1.96\sqrt{\frac{0.345(1-0.345)}{3532}},$$

$$0.345\pm 0.016,$$

$$(0.329, 0.361).$$

by taking the ratio of the number of successes in the sample to the sample size, $\hat{p}=\frac{x}{n}$. The formula for the CI for the population proportion is given in Table 6–6.

The CI for the population proportion takes the same form as the CI for the population mean (i.e., *point estimate + margin of error*). The point estimate for the population proportion is the sample proportion. The margin of error is the product of the z value for the desired confidence level (e.g., $z = 1.96$ for 95% confidence) and the standard error of the point estimate,

$$SE(\hat{p})=\sqrt{\frac{\hat{p}(1-\hat{p})}{n}}\;.$$

The preceding formula is appropriate for large samples, defined as at least five successes ($n\hat{p}$) and at least five failures $[n(1-\hat{p})]$ in the sample. Recall that this was a condition for the Central Limit Theorem for binomial populations. If there are fewer than five successes or failures, then alternative procedures—called exact methods—must be used to estimate the population proportion.[1, 2]

Example 6.3. In Chapter 4, we presented data on $n = 3539$ participants who attended the seventh examination of the Offspring in the Framingham Heart Study. One particular characteristic measured was treatment with antihypertensive medication. There were a total of 1219 participants on treatment and 2313 participants not on treatment (Table 4–3). If we call treatment a success, then $x = 1219$ and $n = 3532$. The sample proportion is

$$\hat{p}=\frac{x}{n}=\frac{1219}{3532}=0.345.$$

Thus, a point estimate for the population proportion is 0.345, or 34.5%. Our best estimate of the proportion of participants in the population on treatment for hypertension is 34.5%. Suppose we now wish to generate a 95% CI. To use the preceding formula, we need to satisfy the sample size criterion—specifically, we need at least five successes and five failures. Here we more than satisfy that requirement, so the CI formula in Table 6–6 can be used.

Thus, we are 95% confident that the true proportion of persons on antihypertensive medication is between 32.9% and 36.1%.

Specific applications of estimation for a single population with a dichotomous outcome involve estimating prevalence and cumulative incidence. In Chapter 3, we generated point estimates for prevalence and incidence data; in the following examples, we will add CI estimates.

Example 6.4. In Example 3.1, we presented data on $n = 3799$ participants who attended the fifth examination of the Offspring in the Framingham Heart Study. Table 6–7 shows the numbers of men and women with diagnosed, or prevalent, cardiovascular disease (CVD) at the fifth examination.

The prevalence of CVD for all participants attending the fifth examination of the Framingham Offspring Study is 379 / 3799 = 0.0998. The prevalence of CVD among men is 244 / 1792 = 0.1362, and the prevalence of CVD among women is 135 / 2007 = 0.0673. These are point estimates. Following, we generate 95% CI estimates for prevalence in the total population and in the populations of men and women. To use the preceding formula, we need to satisfy the sample size criterion—specifically, we need at least five successes and five failures in each sample. In this example, a success is prevalent CVD and a failure is freedom from CVD. Here we more than satisfy that requirement for men, women, and the pooled or total sample. For the total sample,

$$0.0998\pm 1.96\sqrt{\frac{0.0998(1-0.0998)}{3799}},$$

TABLE 6–7 Prevalent CVD in Men and Women

	Free of CVD	Prevalent CVD	Total
Men	1548	244	1792
Women	1872	135	2007
Total	3420	379	3799

$$0.0998 \pm 0.0098,$$

$$(0.089, 0.110).$$

We are 95% confident that the true prevalence of CVD in the population is between 8.9% and 11.0%.

The CI estimates for men and women are as follows. For men:

$$0.1362 \pm 1.96 \sqrt{\frac{0.1362(1-0.1362)}{1792}},$$

$$0.1362 \pm 0.016,$$

$$(0.120, 0.152).$$

For women:

$$0.0673 \pm 1.96 \sqrt{\frac{0.0673(1-0.0673)}{2007}},$$

$$0.0673 \pm 0.012,$$

$$(0.055, 0.079).$$

We are 95% confident that the true prevalence of CVD in men is between 12.0% and 15.2%, and in women, between 5.5% and 7.9%. Each of these CI estimates is very precise (small margins of error) because of the large sample sizes.

6.4 CONFIDENCE INTERVALS FOR TWO INDEPENDENT SAMPLES, CONTINUOUS OUTCOME

There are many applications where it is of interest to compare two groups with respect to their mean scores on a continuous outcome. The comparison groups might be men versus women, patients assigned to an experimental treatment versus a placebo in a clinical trial, patients with a history of cardiovascular disease versus patients free of cardiovascular disease. We could compare mean systolic blood pressures in men versus women, mean BMI or total cholesterol levels in patients assigned to an experimental treatment versus placebo.

A key feature here is that the two comparison groups are independent, or physically separate. The two groups might be determined by a particular attribute or characteristic (e.g., gender, diagnosis of cardiovascular disease) or might be set up by the investigator (e.g., participants assigned to receive an experimental drug or placebo).

Similar to the approach we used to estimate the mean of a continuous variable in a single population (Section 6.2), we first compute descriptive statistics on each of the two samples using the techniques described in Chapter 4. Specifically, we compute the sample size, mean, and standard deviation in each sample. We denote these summary statistics as $n_1, \overline{X}_1$, and s_1 for Sample 1 and $n_2, \overline{X}_2$, and s_2 for Sample 2. (The designation of Sample 1 and Sample 2 is essentially arbitrary. In a clinical trial setting, the convention is to call the experimental treatment Group 1 and the control Group 2. However, when comparing groups such as men and women, either group can be 1 or 2.) The interpretation of the CI estimate will depend on how the samples are assigned, but this is just for interpretation and does not affect the computations. This will be illustrated in the following examples.

In the two independent samples application with a continuous outcome, the parameter of interest is the difference in population means, $\mu_1 - \mu_2$. The point estimate for the difference in population means is the difference in sample means, $\overline{X}_1 - \overline{X}_2$. The form of the CI is again *point estimate ± margin of error*, and the margin of error incorporates a value from either the z or t distribution reflecting the selected confidence level and the standard error of the point estimate. The use of z or t depends on whether the sample sizes are large or small. (The specific guidelines follow.) The standard error of the point estimate will incorporate the variability in the outcome of interest in each of the comparison groups. Table 6–8 contains the formulas for CIs for the difference in population means.

TABLE 6–8 Confidence Intervals for $(\mu_1 - \mu_2)$

$n_1 \geq 30$ and $n_2 \geq 30$	$(\overline{X}_1 - \overline{X}_2) \pm zS_p \sqrt{\dfrac{1}{n_1} + \dfrac{1}{n_2}}$	Find z in Table 1B
$n_1 < 30$ and $n_2 < 30$	$(\overline{X}_1 - \overline{X}_2) \pm tS_p \sqrt{\dfrac{1}{n_1} + \dfrac{1}{n_2}}$	Find t in Table 2 (df $= n_1 + n_2 - 2$)

Note that the formulas in Table 6–8 assume equal variability in the two populations (i.e., that the population variances are equal, or $\sigma_1^2 = \sigma_2^2$). This means that the outcome is equally variable in each of the comparison populations. For analysis, we have samples from each of the comparison populations. If the sample variances are similar, then the assumption about variability in the populations is reasonable. As a guideline, if the ratio of the sample variances, s_1^2/s_2^2, is between 0.5 and 2 (i.e., if one variance is no more than double the other), then the formulas in Table 6–8 are appropriate. If the ratio of the sample variances is greater than 2 or less than 0.5, then alternative formulas must be used to account for the heterogeneity in variances. Specific details can be found in D'Agostino, Sullivan, and Beiser and in Rosner.[3,4]

In the formulas in Table 6–8, $\overline{X}_1$ and $\overline{X}_2$ are the means of the outcome in the independent samples, z or t are values from the z or t distributions reflecting the desired confidence level, and SE($\overline{X}_1 - \overline{X}_2$), the standard error, is the standard deviation of the difference in sample means. Specifically, the standard error is

$$\text{SE}(\overline{X}_1 - \overline{X}_2) = S_p \sqrt{\frac{1}{n_1} + \frac{1}{n_2}},$$

where S_p is the pooled estimate of the common standard deviation (again, assuming that the variances in the populations are similar) computed as the weighted average of the standard deviations in the samples,

$$S_p = \sqrt{\frac{(n_1-1)s_1^2 + (n_2-1)s_2^2}{n_1 + n_2 - 2}}.$$

Because we are assuming equal variances in the groups, we pool the information on variability (sample variances) to generate an estimate of the population variability.

Example 6.5. In Example 6.1, we recapped the data presented in Chapter 4 on $n = 3539$ participants who attended the seventh examination of the Offspring in the Framingham Heart Study. Table 6–9 contains descriptive statistics on the

same continuous characteristics stratified (or generated separately) by gender.

Suppose we want to compare mean systolic blood pressures in men versus women using a 95% CI. The summary statistics shown in Table 6–9 indicate that we have large samples (more than 30) of both men and women, and therefore we can use the CI formula with z as opposed to t. However, before implementing the formula, we will first check whether the assumption of equality of the population variances is reasonable. The guideline suggests investigating the ratio of the sample variances, s_1^2/s_2^2. Suppose we call the men Group 1 and the women Group 2. (Again, this is arbitrary. It only needs to be noted when interpreting the results.) The ratio of the sample variances is $17.52^2 / 20.12^2 = 0.76$, which falls between 0.5 and 2, suggesting that the assumption of equality of the population variances is reasonable. The appropriate CI formula for the difference in mean systolic blood pressures between men and women is:

$$(\overline{X}_1 - \overline{X}_2) \pm zS_p\sqrt{\frac{1}{n_1} + \frac{1}{n_2}}.$$

Before substituting, we will first compute S_p, the pooled estimate of the common standard deviation:

$$S_p = \sqrt{\frac{(n_1-1)s_1^2 + (n_2-1)s_2^2}{n_1 + n_2 - 2}},$$

$$S_p = \sqrt{\frac{(1623-1)(17.5)^2 + (1911-1)(20.1)^2}{1623+1911-2}},$$

$$S_p = \sqrt{359.12} = 19.0.$$

Notice that the pooled estimate of the common standard deviation, S_p, falls between the standard deviations in the comparison groups (i.e., 17.5 and 20.1). S_p is slightly closer in value to the standard deviation in the women (20.1) as there are

TABLE 6–9 Summary Statistics on Men and Women Attending the Seventh Examination of the Framingham Offspring Study

	Men			Women		
	n	$\overline{X}$	s	n	$\overline{X}$	s
Systolic blood pressure	1623	128.2	17.5	1911	126.5	20.1
Diastolic blood pressure	1622	75.6	9.8	1910	72.6	9.7
Total serum cholesterol	1544	192.4	35.2	1766	207.1	36.7
Weight (lbs)	1612	194.0	33.8	1894	157.7	34.6
Height (in.)	1545	68.9	2.7	1781	63.4	2.5
Body mass index (BMI)	1545	28.8	4.6	1781	27.6	5.9

slightly more women in the sample. Recall that S_p is a weighted average of the standard deviations in the comparison groups, weighted by the respective sample sizes.

The 95% CI for the difference in mean systolic blood pressures is:

$$(128.2 - 126.5) \pm 1.96(19.0)\sqrt{\frac{1}{1623} + \frac{1}{1911}},$$

$$1.7 \pm 1.26,$$

$$(0.44, 2.96).$$

The CI is interpreted as follows: We are 95% confident that the difference in mean systolic blood pressures between men and women is between 0.44 and 2.96 units. Our best estimate of the difference, the point estimate, is 1.7 units. The standard error of the difference is 0.641, and the margin of error is 1.26 units.

Note that when we generate estimates for a population parameter in a single sample (e.g., the mean μ or population proportion p), the resulting CI provides a range of likely values for that parameter. In contrast, when there are two independent samples and the goal is to compare means (or proportions, discussed in Section 6.6), the resultant CI does not provide a range of values for the parameters in the comparison populations; instead, the CI provides a range of values for the difference. In this example, we estimate that the difference in mean systolic blood pressures is between 0.44 and 2.96 units, with men having the higher values. The last aspect of the interpretation is based on the fact that the CI is positive and that we called the men Group 1 and the women Group 2. Had we designated the groups the other way (i.e., women as Group 1 and men as Group 2), the CI would have been −2.96 to −0.44, suggesting that women have lower systolic blood pressures (anywhere from 0.44 to 2.96 units lower than men).

Table 6–10 includes 95% CIs for the difference in means in each characteristic, computed using the same formula we used for the CI for the difference in mean systolic blood pressures. Notice that the 95% CI for the difference in mean total cholesterol levels between men and women is −17.16 to −12.24. Men have lower mean total cholesterol levels than women, anywhere from 12.24 to 17.16 units lower. The men have higher mean values on each of the other characteristics considered (indicated by the positive CIs).

Again, the CI for the difference in means provides an estimate of the absolute difference in means of the outcome variable of interest between the comparison groups. It is often of interest to make a judgment as to whether there is a statistically meaningful difference between comparison groups. This judgment is based on whether the observed difference is beyond that expected by chance.

The CIs for the difference in means provide a range of likely values for $(\mu_1 - \mu_2)$. It is important to note that all values in the CI are equally likely estimates of the true value of $(\mu_1 - \mu_2)$. If there is no difference between the population means, then the difference is zero (i.e., $\mu_1 - \mu_2 = 0$). Zero is the no difference or null value of the parameter (in this case, no difference in means). If a 95% CI for the difference in means includes 0 (the null value), then we say that there is no statistically meaningful or statistically significant difference in the means. If the CI does not include 0, then we conclude that there is a statistically significant difference in means. (We will discuss statistical significance in much greater detail in Chapter 7.) For each of the characteristics considered in Example 6.5, there is a statistically significant difference in means between men and women because none of the CIs include the null value, 0. However, notice that some of the means are not very different between men and women (e.g., systolic blood pressure and BMI). Because the 95% CIs do not include 0, we conclude that there are statistically meaningful differences between means.

TABLE 6–10 Confidence Intervals for Differences in Means

	Men		Women		95% CI
	$\overline{X}$	s	$\overline{X}$	s	
Systolic blood pressure	128.2	17.5	126.5	20.1	(0.44, 2.96)
Diastolic blood pressure	75.6	9.8	72.6	9.7	(2.38, 3.67)
Total serum cholesterol	192.4	35.2	207.1	36.7	(−17.16, −12.24)
Weight (lbs)	194.0	33.8	157.7	34.6	(33.98, 38.53)
Height (in.)	68.9	2.7	63.4	2.5	(5.31, 5.66)
Body mass index (BMI)	28.8	4.6	27.6	5.9	(0.76, 1.48)

This is primarily due to the very large sample sizes. We will discuss this in further detail in Chapter 7.

Example 6.6. In Example 6.2, we recapped the data presented in Chapter 4 on the subsample of $n = 10$ participants who attended the seventh examination of the Offspring in the Framingham Heart Study. Table 6–11 contains descriptive statistics on the same continuous characteristics in the subsample stratified (or generated separately) by gender.

Using these data, suppose we wish to construct a 95% CI for the difference in mean systolic blood pressures between men and women. Again, we will call men Group 1 and women Group 2. Because the sample sizes are small (i.e., $n_1 < 30$ and $n_2 < 30$), the CI formula with t is appropriate. However, before implementing the formula we will first check whether the assumption of equality of the population variances is reasonable. The ratio of the sample variances is $9.72^2 / 12.02^2 = 0.65$, which falls between 0.5 and 2, suggesting that the assumption of equality of the population variances is reasonable. The appropriate CI formula for comparing mean systolic blood pressures between men and women is:

$$(\overline{X}_1 - \overline{X}_2) \pm t S_p \sqrt{\frac{1}{n_1} + \frac{1}{n_2}}.$$

Before substituting, we will first compute S_p, the pooled estimate of the common standard deviation:

$$S_p = \sqrt{\frac{(6-1)(9.7)^2 + (4-1)(12.0)^2}{6+4-2}}$$

$$= \sqrt{112.81} = 10.6.$$

Notice that again the pooled estimate of the common standard deviation, S_p, falls between the standard deviations in the comparison groups (i.e., 9.7 and 12.0). We next need to find the appropriate t value for 95% confidence. The degrees of freedom for the two sample procedures are defined as

$df = n_1 + n_2 - 2 = 6 + 4 - 2 = 8$. From Table 2, $t = 2.306$. The 95% CI for the difference in mean systolic blood pressures is:

$$(117.5 - 126.8) \pm 2.306(10.6) \sqrt{\frac{1}{6} + \frac{1}{4}},$$

$$-9.3 \pm 15.77,$$

$$(-25.07, 6.47).$$

We are 95% confident that the difference in mean systolic blood pressures between men and women is between -25.07 and 6.47 units. Our best estimate of the difference, the point estimate, is -9.3 units. The standard error of the difference is 6.84 units, and the margin of error is 15.77 units. In this sample, the men have lower mean systolic blood pressures than women by 9.3 units. However, based on this interval, we cannot conclude that there is a statistically significant difference in mean systolic blood pressures between men and women because the 95% CI includes the null value, 0. Again, the CI is a range of likely values for the difference in means. Because the interval contains some positive values (suggesting men have higher mean blood pressures) and some negative values (suggesting that women have higher values) and therefore also 0 (no difference), we cannot conclude that there is a difference. This 95% CI for the difference in mean blood pressures is much wider than the one based on the full sample derived in Example 6.5. The small sample size produces a very imprecise estimate of the difference in mean systolic blood pressures.

6.5   CONFIDENCE INTERVALS FOR MATCHED SAMPLES, CONTINUOUS OUTCOME

There is an alternative study design to that described in the previous section where again it is of interest to compare two groups with respect to their mean scores on a continuous outcome. Here the two comparison groups are dependent,

TABLE 6–11 Summary Statistics on the Subsample of $n = 10$ Men and Women Attending the Seventh Examination of the Framingham Offspring Study

	Men			Women		
	n	$\overline{X}$	s	n	$\overline{X}$	s
Systolic blood pressure	6	117.5	9.7	4	126.8	12.0
Diastolic blood pressure	6	72.5	7.1	4	69.5	8.1
Total serum cholesterol	6	193.8	30.2	4	215.0	48.8
Weight (lbs)	6	196.9	26.9	4	146.0	7.2
Height (in.)	6	70.2	1.0	4	62.6	2.3
Body mass index (BMI)	6	28.0	3.6	4	26.2	2.0

matched, or paired. One possible scenario involves a single sample of participants and each participant is measured twice, possibly before and after an intervention or under two experimental conditions (e.g., in a crossover trial). The goal of the analysis is to compare the mean score measured before the intervention with the mean measured afterward. Another scenario is one in which matched samples are analyzed. For example, we might be interested in the difference in an outcome between twins or siblings. Again, we have two samples and the goal is to compare the two means. However, the samples are related or dependent. In the first scenario, before and after measurements are taken in the same individual. In the second scenario, measures are taken in pairs of individuals from the same family. When the samples are dependent, we cannot use the techniques described in Section 6.4 to compare means. Because the samples are dependent, statistical techniques that account for the dependency must be used. The technique used focuses on difference scores (e.g., the difference between measures taken before versus after the intervention, or the difference between measures taken in twins or siblings).

In estimation and other statistical inference applications, it is critically important to appropriately identify the unit of analysis. Units of analysis are independent entities. In the one sample and two independent samples applications, participants are the units of analysis. In the two dependent samples application, the pair is the unit and not the number of measurements, which is twice the number of units.

The parameter of interest is the mean difference, μ_d. Again, the first step is to compute descriptive statistics on the sample data. Specifically, descriptive statistics are computed on difference scores. We compute the sample size (which, in this case, is the number of distinct participants or distinct pairs), the mean, and standard deviation of the difference scores. We denote these summary statistics as n, $\overline{X}_d$, and s_d, respectively. The appropriate formula for the CI for the mean difference depends on the sample size. The formulas are shown in Table 6–12 and are identical to those we presented for estimating the mean of a single sample, except here we focus on difference scores.

Here n is the number of participants or pairs, $\overline{X}_d$ and s_d are the mean and standard deviation of the difference scores (where differences are computed on each participant or between members of a matched pair), and z or t are the values from the z or t distributions reflecting the desired confidence level. $s_d/\sqrt{n}$ is the standard error of the point estimate, $\text{SE}(\overline{X}_d)$.

Example 6.7. In the Framingham Offspring Study, participants attend clinical examinations approximately every four years. The data in Table 6–13 are systolic blood pressures measured at the sixth and seventh examinations in a subsample of $n = 15$ randomly selected participants. The first column contains unique identification numbers, assigned only to distinguish individual participants.

Suppose we want to compare systolic blood pressures between examinations (i.e., changes over four years). Because the data in the two samples (Examination 6 and Examination 7) are matched, we compute difference scores. The difference scores can be computed by subtracting the blood pressure measured at Examination 7 from that measured at Examination 6, or vice versa. If we subtract the blood pressure measured at Examination 6 from that measured at Examination 7, then positive differences represent increases over time and negative differences represent decreases over time. Table 6–14 contains the difference scores for each participant.

Notice that several participants' systolic blood pressures decreased over four years (e.g., Participant 1's blood pressure

---

TABLE 6–12 Confidence Intervals for μ_d

$n \geq 30$	$\overline{X}_d \pm z \dfrac{s_d}{\sqrt{n}}$	Find z in Table 1B
$n < 30$	$\overline{X}_d \pm t \dfrac{s_d}{\sqrt{n}}$	Find t in Table 2 (df $= n-1$)

TABLE 6–13 Systolic Blood Pressures Measured at the Sixth and Seventh Examinations of the Framingham Offspring Study

Subject Identification Number	Examination 6	Examination 7
1	168	141
2	111	119
3	139	122
4	127	127
5	155	125
6	115	123
7	125	113
8	123	106
9	130	131
10	137	142
11	130	131
12	129	135
13	112	119
14	141	130
15	122	121

decreased by 27 units from 168 to 141), whereas others increased (e.g., Participant 2's blood pressure increased by 8 units from 111 to 119). We now estimate the mean difference in blood pressures over four years. This is similar to a one sample problem with a continuous outcome (Section 6.2), except here we focus on the difference scores. In this sample, we have $n = 15$, $\overline{X}_d = -5.3$ and $s_d = 12.8$, respectively. The calculations are shown in Table 6–15.

We can now use these descriptive statistics to compute a 95% CI for the mean difference in systolic blood pressures in the population. Because the sample size is small ($n = 15$), we use the following formula:

$$\overline{X}_d \pm t \frac{s_d}{\sqrt{n}}.$$

TABLE 6–14 Difference Scores

Subject Identification Number	Examination 6	Examination 7	Difference
1	168	141	−27
2	111	119	8
3	139	122	−17
4	127	127	0
5	155	125	−30
6	115	123	8
7	125	113	−12
8	123	106	−17
9	130	131	1
10	137	142	5
11	130	131	1
12	129	135	6
13	112	119	7
14	141	130	−11
15	122	121	−1

TABLE 6–15 Summary Statistics on Difference Scores

Subject Identification Number	Difference	Difference-$\overline{X}_d$	(Difference-$\overline{X}_d$)^2
1	−27	−21.7	470.89
2	8	13.3	176.89
3	−17	−11.7	136.89
4	0	5.3	28.09
5	−30	−24.7	610.09
6	8	13.3	176.89
7	−12	−6.7	44.89
8	−17	−11.7	136.89
9	1	6.3	39.69
10	5	10.3	106.09
11	1	6.3	39.69
12	6	11.3	127.69
13	7	12.3	151.29
14	−11	−5.7	32.49
15	−1	4.3	18.49
	−79.0	0	2296.95

We first need the t value for 95% confidence. The degrees of freedom are df $= n-1 = 14$. From Table 2, $t = 2.145$. We can now substitute the descriptive statistics on the difference scores and the t value for 95% confidence:

$$-5.3 \pm 2.145 \frac{12.8}{\sqrt{15}},$$

$$-5.3 + 7.1,$$

$$(-12.4, 1.8).$$

We are 95% confident that the mean difference in systolic blood pressures between Examination 6 and Examination 7 (approximately four years apart) is between -12.4 and 1.8. The null (or no effect) value of the CI for the mean difference is 0. Therefore, based on the 95% CI we cannot conclude that there is a statistically significant difference in blood pressures over time because the CI for the mean difference includes 0.

In Chapter 2, we discussed various study designs, particularly a special case of the randomized trial called the crossover trial (Section 2.3.2). In a crossover trial with two treatments (e.g., an experimental treatment and a control), each participant receives both treatments. Outcomes are measured after each treatment in each participant (see Figure 2.6). A major advantage to the crossover trial is that each participant acts as his or her own control, and therefore fewer participants are required to demonstrate an effect. When the outcome is continuous, the assessment of a treatment effect in a crossover trial is performed using the techniques described here.

Example 6.8. A crossover trial is conducted to evaluate the effectiveness of a new drug designed to reduce the symptoms of depression in adults over 65 years of age following a stroke. Symptoms of depression are measured on a scale of 0 to 100, with higher scores indicative of more frequent and severe symptoms of depression. Patients who suffered a stroke were eligible for the trial. The trial was run as a crossover trial where each patient received both the new drug and a placebo. Patients were blind to the treatment assignment and the order of treatments (e.g., placebo and then new drug or new drug and then placebo) were randomly assigned. After each treatment, depressive symptoms were measured in each patient. The difference in depressive symptoms was measured in each patient by subtracting the depressive symptom score after taking the placebo from the depressive symptom score after taking the new drug. A total of 100 participants completed the trial and the data are summarized in Table 6–16.

The mean difference in the sample is $\overline{X}_d = -12.7$, meaning on average patients scored 12.7 points lower on the depressive symptoms scale after taking the new drug as compared

TABLE 6–16 Summary Statistics on Differences in Depressive Symptoms

	n	Mean Difference	Std Dev Difference
Depressive symptoms after taking the new drug – Depressive symptoms after taking placebo	100	−12.7	8.9

to placebo (i.e., improved by 12.7 points on average). We will now construct a 95% CI for the mean difference in the population. Because the sample size is large, we will use the following formula:

$$\overline{X}_d \pm z \frac{s_d}{\sqrt{n}},$$

$$-12.7 \pm 1.96 \frac{8.9}{\sqrt{100}},$$

$$-12.7 + 1.74,$$

$$(-14.1, -10.7).$$

We are 95% confident that the mean improvement in depressive symptoms after taking the new drug as compared to placebo is between 10.7 and 14.1 units (or alternatively, the depressive symptoms scores are 10.7 to 14.1 units lower after taking the new drug as compared to the placebo). Because we computed the differences by subtracting the scores after taking the placebo from the scores after taking the new drug, and because higher scores are indicative of worse or more severe depressive symptoms, negative differences reflect improvement (i.e., lower depressive symptoms scores after taking the new drug as compared to the placebo). Because the 95% CI for the mean difference does not include 0, we can conclude that there is a statistically significant difference (in this case, a significant improvement) in depressive symptom scores after taking the new drug as compared to the placebo.

6.6 CONFIDENCE INTERVALS FOR TWO INDEPENDENT SAMPLES, DICHOTOMOUS OUTCOME

It is very common to compare two groups in terms of the presence or absence of a particular characteristic or attribute. There are many instances in which the outcome variable is dichotomous (e.g., prevalent cardiovascular disease or diabetes, current smoking status, cancer remission, successful device implant). Similar to the applications described in Section 6.4 for continuous outcomes, we will focus here on the case where there are two comparison groups that are independent or physically separate and the outcome is dichotomous. The two groups might be determined by a particular attribute or characteristic of the participant (e.g., gender, age less than 65 versus age 65 and older) or might be set up by the investigator (e.g., participants assigned to receive an experimental drug or a placebo, a pharmacological versus a surgical treatment). When the outcome is dichotomous, the analysis involves comparing the proportions of successes between the two groups.

We discussed several methods that are used to compare proportions in two independent groups in Chapter 3, including the risk difference, which is computed by taking the difference in proportions between comparison groups and is similar to the estimate of the difference in means for a continuous outcome described in Section 6.4. The *relative risk*, also called the *risk ratio*, is another useful measure to compare proportions between two independent populations, and it is computed by taking the ratio of proportions. Generally, the reference group (e.g., unexposed persons, persons without a risk factor, or persons assigned to the control group in a clinical trial setting) is considered in the denominator of the ratio. The relative risk is often felt to be a better measure of the strength of an effect than the risk difference because it is a relative as opposed to an absolute measure. A third popular measure is the odds ratio. The *odds ratio* is computed by taking the ratio of the odds of success in the comparison groups. The odds is defined as the ratio of the number of successes to the number of failures (see Section 3.4.2 for more details). CI estimates for the risk difference, the relative risk and the odds ratio are described in the following.

6.6.1 Confidence Intervals for the Risk Difference

The *risk difference* (RD) is similar to the difference in means when the outcome is continuous. The parameter of interest is the difference in proportions in the population, RD $= p_1 - p_2$. The point estimate is the difference in sample proportions, $\hat{RD} = \hat{p}_1 - \hat{p}_2$. The sample proportions are computed by taking the ratio of the number of successes (x) to the sample size (n)

in each group, $\hat{p}_1 = x_1/n_1$ and $\hat{p}_2 = x_2/n_2$, respectively. The formula for the CI for the difference in proportions, or the RD, is given in Table 6–17.

The previous formula is appropriate for large samples, defined as at least five successes ($n\hat{p}$) and at least five failures [$n(1-\hat{p})$] in each sample. Recall that this was a condition for the Central Limit Theorem for binomial populations. If there are fewer than five successes or five failures in either comparison group, then alternative procedures called exact methods must be used to estimate the difference in population proportions.[5]

Example 6.9. In Example 3.1, we presented data measured in participants who attended the fifth examination of the Offspring in the Framingham Heart Study. A total of $n = 3799$ participants attended the fifth examination and Table 6–18 contains data on prevalent CVD among participants who were and were not currently smoking cigarettes at the time of the fifth examination in the Framingham Offspring Study.

The outcome is prevalent CVD and the two comparison groups are defined by current smoking status. The point estimate of prevalent CVD among nonsmokers is 298 / 3055 = 0.0975, and the point estimate of prevalent CVD among current smokers is 81 / 744 = 0.1089. When constructing CIs for the RD, the convention is to call the exposed or treated Group 1 and the unexposed or untreated Group 2. Here smoking status defines the comparison groups, and we will call the current smokers Group 1 and the nonsmokers Group 2. A CI for the difference in prevalent CVD (or RD) between smokers and nonsmokers is given below. In this example, we have more than enough successes (cases of prevalent CVD) and failures (persons free of CVD) in each comparison group.

$$\hat{p}_1 - \hat{p}_2 \pm z \sqrt{\frac{\hat{p}_1(1-\hat{p}_1)}{n_1} + \frac{\hat{p}_2(1-\hat{p}_2)}{n_2}},$$

$$(0.1089 - 0.0975 \pm 1.96 \sqrt{\frac{0.1089(1-0.1089)}{744} + \frac{0.0975(1-0.0975)}{3055}},$$

$$0.0114 \pm 0.0247,$$

$$(-0.0133, 0.0361).$$

TABLE 6–17 Confidence Interval for ($p_1 - p_2$)

$\min[n_1\hat{p}_1, n_1(1-\hat{p}_1), n_2\hat{p}_2, n_2(1-\hat{p}_2)] \geq 5$	$\hat{p}_1 - \hat{p}_2 \pm z\sqrt{\frac{\hat{p}_1(1-\hat{p}_1)}{n_1} + \frac{\hat{p}_2(1-\hat{p}_2)}{n_2}}$	Find z in Table 1B

TABLE 6-18 Prevalent CVD in Smokers and Nonsmokers

	Free of CVD	History of CVD	Total
Nonsmoker	2757	298	3055
Current smoker	663	81	744
Total	3420	379	3799

We are 95% confident that the difference in proportions of smokers as compared to nonsmokers with prevalent CVD is between −0.0133 and 0.0361. The null, or no difference, value for the RD is 0. Because the 95% CI includes 0, we cannot conclude that there is a statistically significant difference in prevalent CVD between smokers and nonsmokers.

Example 6.10. A randomized trial is conducted to evaluate the effectiveness of a newly developed pain reliever designed to reduce pain in patients following joint replacement surgery. The trial compares the new pain reliever to the pain reliever currently used (called the standard of care). A total of 100 patients undergoing joint replacement surgery agree to participate in the trial. Patients are randomly assigned to receive either the new pain reliever or the standard pain reliever following surgery. The patients are blind to the treatment assignment. Before receiving the assigned treatment, patients are asked to rate their pain on a scale of 0 to 10 with higher scores indicative of more pain. Each patient is then given the assigned treatment and after 30 minutes is again asked to rate their pain on the same scale. The primary outcome is a reduction in pain of 3 or more scale points (defined by clinicians as a clinically meaningful reduction). The data shown in Table 6–19 are observed in the trial.

A point estimate for the difference in proportions of patients reporting a clinically meaningful reduction in pain between treatment groups is 0.46 − 0.22 = 0.24. (Notice that we call the experimental or new treatment Group 1 and the standard Group 2.) Twenty-four percent more patients

TABLE 6-19 Pain Reduction by Treatment

Treatment Group	n	Reduction of 3+ Points Number	Proportion
New pain reliever	50	23	0.46
Standard pain reliever	50	11	0.22

reported a meaningful reduction in pain with the new pain reliever as compared to the standard pain reliever. We will now construct a 95% CI for the difference in proportions. The sample sizes in each comparison group are adequate—i.e., each treatment group has at least five successes (patients reporting reduction in pain) and at least five failures—therefore the formula for the CI is

$$(0.46-0.22) \pm 1.96 \sqrt{\frac{0.46(1-0.46)}{50} + \frac{0.22(1-0.22)}{50}},$$

$$0.24 \pm 0.180,$$

$$(0.06, 0.42).$$

We are 95% confident that the difference in proportions of patients reporting a meaningful reduction in pain is between 6% and 42% comparing the new and standard pain relievers. Our best estimate is an increase of 24% with the new pain reliever. Because the 95% CI does not contain 0 (the null value), we can conclude that there is a statistically significant difference between pain relievers—in this case, in favor of the new pain reliever.

6.6.2 Confidence Intervals for the Relative Risk

The RD quantifies the absolute difference in risk (or proportions), whereas the relative risk is, as the name indicates, a relative measure. Both measures are useful but they convey different information. A *relative risk* (RR) is computed by taking the ratio of proportions, p_1/p_2. Again, the convention is to place the proportion of successes or the risk for the control or unexposed group in the denominator. The parameter of interest is the relative risk in the population, $RR = p_1/p_2$, and the point estimate is the relative risk in the sample, $\hat{RR} = \hat{p}_1/\hat{p}_2$. The RR is a ratio and does not follow a normal distribution, regardless of the sample sizes in the comparison groups. However, the natural log (ln) of the $\hat{RR}$ is approximately normally distributed and is used to produce a CI for the RR. First, a CI is generated for ln(RR) and then the antilog of the upper and lower limits of the CI for ln(RR) are taken to give the upper and lower limits of the CI for the RR. The two steps are detailed in Table 6–20.

The null or no difference value of the CI for the RR is 1. If a 95% CI for the RR does not include 1, then the risks (or proportions) are said to be statistically significantly different.

Example 6.11. Consider again the data shown in Example 6.18, reflecting the prevalence of CVD among participants who were and were not currently smoking cigarettes at the time of the fifth examination in the Framingham Offspring Study.

TABLE 6–20 Confidence Interval for RR $= p_1/p_2$

CI for ln(RR)	$\ln(\hat{RR}) \pm z \sqrt{\dfrac{(n_1-x_1)/x_1}{n_1} + \dfrac{(n_2-x_2)/x_2}{n_2}}$	Find z in Table 1B
CI for RR	exp(Lower limit), exp (Upper limit)	

The outcome is prevalent CVD and the two comparison groups are defined by current smoking status. In Example 6.9, we generated a point estimate for the difference in prevalence of CVD between smokers and nonsmokers of 0.0114. Smokers had a higher prevalence by 1.14%. We then generated a 95% CI for the difference in prevalent CVD between smokers and non-smokers of $(-0.0133, 0.0361)$. Because the 95% CI included 0, we could not conclude that there was a statistically significant difference in prevalent CVD between smokers and nonsmokers. We will now use these data to generate a point estimate and 95% CI estimate of the RR.

The point estimate for the relative risk is

$$\hat{RR} = \frac{\hat{p}_1}{\hat{p}_2} = \frac{0.1089}{0.0975} = 1.12$$

and the interpretation is as follows: The prevalence of CVD is 1.12 times higher in smokers as compared to nonsmokers. The 95% CI estimate for the RR is computed using the two-step procedure outlined in Table 6–20:

$$\ln(\hat{RR}) \pm z \sqrt{\frac{(n_1-x_1)/x_1}{n_1} + \frac{(n_2-x_2)/x_2}{n_2}},$$

$$\ln(1.12) \pm 1.96 \sqrt{\frac{663/81}{744} + \frac{2757/298}{3055}},$$

$$0.113 \pm 0.231,$$

$$(-0.118, 0.344).$$

A 95% CI for ln(RR) is $(-0.118, 0.344)$. To generate the CI for the RR, we take the antilog (exp) of the lower and upper limts:

$$(\exp(-0.118), \exp(0.344)),$$

$$(0.89, 1.41).$$

Thus, we are 95% confident that the RR of prevalent CVD in smokers as compared to nonsmokers is between 0.89 and 1.41. Because this CI includes the null value (1), we cannot conclude

that there is a difference in prevalent CVD between smokers and nonsmokers.

Example 6.12. Consider again the data shown in Table 6–19 from the randomized trial assessing the effectiveness of a newly developed pain reliever as compared to the standard pain reliever. The primary outcome is reduction in pain of 3 or more scale points (defined by clinicians as a clinically meaningful reduction).

We generated a point estimate for the difference in proportions of patients reporting a clinically meaningful reduction in pain between pain relievers as $0.46 - 0.22 = 0.24$, or 24%, and the 95% CI was (6%, 42%). Because the 95% CI for the RD did not contain 0 (the null value), we concluded that there was a statistically significant difference between pain relievers. We will now use these data to generate a point estimate and 95% CI estimate of the RR.

The point estimate for the relative risk is

$$\hat{RR} = \frac{\hat{p}_1}{\hat{p}_2} = \frac{0.46}{0.22} = 2.09.$$

Patients receiving the new pain reliever are 2.09 times more likely to report a meaningful reduction in pain as compared to patients receiving the standard pain reliever. The 95% CI estimate for the RR is computed using the two-step procedure outlined in Table 6–20.

$$\ln(2.09) \pm 1.96 \sqrt{\frac{27/23}{50} + \frac{39/11}{50}},$$

$$0.737 \pm 0.602,$$

$$(0.135, 1.339).$$

A 95% CI for ln(RR) is (0.135, 1.339). To generate the CI for the RR, we take the antilog (exp) of the lower and upper limits:

$$(\exp(0.135), \exp(1.339)),$$

$$(1.14, 3.82).$$

Thus, we are 95% confident that patients receiving the new pain reliever are between 1.14 and 3.82 times more likely to report a meaningful reduction in pain as compared to patients receiving the standard pain reliever. Because this CI does not include 1 (the null value), we can conclude that this difference is statistically significant.

6.6.3   Confidence Intervals for the Odds Ratio

There are some study designs in which is it not possible to estimate an RR (e.g., a case-control study), and therefore an odds ratio is computed as a relative measure of effect.[6] The odds ratio is similar to the RR in that it is a ratio, as opposed to a difference. An *odds ratio* (OR) is computed by taking the ratio of odds, where the odds in each group is computed by dividing the number of successes (x) by the number of failures ($n - x$) in that group. Similar to the RR, the convention is to place the odds in the control or unexposed group in the denominator. The parameter of interest is the odds ratio in the population, OR, and the point estimate is the odds ratio in the sample,

$$\hat{OR} = \frac{\hat{p}_1/(1-\hat{p}_1)}{\hat{p}_2/(1-\hat{p}_2)}.$$

The odds ratio can also be expressed as

$$\hat{OR} = \frac{x_1/(n_1-x_1)}{x_2/(n_2-x_2)}.$$

Similar to the RR, the OR does not follow a normal distribution and so we use the log transformation to promote normality. We first generate a CI for ln(OR) and then take the antilog of the upper and lower limits of the CI for ln(OR) to determine the upper and lower limits of the CI for the OR. The two steps are detailed in Table 6–21.

The null, or no difference, value of the CI for the OR is 1. If a 95% CI for the OR does not include 1, then the odds are said to be statistically significantly different. We again reconsider Example 6.9 and Example 6.10 and produce estimates of ORs and compare these to our estimates of RDs and RRs.

Example 6.13. Consider again the data shown in Table 6–18 reflecting the prevalence of CVD among participants who were

and were not currently smoking cigarettes at the time of the fifth examination in the Framingham Offspring Study. The outcome is prevalent CVD and the two comparison groups are defined by current smoking status. In Example 6.9, we generated a point estimate for the difference in prevalent CVD between smokers and nonsmokers of 0.0114 and a 95% CI of $(-0.0133, 0.0361)$. Because the 95% CI included 0, we could not conclude that there was a statistically significant difference in prevalent CVD between smokers and nonsmokers. In Example 6.11, we generated a point estimate for the relative risk,

$$\hat{RR} = \frac{\hat{p}_1}{\hat{p}_2} = \frac{0.1089}{0.0975} = 1.12,$$

and a 95% CI of (0.89, 1.41), and because the CI included 1, we concluded that there was no statistically significant difference in prevalent CVD between smokers and nonsmokers.

We will now use these data to estimate an OR. A point estimate of the odds ratio is

$$\hat{OR} = \frac{x_1/(n_1-x_1)}{x_2/(n_2-x_2)} = \frac{81/663}{298/2757} = 1.13,$$

and the interpretation is that the odds that a smoker has prevalent CVD is 1.13 times higher than the odds that a nonsmoker has prevalent CVD. The 95% CI estimate for the OR is computed using the two-step procedure outlined in Table 6–21,

$$\ln(\hat{OR}) \pm z \sqrt{\frac{1}{x_1} + \frac{1}{n_1-x_1} + \frac{1}{x_2} + \frac{1}{n_2-x_2}},$$

$$\ln(1.13) \pm 1.96 \sqrt{\frac{1}{81} + \frac{1}{663} + \frac{1}{298} + \frac{1}{2757}},$$

$$0.122 \pm 0.261,$$

$$(-0.139, 0.383).$$

A 95% CI for ln(OR) is $(-0.139, 0.383)$. To generate the CI for the OR, we take the antilog (exp) of the lower and upper limits,

---

TABLE 6–21 Confidence Interval for OR

CI for ln(OR)	$\ln(\hat{OR}) \pm z \sqrt{\dfrac{1}{x_1} + \dfrac{1}{(n_1-x_1)} + \dfrac{1}{x_2} + \dfrac{1}{(n_2-x_2)}}$	Find z in Table 1B
CI for OR	exp(Lower limit), exp (Upper limit)	

$$(\exp(-0.139), \exp(0.383)),$$

$$(0.870, 1.47).$$

Thus, we are 95% confident that the odds of prevalent CVD in smokers is between 0.87 and 1.47 times the odds of prevalent CVD in nonsmokers. The null value is 1 and because this CI includes 1, we cannot conclude that there is a significant difference in the odds of prevalent CVD between smokers and nonsmokers.

Example 6.14. Consider again the data shown in Table 6–19 from the randomized trial assessing the effectiveness of a newly developed pain reliever as compared to the standard of care. The primary outcome is reduction in pain of 3 or more scale points (defined by clinicians as a clinically meaningful reduction).

We generated a point estimate for the difference in proportions of patients reporting a clinically meaningful reduction in pain between pain relievers as $0.46 - 0.22 = 0.24$, or 24%, and the 95% CI was (6%, 42%). Because the 95% CI for the RD did not contain 0 (the null value), we concluded that there was a statistically significant difference between pain relievers. We then generated a point estimate for the relative risk,

$$\hat{RR} = \frac{\hat{p}_1}{\hat{p}_2} = \frac{0.46}{0.22} = 2.09.$$

and a 95% CI of (1.14, 3.82). Because this CI did not include 1, we concluded that this difference was statistically significant.

We will now use these data to generate a point estimate and 95% CI estimate for the OR. The point estimate for the odds ratio is

$$\hat{OR} = \frac{x_1/(n_1 - x_1)}{x_2/(n_2 - x_2)} = \frac{23/27}{11/39} = 3.02.$$

This suggests that the odds that a patient on the new pain reliever reports a meaningful reduction in pain is 3.02 times the odds that a patient on the standard pain reliever reports a meaningful reduction. The 95% CI estimate for the OR is computed using the two-step procedure outlined in Table 6–21,

$$\ln(3.02) \pm 1.96 \sqrt{\frac{1}{23} + \frac{1}{27} + \frac{1}{11} + \frac{1}{39}},$$

$$1.105 \pm 0.870,$$

$$(0.235, 1.975).$$

A 95% CI for ln(OR) is (0.235, 1.975). To generate the CI for the OR, we take the antilog (exp) of the lower and upper limits,

$$(\exp(0.235), \exp(1.975)),$$

$$(1.26, 7.21).$$

Thus, we are 95% confident that the odds that a patient on the new pain reliever reports a meaningful reduction in pain is between 1.26 and 7.21 times the odds that a patient on the standard pain reliever reports a meaningful reduction. Because this CI does not include 1, we can conclude that this difference is statistically significant.

When the study design allows for the calculation of an RR, it is the preferred measure as it is far more interpretable than an OR. However, the OR is extremely important as it is the only measure of effect that can be computed in a case-control study design. When the outcome of interest is relatively rare (e.g., fewer than 10% successes), then the OR and RR will be very close in magnitude. In such a case, investigators often interpret the OR as if it were a RR—i.e., as a comparison of risks rather than a comparison of odds, which is less intuitive.

6.7   SUMMARY

In this chapter, we presented various formulas for estimating different unknown population parameters. In each application, a random sample or two independent random samples were selected from the target population and sample statistics (e.g., sample sizes, means, and standard deviations, or sample sizes and proportions) were generated. Point estimates are the best single-valued estimates of unknown population parameters. Because these can vary from sample to sample, most investigations start with a point estimate and build in a margin of error. The margin of error quantifies sampling variability and includes a value from the z or t distribution reflecting the selected confidence level as well as the standard error of the point estimate.

It is important to remember that the confidence internal contains a range of likely values for the unknown population parameter; a range of values for the population parameter consistent with the data. It is also possible that the confidence internal does not contain the true population parameter. This is important to remember in interpreting intervals. Confidence internals are also very useful for comparing means or proportions and can be used to assess whether there is a statistically meaningful difference in parameters. This is based on whether the confidence internal includes the null value (e.g., 0 for the difference in means, mean difference, and risk difference or 1 for the relative risk and odds ratio). The precision of a confidence internal is defined by the margin of error (or the width of the interval). A larger margin of error (wider interval) is indicative of a less precise estimate. Table 6–22 summarizes key formulas for confidence internal estimates.

TABLE 6–22 Summary of Key Formulas

Number of Groups, Outcome: Parameter	Confidence Interval*
One sample, continuous: CI for μ	$\overline{X} \pm z\dfrac{s}{\sqrt{n}}$
Two independent samples, continuous: CI for $(\mu_1 - \mu_2)$	$(\overline{X}_1 - \overline{X}_2) \pm zS_p\sqrt{\dfrac{1}{n_1} + \dfrac{1}{n_2}}$
Two matched samples, continuous: CI for μ_d	$\overline{X}_d \pm z\dfrac{s_d}{\sqrt{n}}$
One sample, dichotomous: CI for p	$\hat{p} \pm z\sqrt{\dfrac{\hat{p}(1-\hat{p})}{n}}$
Two independent samples, dichotomous: CI for RD $= (p_1 - p_2)$	$\hat{p}_1 - \hat{p}_2 \pm z\sqrt{\dfrac{\hat{p}_1(1-\hat{p}_1)}{n_1} + \dfrac{\hat{p}_2(1-\hat{p}_2)}{n_2}}$
Two independent samples, dichotomous: CI for RR $= \dfrac{p_1}{p_2}$	$\ln(\hat{RR}) \pm z\sqrt{\dfrac{(n_1 - X_1)/X_1}{n_1} + \dfrac{(n_2 - X_2)/X_2}{n_2}}$ exp(Lower limit), exp (Upper limit)
Two independent samples, dichotomous: CI for OR $= \dfrac{X_1/(n_1 - X_1)}{X_2/(n_2 - X_2)}$	$\ln(\hat{OR}) \pm z\sqrt{\dfrac{1}{X_1} + \dfrac{1}{(n_1 - X_1)} + \dfrac{1}{X_2} + \dfrac{1}{(n_2 - X_2)}}$ exp(Lower limit), exp (Upper limit)

*See Tables 6–3, 6–8, and 6–12 for alternative formulas that are appropriate for small samples.

6.8 PRACTICE PROBLEMS

1. A study is run to estimate the mean total cholesterol level in children 2 to 6 years of age. A sample of nine participants is selected and their total cholesterol levels are measured as follows:

185   225   240   196   175   180   194   147   223

Generate a 95% CI for the true mean total cholesterol levels in children.

2. A clinical trial is planned to compare an experimental medication designed to lower blood pressure to a placebo. Before starting the trial, a pilot study is conducted involving ten participants. The objective of the study is to assess how systolic blood pressure changes over time untreated. Systolic blood pressures are measured at baseline and again 4 weeks later. Compute a 95% CI for the difference in blood pressures over 4 weeks.

Baseline: 120 145 130 160 152 143 126 121 115 135

4 Weeks: 122 142 135 158 155 140 130 120 124 130

3. The main trial for the medication in Problem 2 is conducted and involves a total of 200 patients. Patients are enrolled and randomized to receive either the experimental medication or the placebo. The data shown in Table 6–23 are data collected at the end of the study after 6 weeks on the assigned treatment.
   a. Generate a 95% CI for the difference in mean systolic blood pressures between groups.
   b. Generate a 95% CI for the difference in proportions of patients with hypertension between groups.
   c. Generate a point estimate for the RR of side effects in patients assigned to the experimental group as compared to placebo. Generate a 95% CI for the RR.

TABLE 6–23 Outcome Data by Treatment

	Experimental ($n=100$)	Placebo ($n=100$)
Mean (SD) systolic blood pressure	120.2 (15.4)	131.4 (18.9)
Hypertensive (%)	14	22
Side effects (%)	6	8

TABLE 6–25 Wound Healing by Treatment

Treatment	Number of Patients with Percent Reduction in Size of Wound				
	None	1–25	26–50	51–75	76–100
New compound ($n = 125$)	4	11	37	32	41
Placebo ($n = 125$)	12	24	45	34	10

4. The following data were collected as part of a study of coffee consumption among undergraduate students. The following values reflect cups per day consumed:

   3   4   6   8   2   1   0   2

   a. Compute the sample mean.
   b. Compute the sample standard deviation.
   c. Construct a 95% CI for the mean number of cups of coffee consumed among all undergraduates.

5. A clinical trial is conducted to evaluate a new pain reliever for arthritis. Participants are randomly assigned to receive the new treatment or a placebo. The outcome is pain relief within 30 minutes, and the data are shown in Table 6–24.
   a. Estimate the RD in pain relief between treatments.
   b. Estimate the RR in pain relief between treatments.
   c. Estimate the OR in pain relief between treatments.
   d. Construct a 95% CI for the OR.

6. Data was collected in a clinical trial evaluating a new compound designed to improve wound healing in trauma patients. The new compound was compared against a placebo. After treatment for 5 days with the new compound or placebo, the extent of wound healing was measured and the data are shown in Table 6–25. Suppose that clinicians feel that if the percent reduction in the size of the wound is greater than 50%, then the treatment is a success.
   a. Generate a 95% CI for the percent success in patients receiving the new compound.
   b. Generate a 95% CI for the difference in the percent success between the new compound and placebo.
   c. Generate a 95% CI for the RR of treatment success between treatments.
   d. Generate a 95% CI for the OR of treatment success between treatments.

7. A clinical trial is conducted to compare an experimental medication to placebo to reduce the symptoms of asthma. Two hundred participants are enrolled in the study and randomized to receive either the experimental medication or placebo. The primary outcome is a self-reported reduction of symptoms. Among 100 participants who received the experimental medication, 38 reported a reduction of symptoms as compared to 21 participants of 100 assigned to the placebo.
   a. Generate a 95% CI for the difference in proportions of participants reporting a reduction of symptoms between the experimental and placebo groups.
   b. Estimate the RR for reduction in symptoms between groups.
   c. Estimate the OR for reduction in symptoms between groups.
   d. Generate a 95% CI for the RR.

8. Table 6–26 displays descriptive statistics on the subjects involved in the study described in Problem 7.
   a. Generate a 95% CI for the mean age among persons assigned to the placebo.
   b. Generate a 95% CI for the difference in mean ages in patients assigned to the experimental versus the placebo groups.
   c. Generate a 95% CI for the difference in mean BMI in patients assigned to the experimental versus the placebo groups.

TABLE 6–24 Pain Relief by Treatment

	Pain Relief	No Pain Relief
New medication	44	76
Placebo	21	99

TABLE 6–26 Descriptive Statistics by Treatment

	Experimental Medication ($N=100$)	Placebo ($n=100$)
Mean (SD) age, (years)	47.2 (4.3)	46.1 (5.1)
Men (%)	46%	58%
Mean (SD) educational level, (years)	13.1 (2.9)	14.2 (3.1)
Mean (SD) annual income,	$36,560 ($1054)	$37,470 ($998)
Mean (SD) body mass index (BMI),	24.7 (2.7)	25.1 (2.4)

9. A crossover trial is conducted to compare an experimental medication for migraine headaches to a currently available medication. A total of 50 patients are enrolled in the study and each patient re-ceives both treatments. The outcome is the time, in minutes, until the headache pain resolves. Following each treatment, patients record the time it takes until pain is resolved. Treatments are assigned in random order (i.e., some patients receive the currently available medication first and then the experimental medication, and others receive the experimental medication first and then the currently available medication). The mean difference in times between the experimental and currently available medication is -9.4 minutes with a standard deviation of 2.8 minutes. Construct a 95% CI for the mean difference in times between the experimental and currently available medication.

10. Suppose in the study described in Problem 9 each patient was also asked if the assigned medication caused any stomach upset. Among the 50 patients, 12 reported stomach upset with the experimental medication. Construct a 90% CI for the proportion of patients who experience stomach upset with the experimental medication.

REFERENCES

1. Newcomb, R.G. "Two-sided confidence intervals for the single proportion: Comparison of seven methods." *Statistics in Medicine* 1998; 17(8): 857–872.

2. StatXact Version 7 © 2006 by Cytel, Inc., Cambridge, MA.

3. D'Agostino, R.B., Sullivan, L.M., and Beiser, A. *Introductory Applied Biostatistics*. Belmont, CA: Duxbury-Brooks/Cole, 2004.

4. Rosner, B. *Fundamentals of Biostatistics*. Belmont, CA: Duxbury-Brooks/Cole, 2006.

5. Agresti, A. *Categorical Data Analysis* (2nd ed.). New York: John Wiley & Sons, 2002.

6. Rothman, K.J. and Greenland, S. *Modern Epidemiology* (2nd ed.). Philadelphia: Lippincott-Raven, 1998.

CHAPTER 7

Hypothesis Testing Procedures

The second area of statistical inference is hypothesis testing. In *hypothesis testing,* a specific statement or hypothesis is generated about a population parameter and sample statistics are used to assess the likelihood that the hypothesis is true. This statement or hypothesis is based on available information and the investigator's belief about the parameter. The process of hypothesis testing involves setting up two competing hypotheses: one that reflects no difference, no association, or no effect (called the *null hypothesis*) and the other that reflects the investigator's belief (called the *research* or *alternative hypothesis*). We select a random sample (or multiple samples when there are more comparison groups) and generate summary statistics. We then assess the likelihood that the sample data support the research or alternative hypothesis. Similar to estimation, the process of hypothesis testing is based on probability theory and the Central Limit Theorem.

The techniques for hypothesis testing again depend on the appropriate classification of the key study outcome variable or endpoint as continuous or discrete. The number of comparison groups in the investigation must also be specified. It is again important to determine whether the comparison groups are independent (i.e., physically separate, such as men versus women) or dependent (i.e., matched or paired, such as pre- and post-assessments on the same participants). These issues dictate the appropriate hypothesis testing technique. In estimation, we focused explicitly on techniques for one and two samples. We discussed estimation for a specific parameter (e.g., the mean or proportion of a population), for differences (e.g., difference in means, the risk difference) and ratios (e.g., the relative risk and odds ratio). Here we will focus on procedures for one, two, and more than two samples. Hypothesis

testing can generalize to the situation of more than two groups, whereas estimation is not intuitive when there are more than two groups. Table 7–1 outlines hypothesis testing procedures that we consider here.

7.1 INTRODUCTION TO HYPOTHESIS TESTING

Before discussing the different procedures that are appropriate for each scenario outlined in Table 7–1, we first present the general approach using a simple example. The Centers for Disease Control and Prevention (CDC) reported on trends in weight, height, and body mass index (BMI) from the 1960s through 2002.[1] The data for the report were collected in the National Health Examination and the National Health and Nutrition Examination Surveys, which were conducted between 1960 and 2002. The general trend was that Americans were much heavier and slightly taller in 2002 as compared to 1960. The report indicated that both men and women gained approximately 24 pounds, on average, between 1960 and 2002. In 2002, the mean weight for American men was reported at 191 pounds and the mean weight for women was reported at 163 pounds.

Suppose we focus on the mean weight in men. In 2002, the mean weight for men was reported at 191 pounds. Suppose that an investigator hypothesizes that weights are even higher in 2006 (i.e., that the trend continued over the next 4 years). In hypothesis testing, we set up competing hypotheses about the unknown parameter. One hypothesis is called the null hypothesis and the other is called the alternative or research hypothesis. The research hypothesis is that the mean weight in men in 2006 is more than 191 pounds. The null hypothesis is that there is no change in weight and therefore the mean

TABLE 7–1 Hypothesis Testing Techniques

Number of Samples	Outcome Variable
One sample	Continuous
Two independent samples	
Two dependent, matched samples	
More than two independent samples	
One sample	Dichotomous
Two independent samples	
More than two independent samples	
One sample	Discrete (more than 2 response options)
Two or more independent samples	

weight is still 191 pounds in 2006. The null and research hypotheses are denoted as

Null hypothesis, H_0: $\mu = 191$ (no change),

Research hypothesis, H_1: $\mu > 191$ (investigator's belief).

To test the hypotheses, we select a random sample of American males in 2006 and measure their weights. Suppose we have resources available to recruit $n = 100$ men into our sample. We weigh each participant and compute summary statistics on the sample data. Suppose in the sample we determine the following: $n = 100$, $\overline{X} = 197.1$, $s = 25.6$.

Do the sample data support the null or research hypothesis? The sample mean of 197.1 is numerically higher than 191. However, is this difference more than would be expected by chance? In hypothesis testing, we assume that the null hypothesis holds until proven otherwise. We therefore need to determine the likelihood of observing a sample mean of 197.1 or higher when the true population mean is 191 (i.e., if the null hypothesis is true or under the null hypothesis). We can compute this probability using the Central Limit Theorem. Specifically,

$$P(\overline{X} > 197.1) = P\left(z > \frac{197.1 - 191}{25.6/\sqrt{100}}\right) =$$
$$P(z > 2.38) = 1 - 0.9913 = 0.0087.$$

(Notice that we use the sample standard deviation in computing the z score. This is generally an appropriate substitution as long as the sample size is large, $n > 30$.) Thus, there is less than a 1% probability of observing a sample mean as large as 197.1 when the true population mean is 191. Do you think that the null hypothesis is likely true? Based on how

unlikely it is to observe a sample mean of 197.1 under the null hypothesis (i.e., less than 1% probability), we might infer from our data that the null hypothesis is probably not true.

Suppose that the sample data had turned out differently. Suppose that we instead observed the following in 2006: $n = 100$, $\overline{X} = 192.1$, $s = 25.6$. How likely is it to observe a sample mean of 192.1 or higher when the true population mean is 191 (i.e., if the null hypothesis is true)? We can again compute this probability using the Central Limit Theorem. Specifically,

$$P(\overline{X} > 192.1) = P\left(z > \frac{197.1 - 191}{25.6/\sqrt{100}}\right) =$$
$$P(z > 0.43) = 1 - 0.6664 = 0.3336.$$

There is a 33.4% probability of observing a sample mean as large as 192.1 when the true population mean is 191. Do you think that the null hypothesis is likely true?

We need to determine a threshold or cutoff point (called the *critical value*) to decide when to believe the null hypothesis and when to believe the research hypothesis. It is important to note that although it is possible to observe any sample mean when the true population mean is 191, some are very unlikely. Based on the previous two samples, it would seem reasonable to believe the research hypothesis when $\overline{X} = 197.1$, but to believe the null hypothesis when $\overline{X} = 192.1$. What we need is a threshold value such that if $\overline{X}$ is above that threshold, we believe that H_1 is true and if $\overline{X}$ is below that threshold, we believe H_0 is true. The difficulty in determining a threshold for $\overline{X}$ is that it depends on the scale of measurement. In this example, the critical value might be 195 (i.e., if the sample mean is 195 or more, we believe that H_1 is true and if the sample mean is less than 195, we believe that H_0 is true). Suppose we are interested in assessing an increase in blood pressure over time. The critical value would be different because blood pressures are measured in millimeters of mercury (mmHg) as opposed to in pounds. In the following, we will explain how the critical value is determined and how we handle the issue of scale.

First, to address the issue of scale in determining the critical value we convert our sample data (in particular, the sample mean) into a z score. We know from Chapter 4 that the center of the z distribution is 0 and extreme values are those that exceed 2 or fall below -2 (values above 2 and below -2 represent approximately 5% of all z values). If the observed sample mean is close to the mean specified in H_0 ($\mu = 191$), then z will be close to 0. If the observed sample mean is much larger than the mean specified in H_0, then z will be large.

In hypothesis testing, we select a critical value from the z distribution. This is done by first determining what is called the level of significance, denoted α. Remember that if the null hypothesis is true, it is possible to observe any sample mean. What we are doing here is drawing a line at extreme values. The level of significance is the probability that we reject the null hypothesis (in favor of the alternative) when it is actually true:

$$\alpha = \text{Level of significance} = P(\text{reject } H_0 \mid H_0 \text{ is true}).$$

Because α is a probability, it ranges between 0 and 1. The usual value for α is 0.05, or 5%. If an investigator selects $\alpha = 0.05$, they are allowing a 5% probability of incorrectly rejecting the null hypothesis in favor of the alternative when the null is true. The typical values for α are 0.01, 0.05, and 0.10, with $\alpha = 0.05$ the most commonly used value.

Suppose in our weight study we select $\alpha = 0.05$. We need to determine the value of z that holds 5% of the values above it (Figure 7–1). The critical value of z for $\alpha = 0.05$ is $z = 1.645$ (i.e., 5% of the distribution is above 1.645). With this value, we can set up what is called our decision rule for the test. The rule is to reject H_0 if the z score is 1.645 or more.

With the first sample, we have $\overline{X} = 197.1$ and $z = 2.38$. Because $2.38 > 1.645$, we reject the null hypothesis. (The same conclusion can be drawn by comparing the 0.0087 probability of observing a sample mean as extreme as 197.1 to the level

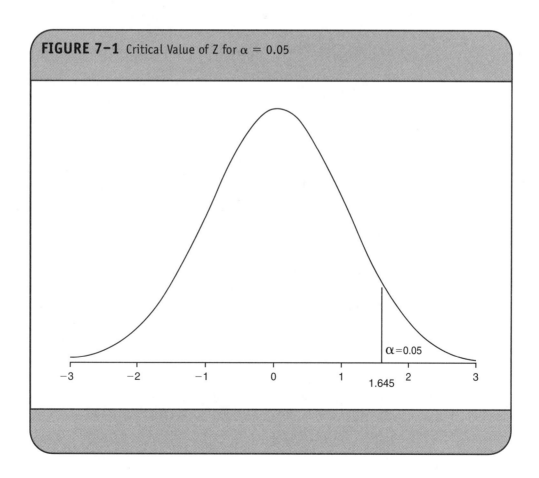

FIGURE 7–1 Critical Value of Z for $\alpha = 0.05$

of significance of 0.05. If the observed probability is smaller than the level of significance, we reject H₀.) Because the *z* score exceeds the critical value, we conclude that the mean weight for men in 2006 is more than 191 pounds, the value reported in 2002. If we observed the second sample ($\overline{X}=192.1$), we would not reject the null hypothesis because the *z* score is 0.43, which is not in the rejection region (i.e., the region in the tail end of the curve above 1.645). With the second sample we do not have evidence to conclude that weights have increased. (Again, the same conclusion can be reached by comparing probabilities. The probability of observing a sample mean as extreme as 192.1 is 33.4%, which is not below our 5% level of significance.)

The procedure for hypothesis testing is based on the ideas described previously. Specifically, we set up competing hypotheses, select a random sample from the population of interest, and compute summary statistics. We then determine whether the sample data supports the null or alternative hypotheses. The procedure can be broken down into the following five steps. We will use this five-step approach in performing tests of hypotheses for all of the scenarios in Table 7–1.

Step 1: Set up hypotheses and determine the level of significance.

H₀: Null hypothesis (no change, no difference),

H₁: Research hypothesis (investigator's belief),

$\alpha = 0.05.$

The research or alternative hypothesis can take one of three forms. An investigator might believe that the parameter has increased, decreased, or changed. For example, an investigator might hypothesize:

1. H₁: $\mu > \mu_0$, where μ_0 is the comparator or null value (e.g., $\mu_0 = 191$ in our example about weight in men in 2006) and an increase is hypothesized—this type of test is called an *upper-tailed test.*
2. H₁: $\mu < \mu_0$, where a decrease is hypothesized—this is called a *lower-tailed test.*
3. H₁: $\mu \neq \mu_0$, where a difference is hypothesized—this is called a *two-tailed test.*

The exact form of the research hypothesis depends on the investigator's belief about the parameter of interest and whether it has possibly increased, decreased, or is different from the null value. The research hypothesis is set up by the investigator before any data are collected.

Step 2: Select the appropriate test statistic.

The test statistic is a single number that summarizes the sample information. An example of a test statistic is the *z* statistic computed as

$$z = \frac{\overline{X}-\mu_0}{s/\sqrt{n}}.$$

When the sample size is small, we will use *t* statistics (just as we did in estimation in Chapter 6). As we present each scenario, alternative test statistics are provided along with conditions for their appropriate use.

Step 3: Set up the decision rule.

The decision rule is a statement that tells under what circumstances to reject the null hypothesis. The decision rule is based on specific values of the test statistic (e.g., reject H₀ if $z \geq 1.645$). The decision rule for a specific test depends on three factors: the research hypothesis, the test statistic, and the level of significance.

The decision rule depends on whether an upper-tailed, lower-tailed, or two-tailed test is proposed. In an upper-tailed test, the decision rule has investigators reject H₀ if the test statistic is larger than the critical value. In a lower-tailed test, the decision rule has investigators reject H₀ if the test statistic is smaller than the critical value. In a two-tailed test, the decision rule has investigators reject H₀ if the test statistic, is extreme, either larger than an upper critical value or smaller than a lower critical value.

The exact form of the test statistic is also important in determining the decision rule. If the test statistic follows the standard normal distribution (*z*), then the decision rule will be based on the standard normal distribution. If the test statistic follows the *t* distribution, then the decision rule will be based on the *t* distribution. The appropriate critical value will be selected from the *t* distribution again depending on the specific alternative hypothesis and the level of significance.

The third factor is the level of significance which is selected in Step 1 (e.g., $\alpha = 0.05$). For example, in an upper-tailed *z* test, if $\alpha = 0.05$, then the critical value is $z = 1.645$.

Figures 7–2 through Figure 7–4 illustrate the rejection regions defined by the decision rule for upper-, lower-, and two-tailed *z* tests with $\alpha = 0.05$. Notice that the rejection regions are in the upper, lower, and both tails of the curves, respectively. Notice in the two-tailed test that the rejection region is split into two equal parts. The total area in the rejection region is still equal to α. In Figure 7–4, $\alpha = 0.05$ and the area in each tail is 0.025.

Critical values of *z* for upper-, lower-, and two-tailed tests can be found in Table 1C in the Appendix. Critical values

FIGURE 7–2 Rejection Region for Upper-Tailed Z Test ($H_1: \mu \neq \mu_0$) with $\alpha = 0.05$

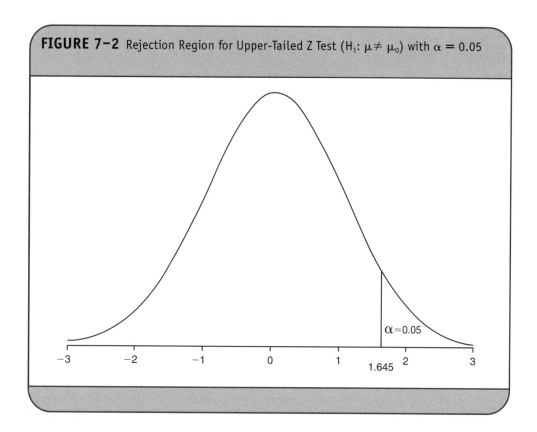

FIGURE 7–3 Rejection Region for Lower-Tailed Z Test ($H_1: \mu < \mu_0$) with $\alpha = 0.05$

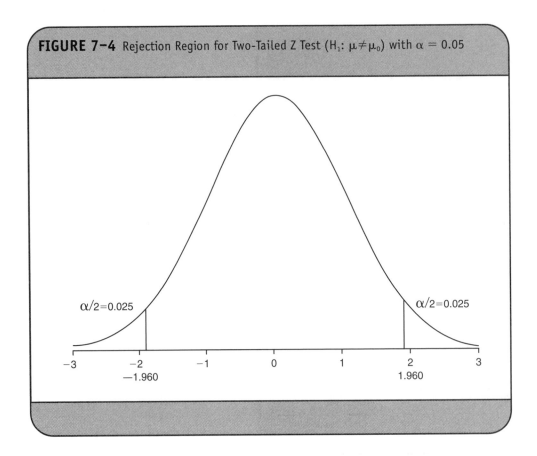

FIGURE 7–4 Rejection Region for Two-Tailed Z Test (H$_1$: $\mu \neq \mu_0$) with $\alpha = 0.05$

of t for upper, lower, and two-tailed tests can be found in Table 2 in the Appendix.

Step 4: Compute the test statistic.

Here we compute the test statistic by substituting the observed sample data into the test statistic identified in Step 2.

Step 5: Conclusion.

The final conclusion is made by comparing the test statistic (which is a summary of the information observed in the sample) to the decision rule. The final conclusion will be either to reject the null hypothesis (because the sample data are very unlikely if the null hypothesis is true) or not to reject the null hypothesis (because the sample data are not very unlikely).

If the null hypothesis is rejected, an exact significance level is computed to describe the likelihood of observing the sample data assuming that the null hypothesis is true. The exact level of significance is called the p-value and it will be less than the chosen level of significance. Statistical computing packages provide exact p-values as part of their standard output for hypothesis tests. We will approximate p-values using Table 1C for tests involving z statistics and Table 2 for tests involving t statistics.

We now use the five-step procedure to test the research hypothesis that the mean weight in men in 2006 is more than 191 pounds. We will assume the sample data are as follows: $n = 100$, $\overline{X} = 197.1$ and $s = 25.6$.

Step 1: Set up hypotheses and determine the level of significance.

$$H_0: \mu = 191,$$

$$H_1: \mu > 191,$$

$$\mu = 0.05.$$

The research hypothesis is that weights have increased, and therefore an upper-tailed test is used.

Step 2: Select the appropriate test statistic.

Because the sample size is large ($n > 30$) the appropriate test statistic is

$$z = \frac{\overline{X} - \mu_0}{s/\sqrt{n}}.$$

(In Section 7.2, we present alternative test statistics appropriate for small samples.)

Step 3: Set up the decision rule.

In this example, we are performing an upper-tailed test ($H_1: \mu > 191$), with a z test statistic and selected $\alpha = 0.05$. The decision rule is shown in Figure 7–2,

$$\text{Reject } H_0 \text{ if } z \geq 1.645.$$

Step 4: Compute the test statistic.

We now substitute the sample data into the formula for the test statistic identified in Step 2,

$$z = \frac{\overline{X} - \mu_0}{s/\sqrt{n}} = \frac{195.3 - 191}{25.6/\sqrt{200}} = 2.38.$$

Step 5: Conclusion.

We reject H_0 because $2.38 > 1.645$. We have statistically significant evidence at $\alpha = 0.05$ to show that the mean weight in men in 2006 is more than 191 pounds. Because we rejected the null hypothesis, we now approximate the p-value, which is the likelihood of observing the sample data if the null hypothesis is true. An alternative definition of the p-value is the smallest level of significance where we can still reject H_0.

In this example, we observed $z = 2.38$ and for $\alpha = 0.05$, the critical value was 1.645. Because 2.38 exceeded 1.645, we rejected H_0. In our conclusion, we reported a statistically significant increase in mean weight at a 5% level of significance. The data actually provide stronger evidence. Table 7–2 is a copy of Table 1C in the Appendix which contains critical values for upper-tailed tests.

What is the smallest level of significance we could choose and still reject H_0? If we select $\alpha = 0.025$, the critical value is 1.96, and we still reject H_0 because $2.38 > 1.960$. If we select $\alpha = 0.010$ the critical value is 2.326, and we still reject H_0 because $2.38 > 2.326$. However, if we select $\alpha = 0.005$, the critical value is 2.576 and we cannot reject H_0 because $2.38 < 2.576$. Therefore, the smallest α where we still reject H_0 is 0.010.

TABLE 7–2 Critical Values for Upper-Tailed Z Tests

Upper-Tailed Test α	Critical Value of z
0.10	1.282
0.05	1.645
0.025	1.960
0.010	2.326
0.005	2.576
0.001	3.090
0.0001	3.719

This is the p-value. A statistical computing package would produce a more precise p-value, which would be between 0.005 and 0.010. Here we are approximating the p-value using Table 1C in the Appendix, and we report p < 0.010.

p-values reflect the exact significance of tests of hypothesis. In this example, we found p < 0.010, indicating that there is less than a 1% chance that we are incorrectly rejecting the null hypothesis if the null hypothesis is true. Suppose in this example that the test statistic was $z = 1.70$. We would still reject H_0 at $\alpha = 0.05$ because $1.70 > 1.645$. However, with $z = 1.70$, the p-value would be reported as $p < 0.05$. The p-value is shown graphically in Figure 7–5.

Smaller p-values are indicative of more evidence in support of the research hypothesis. In the literature, investigators often report p-values to summarize tests of hypothesis. The following rule can be used to interpret p-values:

$$\text{Reject } H_0 \text{ if } p \leq \alpha,$$

where p is the p-value and α is the level of significance selected by the investigator.

For example, suppose we wish to test $H_0: \mu = 100$ versus $H_1: \alpha > 100$ at $\alpha = 0.05$. Data are collected and analyzed with a statistical computing package that reports $p = 0.0176$. Because $p = 0.0176 < \alpha = 0.05$, we reject H_0. However, if we had selected $\alpha = 0.01$, we would not reject H_0. In the examples that follow, we will approximate p-values using Table 1C in the Appendix for tests involving z statistics and Table 2 in the Appendix for tests involving t statistics. We will also discuss appropriate interpretation.

In all tests of hypothesis (for continuous, dichotomous, and discrete outcomes, with one, two, or more than two samples), there are two errors that can be committed. The first is called a *Type I error* and refers to the situation where we incorrectly reject H_0 when, in fact, it is true. This is also called a false positive result (as we incorrectly conclude that the research hypothesis is true when it is not). When we run a test of hypothesis and decide to reject H_0 (e.g., because the test statistic exceeds the critical value in an upper-tailed test), either we make a correct decision because the research hypothesis is true or we commit a Type I error. The different conclusions are summarized in the following. Note that we will never know whether the null hypothesis is really true or false (i.e., we will never know which row of Table 7–3 reflects reality).

In the first step of the hypothesis test, we select a level of significance, α, and $\alpha = P(\text{Type I error})$. Because we purposely select a small value for α, we control the probability of committing a Type I error. For example, if we select $\alpha = 0.05$ and

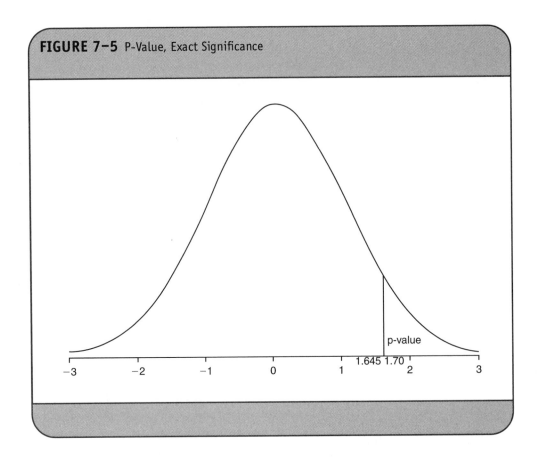

FIGURE 7–5 P-Value, Exact Significance

our test tells us to reject H_0, then there is a 5% probability that we may commit a Type I error. Most investigators are very comfortable with this and are confident when rejecting H_0 that the research hypothesis is true, as it is the more likely scenario when we reject H_0.

When we run a test of hypothesis and decide not to reject H_0 (e.g., because the test statistic is below the critical value in an upper-tailed test), then either we make a correct decision because the null hypothesis is true or we commit a *Type II error*. β represents the probability of a Type II error and is defined as

$$\beta = P(\text{Type II error}) = P(\text{do not reject } H_0 \mid H_0 \text{ is false}).$$

TABLE 7–3 Errors in Tests of Hypothesis

	Conclusion in Test of Hypothesis	
	Do Not Reject H_0	Reject H_0
H_0 is true	Correct decision	Type I error
H_0 is false	Type II error	Correct decision

Unfortunately, we cannot choose β to be small (e.g., 0.05) to control the probability of committing a Type II error because β depends on several factors, including the sample size, β, and the research hypothesis. These issues will be discussed in much further detail in Chapter 8. For now, we must recognize that when we do not reject H_0, it may be very likely that we are committing a Type II error (i.e., failing to reject H_0 when it is false). Therefore, when tests are run and the null hypothesis is not rejected, we often make a weak concluding statement allowing for the possibility that we might be committing a Type II error. If we do not reject H_0, we conclude that we do not have significant evidence to show that H_1 is true. We do not conclude that H_0 is true. The most common reason for a Type II error is a small sample size.

7.2 TESTS WITH ONE SAMPLE, CONTINUOUS OUTCOME

Hypothesis testing applications with a continuous outcome variable in a single population are performed according to the five-step procedure outlined earlier. A key component is setting up the null and research hypotheses. The objective is to compare the mean in a single population to a known mean (μ_0). The known value is generally derived from another

TABLE 7–4 Test Statistics for Testing $H_0: \mu = \mu_0$

$n \geq 30$	$z = \dfrac{\bar{X} - \mu_0}{s/\sqrt{n}}$	Find critical value in Table 1B
$n < 30$	$t = \dfrac{\bar{X} - \mu_0}{s/\sqrt{n}}$	Find critical value in Table 2 (df $= n - 1$)

study or report—for example, a study in a similar but not identical population or a study performed some years ago. The latter is called an historical control ("control" here referring to the fact that the historical study is the comparator). It is important in setting up the hypotheses in a one-sample test that the mean specified in the null hypothesis is a fair and reasonable comparator. This will be discussed in the examples that follow.

In one-sample tests for a continuous outcome, we set up our hypotheses against an appropriate comparator. We select a sample and compute descriptive statistics on the sample data using the techniques described in Chapter 4. Specifically, we compute the sample size (n), the sample mean ($\bar{X}$), and the sample standard deviation (s). We then determine the appropriate test statistic (Step 2) for the hypothesis test. The formulas for test statistics depend on the sample size and are given in Table 7–4.

The National Center for Health Statistics (NCHS) published a report in 2005 entitled "Health, United States," and it contains extensive information on major trends in the health of Americans.[2] Data are provided for the U.S. population as a whole and for specific ages, genders, and races. We use some of the national statistics here as comparative values in one-sample tests in this section for means of continuous outcomes and in Section 7.2 and Section 7.3 for proportions of dichotomous and discrete variable respectively.

Example 7.1. The NCHS report indicated that in 2002, Americans paid an average of $3302 per year on health care and prescription drugs. An investigator hypothesizes that in 2005, expenditures have decreased primarily due to the availability of generic drugs. To test the hypothesis, a sample of 100 Americans is selected and their expenditures on health care and prescription drugs in 2005 are measured. The sample data are summarized as follows: $n = 100$, $\bar{X} = \$3190$, and $s = \$890$. Is there statistical evidence of a reduction in expenditures on health care and prescription drugs in 2005?

Is the sample mean of $3190 evidence of a true reduction in the mean or is it within chance fluctuation? We will run the test using the five-step approach.

Step 1: Set up hypotheses and determine the level of significance.

$$H_0: \mu = 3302,$$

$$H_1: \mu < 3302,$$

$$\alpha = 0.05.$$

The research hypothesis is that expenditures have decreased, and therefore a lower-tailed test is used.

Step 2: Select the appropriate test statistic.
Because the sample size is large ($n > 30$), the appropriate test statistic is

$$z = \frac{\bar{X} - \mu_0}{s/\sqrt{n}}.$$

Step 3: Set up the decision rule.
This is a lower-tailed test, using a z statistic and a 5% level of significance. The appropriate critical value can be found in Table 1C in the Appendix and the decision rule is

$$\text{Reject } H_0 \text{ if } z \leq -1.645.$$

Step 4: Compute the test statistic.
We now substitute the sample data into the formula for the test statistic identified in Step 2:

$$z = \frac{\bar{X} - \mu_0}{s/\sqrt{n}} = \frac{3190 - 3302}{890/\sqrt{100}} = -1.26.$$

Step 5: Conclusion.
We do not reject H_0 because $-1.26 > -1.645$. We do not have statistically significant evidence at $\alpha = 0.05$ to show that the mean expenditures on health care and prescription drugs are lower in 2005 than the mean of $3302 reported in 2002.

Recall that when we fail to reject H_0 in a test of hypothesis that either the null hypothesis is true (the mean expenditures in 2005 are the same as those in 2002 and equal to $3302) or we committed a Type II error (we failed to reject H_0 when in fact it is false). In summarizing this test, we conclude that we do not have sufficient evidence to reject H_0. We do not conclude that H_0 is true because there may be a moderate to high probability that we committed a Type II error. It is possible that the sample size is not large enough to detect a difference in mean expenditures (see Chapter 8 for more details).

Example 7.2. The NCHS reported that the mean total cholesterol level in 2002 for all adults was 203. In Chapter 4, we presented data on $n = 3539$ participants who attended the seventh examination of the Offspring in the Framingham Heart Study. Descriptive statistics on variables measured in the sample were presented in Table 4.20 and included the following statistics on total cholesterol levels of participants: $n = 3310, \overline{X} = 200.3$, and $s = 36.8$. Is there statistical evidence of a difference in mean cholesterol levels in the Framingham Offspring as compared to the national mean? Here we want to assess whether the sample mean of 200.3 in the Framingham sample is statistically significantly different from 203 (i.e., beyond what we would expect by chance). We will run the test using the five-step approach.

Step 1: Set up hypotheses and determine the level of significance

$$H_0: \mu = 203,$$

$$H_1: \mu \neq 203,$$

$$\alpha = 0.05.$$

The research hypothesis is that cholesterol levels are different in the Framingham Offspring, and therefore a two-tailed test is used.

Step 2: Select the appropriate test statistic.
Because the sample size is large ($n > 30$), the appropriate test statistic is

$$z = \frac{\overline{X} - \mu_0}{s/\sqrt{n}}.$$

Step 3: Set up the decision rule.
This is a two-tailed test, using a z statistic and a 5% level of significance. The appropriate critical values can be found in Table 1C in the Appendix and the decision rule is

Reject H_0 if $z \leq -1.960$ or if $z \geq 1.960$.

Step 4: Compute the test statistic.
We now substitute the sample data into the formula for the test statistic identified in Step 2:

$$z = \frac{\overline{X} - \mu_0}{s/\sqrt{n}} = \frac{200.3 - 203}{36.8/\sqrt{3310}} = -4.22.$$

Step 5: Conclusion.
We reject H_0 because $-4.22 \leq -1.960$. We have statistically significant evidence at $\alpha = 0.05$ to show that the mean total cholesterol level in the Framingham Offspring is different from the national mean of 203 reported in 2002. Because we reject H_0,

we also approximate a p-value. Using the two-sided significance levels in Table 1C in the Appendix, $p < 0.0001$.

Example 7.2 raises an important concept of statistical versus clinical or practical significance. From a statistical standpoint, the total cholesterol levels in the Framingham sample are highly statistically significantly different from the national average with $p < 0.0001$ (i.e., there is less than a 0.01% chance that we are incorrectly rejecting the null hypothesis given the observed data). However, the sample mean in the Framingham Offspring study is 200.3, less than 3 units different from the national mean of 203. The reason the data are so highly statistically significant is the very large sample size. It is always important to assess both statistical and practical significance of data. This is particularly relevant when the sample size is large. The five-step procedure allows for an assessment of statistical significance. Investigators must also assess practical significance. Is a 3-unit difference in total cholesterol a meaningful difference?

Example 7.3. Consider again the NCHS-reported mean total cholesterol level of 203 in 2002 for all adults. Suppose a new drug is proposed to lower total cholesterol, and a study is designed to evaluate the efficacy of the drug in lowering cholesterol. Fifteen patients are enrolled in the study and asked to take the new drug for 6 weeks. At the end of 6 weeks, each patient's total cholesterol level is measured and the sample statistics are as follows: $n = 15, \overline{X} = 195.9$, and $s = 28.7$. Is there statistical evidence of a reduction in mean total cholesterol in patients after using the new drug for 6 weeks? We will run the test using the five-step approach.

Step 1: Set up hypotheses and determine the level of significance.

$$H_0: \mu = 203,$$

$$H_1: \mu < 203,$$

$$\alpha = 0.05.$$

Step 2: Select the appropriate test statistic.
Because the sample size is small ($n < 30$), the appropriate test statistic is

$$t = \frac{\overline{X} - \mu_0}{s/\sqrt{n}}.$$

Step 3: Set up the decision rule.
This is a lower-tailed test, using a t statistic and a 5% level of significance. The appropriate critical value can be found in Table 2 in the Appendix. To determine the critical value of t, we need degrees of freedom, df, defined as df $= n - 1$. In this

example, df $= 15 - 1 = 14$. The critical value for a lower-tailed test with df $= 14$ and $\alpha = 0.05$ is -2.145 and the decision rule is

$$\text{Reject } H_0 \text{ if } t \leq -2.145.$$

Step 4: Compute the test statistic.
We now substitute the sample data into the formula for the test statistic identified in Step 2.

$$t = \frac{\overline{X} - \mu_0}{s/\sqrt{n}} = \frac{195.9 - 203}{28.7/\sqrt{15}} = -0.96.$$

Step 5: Conclusion.
We do not reject H_0 because $-0.96 > -2.145$. We do not have statistically significant evidence at $\alpha = 0.05$ to show that the mean total cholesterol level is lower than the national mean in patients taking the new drug for 6 weeks. Again, because we failed to reject the null hypothesis, we make a weaker concluding statement, allowing for the possibility that we may have committed a Type II error (i.e., failed to reject H_0 when the drug is efficacious).

Example 7.3 raises an important issue in terms of study design. In this example, we assume in the null hypothesis that the mean cholesterol level is 203. This is taken to be the mean cholesterol level in patients without treatment. Is this an appropriate comparator? Alternative and potentially more efficient study designs to evaluate the effect of the new drug could involve two treatment groups, where one group receives the new drug and the other does not, or we could measure each patient's baseline or pre-treatment cholesterol level and then assess changes from baseline to 6 weeks post-treatment. These designs will be discussed in Section 7.5 and Section 7.6, respectively.

7.3   TESTS WITH ONE SAMPLE, DICHOTOMOUS OUTCOME

Hypothesis testing applications with a dichotomous outcome variable in a single population are also performed according to the five-step procedure. Similar to tests for means described in Section 7.2, a key component is setting up the null and research hypotheses. The objective is to compare the proportion of successes in a single population to a known proportion (p_0). That known proportion is generally derived from another study or report and is sometimes called a historical control. It is important in setting up the hypotheses in a one-sample test that the proportion specified in the null hypothesis is a fair and reasonable comparator.

In one-sample tests for a dichotomous outcome, we set up our hypotheses against an appropriate comparator. We

select a sample and compute descriptive statistics on the sample data using the techniques described in Chapter 4. Specifically, we compute the sample size (n) and the sample proportion ($\hat{p}$), which is computed by taking the ratio of the number of successes to the sample size, $\hat{p} = x/n$. We then determine the appropriate test statistic (Step 2) for the hypothesis test. The formula for the test statistic is given in Table 7–5.

The preceding formula is appropriate for large samples, defined when the smaller of np_0 and $n(1 - p_0)$ is at least 5. This is similar, but not identical, to the condition required for appropriate use of the confidence interval formula for a population proportion specified in Table 6.6—i.e., $\min[n\hat{p}, n(1 - \hat{p})] > 5$. Here we use the proportion specified in the null hypothesis (p_0) as the true proportion of successes rather than the sample proportion ($\hat{p}$). If we fail to satisfy the condition, then alternative procedures called exact methods must be used to test the hypothesis about the population proportion.[3,4]

Example 7.4. The NCHS report indicated that in 2002 the prevalence of cigarette smoking among American adults was 21.1%. In Chapter 4, we presented data on prevalent smoking in $n = 3536$ participants who attended the seventh examination of the Offspring in the Framingham Heart Study. Suppose we want to assess whether the prevalence of smoking is lower in the Framingham Offspring sample due to the focus on cardiovascular health in that community. Data from the Framingham Offspring study were summarized in Table 4.11 and indicated that $482 / 3536 = 13.6\%$ of the respondents were currently smoking at the time of the exam. Is there evidence of a statistically lower prevalence of smoking in the Framingham Offspring study as compared to the prevalence among all Americans?

Step 1: Set up hypotheses and determine the level of significance.

$$H_0: p = 0.211,$$
$$H_1: p < 0.211,$$
$$\alpha = 0.05.$$

TABLE 7–5 Test Statistic for Testing H_0: $p = p_0$

$\min[np_0, n(1 - p_0)] \geq 5$	$z = \dfrac{\hat{p} - p_0}{\sqrt{p_0(1 - p_0)/n}}$	Find critical value in Table 1C

Step 2: Select the appropriate test statistic.

The formula for the test statistic is in Table 7–5. We must first check that the sample size is adequate. Specifically, we need to check

$$\min[np_0, n(1-p_0)] = \min[3536(0.211), 3536(1-0.211)] = \min(746, 2790) = 746$$

The sample size is more than adequate so the following formula can be used:

$$z = \frac{\hat{p}-p_0}{\sqrt{p_0(1-p_0)/n}}.$$

Step 3: Set up the decision rule.

This is a lower-tailed test, using a z statistic and a 5% level of significance. The appropriate critical value can be found in Table 1C in the Appendix, and the decision rule is

Reject H_0 if $z \le -1.645$.

Step 4: Compute the test statistic.

We now substitute the sample data into the formula for the test statistic identified in Step 2:

$$z = \frac{\hat{p}-p_0}{\sqrt{p_0(1-p_0)/n}} = \frac{0.136-0.211}{\sqrt{0.211(1-0.211)/3536}} = -10.93.$$

Step 5: Conclusion.

We reject H_0 because $-10.93 \le -1.645$. We have statistically significant evidence at $\alpha = 0.05$ to show that the prevalence of smoking in the Framingham Offspring is lower than the national prevalence (21.1%). Using Table 1C in the Appendix, the *p*-value is $p < 0.0001$.

Example 7.5. The NCHS report indicated that in 2002, 75% of children aged 2 to 17 saw a dentist in the past year. An investigator wants to assess whether use of dental services is different in children living in the city of Boston. A sample of 125 children aged 2 to 17 living in Boston is surveyed and 64 reported seeing a dentist over the past 12 months. Is there a significant difference in use of dental services between children living in Boston and the national data?

Step 1: Set up hypotheses and determine the level of significance.

$$H_0: p = 0.75,$$

$$H_1: p \ne 0.75,$$

$$\alpha = 0.05.$$

Step 2: Select the appropriate test statistic.

The formula for the test statistic is in Table 7–5. We must first check that the sample size is adequate. Specifically, we need to check

$$\min[np_0, n(1-p_0)] = \min[125(0.75), 125(1-0.75)] = \min(94, 31) = 31.$$

The sample size is more than adequate, so the following formula can be used:

$$z = \frac{\hat{p}-p_0}{\sqrt{p_0(1-p_0)/n}}.$$

Step 3: Set up the decision rule.

This is a two-tailed test, using a z statistic and a 5% level of significance. The appropriate critical value can be found in Table 1C in the Appendix and the decision rule is

Reject H_0 if $z \le -1.960$ or if $z \ge 1.960$.

Step 4: Compute the test statistic.

We now substitute the sample data into the formula for the test statistic identified in Step 2. The sample proportion is $\hat{p} = 64 / 125 = 0.512$, and

$$z = \frac{\hat{p}-p_0}{\sqrt{p_0(1-p_0)/n}} = \frac{0.512-0.75}{\sqrt{0.75(1-0.75)/125}} = -6.15.$$

Step 5: Conclusion.

We reject H_0 because $-6.15 \le -1.960$. We have evidence at $\alpha = 0.05$ to show that there is a statistically significant difference in the use of dental service by children living in Boston as compared to the national data. Using Table 1C in the Appendix, the *p*-value is $p < 0.0001$.

7.4   TESTS WITH ONE SAMPLE, DISCRETE OUTCOME

Hypothesis testing with a discrete outcome variable in a single population is again performed according to the five-step procedure. Similar to tests for means and proportions described in Section 7.2 and Section 7.3, a key component is setting up the null and research hypotheses. Discrete variables are variables that take on more than two distinct responses or categories. The responses can be ordered or unordered (i.e., the outcome can be ordinal or categorical). The procedure we describe here can be used for ordinal or categorical discrete outcomes, and the objective is to compare the distribution of responses—or the proportions of participants in each response category—to a known distribution. The known distribution is derived from another study or report and it is again important in setting up the hypotheses that the comparator distribution specified in the null hypothesis is a fair comparison.

In one-sample tests for a discrete outcome, we set up our hypotheses against an appropriate comparator. We select a sample and compute descriptive statistics on the sample data using the techniques described in Chapter 4. Specifically, we compute the sample size (n) and the proportions of participants in each response category ($\hat{p}_1$, $\hat{p}_2$, ... $\hat{p}_k$) where k represents the number of response categories. We then determine the appropriate test statistic (Step 2) for the hypothesis test. The formula for the test statistic follows in Table 7–6.

With the χ^2 statistic, we compare the observed frequencies in each response category (O) to the frequencies we would expect (E) if the null hypothesis were true. These expected frequencies are determined by allocating the sample to the response categories according to the distribution specified in H_0. This is done by multiplying the observed sample size (n) by the proportions specified in the null hypothesis (p_{10}, p_{20}, ..., p_{k0}). To ensure that the sample size is appropriate for the use of the test statistic in Table 7–6, we need to ensure that

$$\min(np_{10}, np_{20},..., np_{k0}) \geq 5.$$

The test of hypothesis with a discrete outcome measured in a single sample, where the goal is to assess whether the distribution of responses follows a known distribution, is called the χ^2 *goodness-of-fit test*. As the name indicates, the idea is to assess whether the distribution of responses in the sample "fits" a specified population distribution. In the next example, we illustrate the test using the five-step approach. As we work through the example, we provide additional details related to the use of this new test statistic.

Example 7.6. A university conducted a survey of its recent graduates to collect demographic and health information for future planning purposes, as well as to assess students' satisfaction with their undergraduate experiences. The survey revealed that a substantial proportion of students were not engaging in regular exercise, many felt their nutrition was

poor, and a substantial number were smoking. In response to a question on regular exercise, 60% of all graduates reported getting no regular exercise, 25% reported exercising sporadically, and 15% reported exercising regularly as undergraduates. The next year, the university launched a health promotion campaign on campus in an attempt to increase health behaviors among undergraduates. The program included modules on exercise, nutrition, and smoking cessation. To evaluate the impact of the program, the university again surveyed graduates and asked the same questions. The survey was completed by 470 graduates and the data shown in Table 7–7 were collected on the exercise question. Based on the data, is there evidence of a shift in the distribution of responses to the exercise question following the implementation of the health promotion campaign on campus? Run the test at a 5% level of significance.

In this example, we have one sample and a discrete outcome variable (with three response options). We specifically want to compare the distribution of responses in the sample to the distribution reported the previous year (i.e., 60%, 25%, and 15% reporting no, sporadic, and regular exercise, respectively). We now run the test using the five-step approach.

Step 1: Set up hypotheses and determine the level of significance.

The null hypothesis again represents the "no change" or "no difference" situation. If the health promotion campaign has no impact, then we expect the distribution of responses to the exercise question to be the same as that measured prior to the implementation of the program.

$$H_0: p_1 = 0.60, p_2 = 0.25, p_3 = 0.15 \text{ or, equivalently,}$$

$$H_0: \text{Distribution of responses is } 0.60, 0.25, 0.15,$$

$$H_1: H_0 \text{ is false,}$$

$$\alpha = 0.05.$$

TABLE 7–6 Test Statistic for Testing
$H_0: p_1 = p_{10}, p_2 = p_{20}, ..., p_k = p_{k0}$

$\chi^2 = \sum \dfrac{(O - E)^2}{E}$	Find critical value in Table 3 (df = $k - 1$)

TABLE 7–7 Survey Results on Regular Exercise

	No Regular Exercise	Sporadic Exercise	Regular Exercise	Total
Number of students	255	125	90	470

Notice that the research hypothesis is written in words rather than in symbols. The research hypothesis as stated captures any difference in the distribution of responses from that specified in the null hypothesis. We do not specify a specific alternative distribution; instead, we are testing whether the sample data "fit" the distribution in H_0 or not. With the χ^2 goodness-of-fit test, there is no upper- or lower-tailed version of the test.

Step 2: Select the appropriate test statistic.

The formula for the test statistic is in Table 7–6 and is

$$\chi^2 = \sum \frac{(O-E)^2}{E}.$$

We must first assess whether the sample size is adequate. Specifically, we need to check $\min(np_{10},...,np_{k0}) \geq 5$. The sample size here is $n = 470$ and the proportions specified in the null hypothesis are 0.60, 0.25, and 0.15. Thus,

$$\min[470(0.60), 470(0.25), 470(0.15)] = \min(282, 117.5, 70.5) = 70.5.$$

The sample size is more than adequate, so the test statistic can be used.

Step 3: Set up the decision rule.

The decision rule for the χ^2 test is set up in a similar way to decision rules we established for z and t tests. The decision rule depends on the level of significance and the degrees of freedom, defined as $df = k - 1$, where k is the number of response categories. Again, with χ^2 tests there are no upper-, lower-, or two-tailed distinctions. If the null hypothesis is true, the observed and expected frequencies will be close in value and the χ^2 statistic will be close to 0. If the null hypothesis is false, then the χ^2 statistic will be large. The rejection region for the χ^2 test is always in the upper-tail (right), as shown in Figure 7–6.

Table 3 in the Appendix contains critical values for the χ^2 test, indexed by degrees of freedom and the desired level of significance. Here we have $df = k - 1 = 3 - 1 = 2$ and a 5% level of significance. The appropriate critical value from Table 3 is 5.99, and the decision rule is

$$\text{Reject } H_0 \text{ if } \chi^2 \geq 5.99.$$

Step 4: Compute the test statistic.

We now compute the expected frequencies using the sample size and the proportions specified in the null hypothesis. We then substitute the sample data (observed frequencies) and the expected frequencies into the formula for the test statistic identified in Step 2. The computations can be organized as shown in Table 7–8. Notice that the expected frequencies are taken to one decimal place and that the sum of the observed

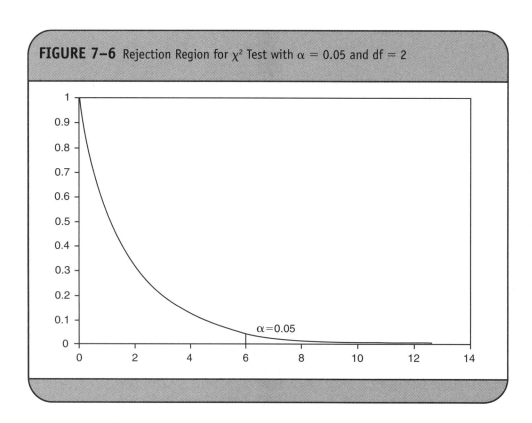

FIGURE 7–6 Rejection Region for χ^2 Test with $\alpha = 0.05$ and $df = 2$

frequencies is equal to the sum of the expected frequencies. The test statistic is computed as

$$\chi^2 = \frac{(255-282)^2}{282} + \frac{(125-1175)^2}{117.5} + \frac{(90-70.5)^2}{70.5},$$

$$\chi^2 = 2.59 + 0.48 + 5.39 = 8.46.$$

Step 5: Conclusion.

We reject H_0 because $8.46 \geq 5.99$. We have statistically significant evidence at $\alpha = 0.05$ to show that H_0 is false, or that the distribution of responses is not 0.60, 0.25, and 0.15. Using Table 3 in the Appendix, we can approximate the p-value. We need to look at critical values for smaller levels of significance with df = 2. Using Table 3 in the Appendix, the p-value is $p < 0.025$.

In the χ^2 goodness-of-fit test, we conclude that either the distribution specified in H_0 is false (when we reject H_0) or that we do not have sufficient evidence to show that the distribution specified in H_0 is false (when we fail to reject H_0). In Example 7.6, we rejected H_0 and concluded that the distribution of responses to the exercise question following the implementation of the health promotion campaign was not the same as the distribution prior. The test itself does not provide details of how the distribution has shifted. A comparison of the observed and expected frequencies will provide some insight into the shift (when the null hypothesis is rejected). In Example 7.6, we observed the data shown in the

first row of Table 7–8. If the null hypothesis were true, we would have expected more students to fall in the *No Regular Exercise* category and fewer in the *Regular Exercise* categories. In the sample, 255 / 470 5 54% reported no regular exercise and 90 / 470 = 19% reported regular exercise. Thus, there is a shift toward more regular exercise following the implementation of the health promotion campaign.

Example 7.7. The NCHS provided data on the distribution of weight (in categories) among Americans in 2002. The distribution was based on specific values of body mass index (BMI) computed as weight in kilograms over height in meters squared. Underweight was defined as a BMI less than 18.5, normal weight as a BMI between 18.5 and 24.9, overweight as a BMI between 25 and 29.9, and obese as a BMI of 30 or greater. Americans in 2002 were distributed as follows: 2% underweight, 39% normal weight, 36% overweight, and 23% obese. Suppose we want to assess whether the distribution of BMI is different in the Framingham Offspring sample. Using data from the $n = 3536$ participants who attended the seventh examination of the Offspring in the Framingham Heart Study, we created the BMI categories as defined and observed the data shown in Table 7–9.

Step 1: Set up hypotheses and determine the level of significance.

$$H_0: p_1 = 0.02, p_2 = 0.39, p_3 = 0.36, p_4 = 0.23 \text{ or, equivalently,}$$

TABLE 7–8 Computing Expected Frequencies

	No Regular Exercise	Sporadic Exercise	Regular Exercise	Total
Observed frequencies (O)	255	125	90	470
Expected frequencies (E)	470(0.60) = 282	470(0.25) = 117.5	470(0.15) = 70.5	470

TABLE 7–9 Distribution of BMI of Framingham Offspring

	Underweight BMI < 18.5	Normal Weight BMI 18.5–24.9	Overweight BMI 25.0–29.9	Obese BMI 30+	Total
Number of participants	20	932	1374	1000	3326

H_0: Distribution of responses is 0.02, 0.39, 0.36, 0.23,

H_1: H_0 is false,

$\alpha = 0.05$.

Step 2: Select the appropriate test statistic.

The formula for the test statistic is in Table 7–6 and is

$$\chi^2 = \sum \frac{(O-E)^2}{E}.$$

We must assess whether the sample size is adequate. Specifically, we need to check $\min(np_{10}, ..., np_{k0}) \geq 5$. The sample size here is $n = 3326$ and the proportions specified in the null hypothesis are 0.02, 0.39, 0.36, and 0.23. Thus,

$$\min[3326(0.02), 3326(0.39), 3326(0.36), 3326(0.23)] =$$
$$\min(66.5, 1297.1, 1197.4, 765.0) = 66.5.$$

The sample size is more than adequate, so the test statistic can be used.

Step 3: Set up the decision rule.

Here we have df $= k - 1 = 4 - 1 = 3$ and a 5% level of significance. The appropriate critical value from Table 3 in the Appendix is 7.81, and the decision rule is

Reject H_0 if $\chi^2 \geq 7.81$.

Step 4: Compute the test statistic.

We now compute the expected frequencies using the sample size and the proportions specified in the null hypothesis. We then substitute the sample data (observed frequencies) into the formula for the test statistic identified in Step 2. We organize the computations in Table 7–10.

The test statistic is computed as

$$\chi^2 = \frac{(20-66.5)^2}{66.5} + \frac{(932-1297.1)^2}{1297.1} +$$

$$\frac{(1374-1197.4)^2}{1197.4} + \frac{(1000-765.0)^2}{765.0},$$

$$\chi^2 = 32.52 + 102.77 + 26.05 + 72.19 = 233.53.$$

Step 5: Conclusion.

We reject H_0 because $233.53 \geq 7.81$. We have statistically significant evidence at $\alpha = 0.05$ to show that H_0 is false or that the distribution of BMI in Framingham is different from the national data reported in 2002. Using Table 3 in the Appendix, we can approximate the p-value. We need to look at critical values for smaller levels of significance for df = 4. Using Table 3, the p-value is $p < 0.005$.

Again, the χ^2 goodness-of-fit test allows us to assess whether the distribution of responses "fits" a specified distribution. In Example 7.7, we showed that the distribution of BMI in the Framingham Offspring Study is different from the national distribution. To understand the nature of the difference, we can compare observed and expected frequencies or observed and expected proportions (or percentages). In Example 7.7, the frequencies are large because of the large sample size—the observed percentages of patients in the Framingham sample are 0.6% underweight, 28% normal weight, 41% overweight, and 30% obese. In the Framingham Offspring sample, there are higher percentages of overweight and obese persons (41% and 30% in Framingham as compared to 36% and 23% nationally) and lower proportions of underweight and normal weight persons (0.6% and 28% in Framingham as compared to 2% and 39% nationally).

7.5   TESTS WITH TWO INDEPENDENT SAMPLES, CONTINUOUS OUTCOME

There are many applications where it is of interest to compare two independent groups with respect to their mean scores on a continuous outcome. In Chapter 6, we presented techniques to estimate the difference in means. Here we will again compare means between groups but rather than generating an estimate of the difference, we will test whether the observed difference (increase, decrease, or difference) is statistically significant or not.

In this section, we discuss the comparison of means when the two comparison groups are independent or physically

---

TABLE 7–10 Observed and Expected Frequencies

	Underweight BMI < 18.5	Normal Weight BMI 18.5–24.9	Overweight BMI 25.0–29.9	Obese BMI 30+	Total
Observed frequencies (O)	20	932	1374	1000	3326
Expected frequencies (E)	66.5	1297.1	1197.4	765.0	3326

separate. The two groups might be determined by a particular attribute (e.g., gender, history of cardiovascular disease) or might be set up by the investigator (e.g., participants assigned to receive an experimental drug or placebo). The first step in the analysis involves computing descriptive statistics on each of the two samples using the techniques described in Chapter 4. Specifically, we compute the sample size, mean and standard deviation in each sample and we denote these summary statistics as follows: n_1, $\overline{X}_1$, and s_1 for Sample 1 and n_2, $\overline{X}_2$, and s_2 for Sample 2. The designation of Sample 1 and Sample 2 is essentially arbitrary. In a clinical trial setting, the convention is to call the treatment Group 1 and the control Group 2. However, when comparing men and women either group can be 1 or 2.

In the two independent samples application with a continuous outcome, the parameter of interest in the test of hypothesis is the difference in population means, $\mu_1 - \mu_2$. The null hypothesis is always that there is no difference between groups with respect to means, i.e., $H_0: \mu_1 - \mu_2 = 0$. The null hypothesis can also be written as $H_0: \mu_1 = \mu_2$. In the research hypothesis, an investigator can hypothesize that the first mean is larger than the second ($H_1: \mu_1 > \mu_2$), that the first mean is smaller than the second ($H_1: \mu_1 < \mu_2$), or that the means are different ($H_1: \mu_1 \neq \mu_2$). The three different alternatives represent upper-, lower-, and two-tailed tests, respectively. Table 7–11 contains the formulas for test statistics for the difference in population means.

In the formulas in Table 7–11, $\overline{X}_1$ and $\overline{X}_2$ are the means of the outcome in the independent samples and S_p is the pooled estimate of the common standard deviation (again assuming that the variances in the populations are similar) computed as the weighted average of the standard deviations in the samples,

$$S_p = \sqrt{\frac{(n_1 - 1)s_1^2 + (n_2 - 1)s_2^2}{n_1 + n_2 - 2}}.$$

Because we are assuming equal variances between groups, we pool the information on variability (sample variances) to generate an estimate of the variability in the population. As a guideline, if the ratio of the sample variances is between 0.5 and 2, the assumption of equality of population variances is taken to be appropriate. (Note that because S_p is a weighted average of the standard deviations in the sample, S_p will always be between s_1 and s_2.)

Example 7.8. In Example 6.5, we used data presented in Chapter 4 on $n = 3539$ participants who attended the seventh examination of the Offspring in the Framingham Heart Study and constructed a 95% confidence interval for the difference in mean systolic blood pressures between men and women. Table 7–12 contains descriptive statistics on the characteristics measured in men and women. Suppose we now wish to assess whether there is a statistically significant difference in mean systolic blood pressures between men and women using a 5% level of significance.

Step 1: Set up hypotheses and determine the level of significance.

$$H_0: \mu_1 = \mu_2,$$

$$H_1: \mu_1 \neq \mu_2,$$

$$\alpha = 0.05.$$

Step 2: Select the appropriate test statistic.

Because both samples are large ($n_1 \geq 30$ and $n_2 \geq 30$), we can use the z test statistic as opposed to t. Before implementing the formula, we first check whether the assumption of equality of population variances is reasonable. The guideline suggests investigating the ratio of the sample variances, s_1^2 / s_2^2. Suppose we call the men Group 1 and the women Group 2. Again, this is arbitrary; it only needs to be noted when interpreting the results. The ratio of the sample variances is $17.52^2 / 20.12^2 = 0.76$, which falls in between 0.5 and 2, suggesting that the

---

TABLE 7–11 Test Statistics for Testing $H_0: \mu_1 = \mu_2$

$n_1 \geq 30$ and $n_2 \geq 30$	$z = \dfrac{\overline{X}_1 - \overline{X}_2}{S_p \sqrt{1/n_1 + 1/n_2}}$	Find critical value of z in Table 1B
$n_1 < 30$ or $n_2 < 30$	$t = \dfrac{\overline{X}_1 - \overline{X}_2}{S_p \sqrt{1/n_1 + 1/n_2}}$	Find critical value of t in Table 2 (df $= n_1 + n_2 - 2$)

TABLE 7–12 Descriptive Statistics in Men and Women

	Men			Women		
	n	$\overline{X}$	s	n	$\overline{X}$	s
Systolic blood pressure	1623	128.2	17.5	1911	126.5	20.1
Diastolic blood pressure	1622	75.6	9.8	1910	72.6	9.7
Total serum cholesterol	1544	192.4	35.2	1766	207.1	36.7
Weight (lbs)	1612	194.0	33.8	1894	157.7	34.6
Height (in.)	1545	68.9	2.7	1781	63.4	2.5
Body mass index (BMI)	1545	28.8	4.6	1781	27.6	5.9

assumption of equality of population variances is reasonable. The appropriate test statistic is

$$z = \frac{\overline{X}_1 - \overline{X}_2}{S_p \sqrt{1/n_1 + 1/n_2}}.$$

Step 3: Set up the decision rule.

This is a two-tailed test, using a z statistic and a 5% level of significance. The appropriate critical values can be found in Table 1C in the Appendix and the decision rule is

Reject H_0 if $z \le -1.960$ or if $z \ge 1.960$.

Step 4: Compute the test statistic.

We now substitute the sample data into the formula for the test statistic identified in Step 2. Before substituting, we first compute S_p, the pooled estimate of the common standard deviation.

$$S_p = \sqrt{\frac{(n_1-1)s_1^2 + (n_2-1)s_2^2}{n_1 + n_2 - 2}},$$

$$S_p = \sqrt{\frac{(1623-1)(17.5)^2 + (1911-1)(20.1)^2}{1623 + 1911 - 2}} = \sqrt{359.12} = 19.0.$$

Notice that the pooled estimate of the common standard deviation, S_p, falls between the standard deviations in the comparison groups (i.e., 17.5 and 20.1). S_p is slightly closer in value to the standard deviation in the women (20.1) as there were slightly more women in the sample. Recall that S_p is a weighted average of the standard deviations in the comparison groups, weighted by the respective sample sizes.

We now calculate the test statistic,

$$z = \frac{128.2 - 126.5}{19.0 \sqrt{1/1623 + 1/1911}} = \frac{1.7}{0.64} = 2.66.$$

Step 5: Conclusion.

We reject H_0 because $2.66 \ge 1.960$. We have statistically significant evidence at $\alpha = 0.05$ to show that there is a difference in mean systolic blood pressures between men and women. The p-value can be found in Table 1C in the Appendix and is equal to $p < 0.010$.

In Example 7.8, we find that there is a statistically significant difference in mean systolic blood pressures between men and women at $p < 0.010$. Notice that there is a very small difference in the sample means ($128.2 - 126.5 = 1.7$ units) but this difference is beyond what would be expected by chance. The large sample sizes in this example are driving the statistical significance. In Example 6.5, we computed a 95% confidence interval for the difference in mean systolic blood pressures as 1.7 ± 1.26, or $(0.44, 2.96)$. The confidence interval provides an assessment of the magnitude of the difference between means, whereas the test of hypothesis and p-value provides an assessment of the significance of the difference. From the confidence interval in Example 6.5, we already knew that the difference in means was significant at the 5% level of significance because the 95% confidence interval did not include the null value of 0. The formal test is needed to compute the exact significance of the difference or the p-value.

In Example 7.3, we analyzed data from a study to evaluate a new drug designed to lower total cholesterol. The study involved one sample of patients, each patient took the new drug for 6 weeks and had their cholesterol measured. As a means of evaluating the efficacy of the new drug, the mean total cholesterol following 6 weeks of treatment was compared to a national mean of 203 based on the NCHS. At the end of the example, we discussed the appropriateness of the historical comparator as well as an alternative study design to evaluate the effect of the new drug involving two treatment groups, where one group receives the new drug and the other does not. In Example 7.9, we revisit this example with a concurrent or parallel control group, which is very typical in randomized controlled trials or clinical trials (for more details, see Section 2.3.1).

Example 7.9. A new drug is proposed to lower total cholesterol. A randomized controlled trial is designed to evaluate the efficacy of the drug in lowering cholesterol. Thirty participants are enrolled in the trial and are randomly assigned to receive either the new drug or a placebo. The participants do not know which treatment they are assigned. Each participant is asked to take the assigned treatment for 6 weeks. At the end of 6 weeks, each patient's total cholesterol level is measured and the sample statistics are shown in Table 7–13. Is there statistical evidence of a reduction in mean total cholesterol in patients taking the new drug for 6 weeks as compared to participants taking a placebo? We will run the test using the five-step approach.

Step 1: Set up hypotheses and determine the level of significance.

$$H_0: \mu_1 = \mu_2,$$

$$H_1: \mu_1 < \mu_2,$$

$$\alpha = 0.05.$$

Step 2: Select the appropriate test statistic.

Because both samples are small ($n_1 < 30$ and $n_2 < 30$), we use the t test statistic. Before implementing the formula, we first check whether the assumption of equality of population variances is reasonable. The ratio of the sample variances, $s_1^2 / s_2^2 = 28.72^2 / 30.32^2 = 0.90$, which falls between 0.5 and 2, suggesting that the assumption of equality of population variances is reasonable. The appropriate test statistic is

$$t = \frac{\overline{X}_1 - \overline{X}_2}{S_p \sqrt{1/n_1 + 1/n_2}}.$$

Step 3: Set up the decision rule.

This is a lower-tailed test, using a t statistic and a 5% level of significance. The appropriate critical value can be found in

TABLE 7–13 Cholesterol Levels by Treatment

	Sample Size	Mean	Standard Deviation
New drug	15	195.9	28.7
Placebo	15	217.4	30.3

Table 2 in the Appendix. To determine the critical value of t, we need degrees of freedom, df, defined as $df = n_1 + n_2 - 2$. In this example, $df = 15 + 15 - 2 = 28$. The critical value for a lower-tailed test with $df = 28$ and $\alpha = 0.05$ is -2.048, and the decision rule is

$$\text{Reject } H_0 \text{ if } t \le -2.048.$$

Step 4: Compute the test statistic.

We now substitute the sample data into the formula for the test statistic identified in Step 2. Before substituting, we will first compute S_p, the pooled estimate of the common standard deviation:

$$S_p = \sqrt{\frac{(15-1)(28.7)^2 + (15-1)(30.3)^2}{15 + 15-2}} = \sqrt{870.89} = 29.5.$$

Now calculate the test statistic,

$$t = \frac{195.9 - 227.4}{29.5 \sqrt{1/15 + 1/15}} = \frac{-31.5}{10.77} = -2.92.$$

Step 5: Conclusion.

We reject H_0 because $-2.92 \le -2.048$. We have statistically significant evidence at $\alpha = 0.05$ to show that the mean total cholesterol level is lower in patients taking the new drug for 6 weeks as compared to patients taking a placebo. Using Table 2 in the Appendix, the p-value is $p < 0.005$.

The clinical trial in Example 7.9 finds a statistically significant reduction in total cholesterol, whereas in Example 7.3 we did not demonstrate the efficacy of the new drug. Notice that the mean total cholesterol level in patients taking a placebo is 217.4, which is very different from the mean cholesterol of 203 reported among all Americans in 2002 and used as the comparator. The historical control value may not have been the most appropriate comparator as cholesterol levels have been increasing over time. In Section 7.6, we will present another design that can be used to assess the efficacy of the new drug.

7.6   TESTS WITH MATCHED SAMPLES, CONTINUOUS OUTCOME

An alternative study design to that described in the previous section, to compare two groups with respect to their mean scores on a continuous outcome, is one based on matched or paired samples. The two comparison groups are said to be dependent and the data can arise from a single sample of participants where each participant is measured twice, possibly before and after an intervention, or from two samples that are matched on specific characteristics (e.g., siblings). When the samples are dependent, we focus on difference scores in each participant or between members of a pair, and the test of hypothesis is based on the mean difference, μ_d. The null hypothesis again reflects "no difference" and is stated as $\mu_d = 0$. Note that there are some instances where it is of interest to test whether there is a difference of a particular magnitude (e.g., $\mu_d = 5$) but in most instances, the null hypothesis reflects no difference (i.e., $\mu_d = 0$). The appropriate formula for the test of hypothesis depends on the sample size. The formulas are shown in Table 7–14 and are identical to those we presented for estimating the mean of a single sample presented in Section 7.2, except here we focus on difference scores.

Example 7.10. In Example 6.7, we compared systolic blood pressures measured at the sixth and seventh examinations (approximately 4 years apart) of the Framingham Offspring Study in a subsample of $n = 15$ randomly selected participants. The data are shown in Example 6.7, where we generated a 95% confidence interval for the mean difference in systolic blood pressures over a 4-year period. Using the same data, we will now test whether there is a statistically significant difference in systolic blood pressures over 4 years using the five-step approach.

Step 1: Set up hypotheses and determine the level of significance.

$$H_0: \mu_d = 0,$$

$$H_1: \mu_d \neq 0,$$

$$\alpha = 0.05.$$

Step 2: Select the appropriate test statistic.
Because the sample is small ($n < 30$), we use the t test statistic,

$$t = \frac{\overline{X}_d - \mu_d}{s_d / \sqrt{n}}.$$

Step 3: Set up the decision rule.
This is a two-tailed test, using a t statistic and a 5% level of significance. The appropriate critical value can be found in Table 2 in the Appendix with degrees of freedom, df, defined as df $= n - 1 = 15 - 1 = 14$. The critical value is 2.145 and the decision rule is

Reject H_0 if $t \leq -2.145$ or if $t \geq 2.145$.

Step 4: Compute the test statistic.
We now substitute the sample data into the formula for the test statistic identified in Step 2. In Example 6.7, we had: $n = 15$, $\overline{X}_d = -5.3$, and $s_d = 12.8$. The test statistic is

$$t = \frac{\overline{X}_d - \mu_d}{s_d / \sqrt{n}} = \frac{-5.3 - 0}{12.8 / \sqrt{15}} = -1.60.$$

Step 5: Conclusion.
We do not reject H_0 because $-2.145 < -1.60 < 2.145$. We do not have statistically significant evidence at $\alpha = 0.05$ to show that there is a difference in systolic blood pressures over time.

In Example 6.7, we estimated a confidence interval and were 95% confident that the mean difference in systolic blood pressures between Examination 6 and Examination 7 (approximately 4 years apart) was between -12.4 and 1.8. Because the null value of the confidence interval for the mean difference is 0, we concluded that there was no statistically significant difference in blood pressures over time because the confidence interval for the mean difference included 0. The test of hypothesis gives the same result.

In Example 7.11 we revisit Example 7.3 and Example 7.9 where we evaluated a new drug designed to lower total cholesterol. In Example 7.3, we collected data on a sample of patients who took the new drug and we compared their mean total cholesterol level to a historical control. In Example 7.9, we evaluated the efficacy of the new drug but we involved a concurrent or parallel placebo control group. In Example 7.11, we will again evaluate the efficacy of the new drug using a matched design.

Example 7.11. A new drug is proposed to lower total cholesterol and a study is designed to evaluate the efficacy of the drug in lowering cholesterol. Fifteen patients agree to participate in the study and each is asked to take the new drug for 6 weeks. However, before starting the treatment each patient's total cholesterol level is measured. The initial measurement is a pretreatment or baseline value. After taking the drug for 6 weeks,

TABLE 7–14 Test Statistics for Testing $H_0: \mu_d = 0$		
$n \geq 30$	$z = \dfrac{\overline{X}_d - \mu_d}{s_d / \sqrt{n}}$	Find critical value of z in Table 1B
$n < 30$	$t = \dfrac{\overline{X}_d - \mu_d}{s_d / \sqrt{n}}$	Find critical value of t in Table 2 (df $= n - 1$)

each patient's total cholesterol level is measured again and the data are shown in Table 7–15. The right column contains difference scores for each patient, computed by subtracting the 6-week cholesterol level from the baseline level. The differences represent the reduction in total cholesterol over 4 weeks. (The differences could have been computed by subtracting the baseline total cholesterol level from the level measured at 6 weeks. The way in which the differences are computed does not affect the outcome of the analysis, only the interpretation.)

Because the differences are computed by subtracting the cholesterols measured at 6 weeks from the baseline values, positive differences indicate reductions and negative differences indicate increases (e.g., Participant 12 increases by 2 units over 6 weeks). The goal here is to test whether there is a statistically significant reduction in cholesterol. Because of the way in which we computed the differences, we want to look for an increase in the mean difference (i.e., a positive reduction). To conduct the test, we need to summarize the differences. In this sample, we have $n = 15$, $\overline{X}_d = 16.9$, and $s_d = 14.2$, respectively. The data necessary to compute the sample statistics is shown in Table 7–16.

$$\overline{X}_d = \frac{\Sigma X}{n} = \frac{254}{15} = 16.9$$

and

$$s_d = \sqrt{\frac{\Sigma \text{Differences} - \Sigma \text{Differences}^2/n}{n-1}},$$

$$s_d = \sqrt{\frac{7110 - {(254)^2}/{15}}{15-1}} = \sqrt{200.64} = 14.2.$$

Is there statistical evidence of a reduction in mean total cholesterol in patients after using the new medication for 6 weeks? We will run the test using the five-step approach.

Step 1: Set up hypotheses and determine the level of significance.

$$H_0: \mu_d = 0,$$

$$H_1: \mu_d > 0,$$

$$\alpha = 0.05.$$

Note that if we had computed differences by subtracting the baseline level from the level measured at 6 weeks, then negative differences would have reflected reductions and the research hypothesis would have been $H_1: \mu_d < 0$.

Step 2: Select the appropriate test statistic.

Because the sample size is small ($n < 30$) the appropriate test statistic is

$$t = \frac{\overline{X}_d - \mu_d}{s_d / \sqrt{n}}.$$

TABLE 7–15 Differences in Cholesterol over 6 Weeks

Subject Identification Number	Baseline	6 Weeks	Difference
1	215	205	10
2	190	156	34
3	230	190	40
4	220	180	40
5	214	201	13
6	240	227	13
7	210	197	13
8	193	173	20
9	210	204	6
10	230	217	13
11	180	142	38
12	260	262	−2
13	210	207	3
14	190	184	6
15	200	193	7

TABLE 7–16 Summary Statistics on Difference Scores

Subject Identification Number	Difference	Difference²
1	10	100
2	34	1156
3	40	1600
4	40	1600
5	13	169
6	13	169
7	13	169
8	20	400
9	6	36
10	13	169
11	38	1444
12	−2	4
13	3	9
14	6	36
15	7	49
Total	254	7110

Step 3: Set up the decision rule.
This is an upper-tailed test, using a t statistic and a 5% level of significance. The appropriate critical value can be found in Table 2 in the Appendix. To determine the critical value of t we need degrees of freedom, df, defined as df $= n - 1$. In this example, df $= 15 - 1 = 14$. The critical value for an upper-tailed test with df $= 14$ and $\alpha = 0.05$ is 2.145, and the decision rule is

$$\text{Reject H}_0 \text{ if } t \geq 2.145.$$

Step 4: Compute the test statistic.
We now substitute the sample data into the formula for the test statistic identified in Step 2:

$$t = \frac{\overline{X}_d - \mu_d}{s_d/\sqrt{n}} = \frac{16.9 - 0}{14.2/\sqrt{15}} = 4.61.$$

Step 5: Conclusion.
We reject H$_0$ because $4.61 \geq 2.145$. We have statistically significant evidence at $\alpha = 0.05$ to show that there is a reduction in cholesterol levels over 6 weeks.

In Example 7.9 and Example 7.11, using parallel samples and matched designs, respectively, we find statistically significant reductions in total cholesterol. In Example 7.3, using a historical comparator, we do not. It is extremely important to design studies that are best suited to detect a meaningful difference when one exists. There are often several alternatives, and investigators work with biostatisticians to determine the best design for each application. It is worth noting that the matched design used in Example 7.11 can be problematic in that observed differences may only reflect a "placebo" effect. All participants took the assigned medication but is the observed reduction attributable to the medication or a result of this participation in a study?

7.7 TESTS WITH TWO INDEPENDENT SAMPLES, DICHOTOMOUS OUTCOME

Techniques presented in Sections 7.5 are appropriate when there are two independent comparison groups and the outcome of interest is continuous (e.g., blood pressure, total cholesterol, weight loss). Here we consider the situation where there are two independent comparison groups and the outcome of interest is dichotomous (e.g., success/failure). The goal of the analysis is to compare proportions of successes between the two groups. The relevant sample data are the sample sizes in each comparison group (n_1 and n_2) and the sample proportions ($\hat{p}_1$ and $\hat{p}_2$), which are computed by taking the ratios of the numbers of successes to the sample sizes in each group, e.g., $\hat{p}_1 = x_1/n_1$ and $\hat{p}_2 = x_2/n_2$.

In Chapter 3, we introduced the risk difference, relative risk and odds ratio, which are different measures to compare proportions in two independent groups. We developed confidence intervals for each of these measures in Chapter 6 in Section 6.6.1, Section 6.6.2, and Section 6.6.3, respectively. The confidence interval formulas were different and depended on the specific measure.

In tests of hypothesis comparing proportions between two independent groups, one test is performed and it can be interpreted relative to a risk difference, relative risk, or odds ratio. As a reminder, the risk difference is computed by taking the difference in proportions between comparison groups, the relative risk is computed by taking the ratio of proportions and the odds ratio is computed by taking the ratio of the odds of success in the comparison groups (see Section 3.4.2 for more details). Because the null values for the risk difference, the relative risk, and the odds ratio are different, the hypotheses in tests of hypothesis look slightly different depending on which measure is used. When performing tests of hypothesis for the risk difference, relative risk, or odds ratio, the convention is to label the exposed or treated Group 1 and the unexposed or control Group 2.

For example, suppose a study is designed to assess whether there is a significant difference in proportions in two independent comparison groups. The test of interest is

$$H_0: p_1 = p_2 \text{ versus } H_1: p_1 \neq p_2.$$

The following are the hypotheses for testing for a difference in proportions using the risk difference (RD), the relative risk (RR), and the odds ratio (OR). First, the previous hypotheses are equivalent to

$$H_0: p_1 - p_2 = 0 \text{ versus } H_1: p_1 - p_2 \neq 0,$$

which are, by definition, equal to

$$H_0: RD = 0 \text{ versus } H_1: RD \neq 0.$$

If an investigator wants to focus on the relative risk, the equivalent hypotheses are

$$H_0: RR = 1 \text{ versus } H_1: RR \neq 1,$$

and if the investigator wants to focus on the odds ratio, the equivalent hypotheses are

$$H_0: OR = 1 \text{ versus } H_1: OR \neq 1.$$

Suppose a test is performed to test

$$H_0: RD = 0 \text{ versus } H_1: RD \neq 0,$$

and the test rejects H_0 at $\alpha = 0.05$. Based on this test, we can conclude that there is significant evidence ($\alpha = 0.05$) of a difference in proportions, significant evidence that the risk difference is not 0, and significant evidence that the relative risk and odds ratio are not 1.

The risk difference is analogous to the difference in means when the outcome is continuous. The test for the difference in means was described in Section 7.5. Here the parameter of interest is the difference in proportions in the population, $RD = p_1 - p_2$, and the null value for the risk difference is 0. In a test of hypothesis for the risk difference, the null hypothesis is always

$$H_0: RD = 0.$$

This is equivalent to

$$H_0: RR = 1 \text{ and } H_0: OR = 1.$$

In the research hypothesis, an investigator can hypothesize that the first proportion is larger than the second,

$$H_1: p_1 > p_2, \text{ which is equivalent to } H_1: RD > 0, H_1: RR > 1 \text{ and } H_1: OR > 1,$$

that the first proportion is smaller than the second,

$$H_1: p_1 < p_2, \text{ which is equivalent to } H_1: RD < 0, H_1: RR < 1 \text{ and } H_1: OR < 1,$$

or that the proportions are different,

$$H_1: p_1 \neq p_2, \text{ which is equivalent to } H_1: RD \neq 0, H_1: RR \neq 1 \text{ and } H_1: OR \neq 1.$$

The three different alternatives represent upper-, lower-, and two-tailed tests, respectively.

The formula for the test of hypothesis for the difference in proportions is given in Table 7–17. The preceding formula is appropriate for large samples, defined as at least five successes

($n\hat{p}$) and at least five failures [$n(1 - \hat{p})$] in each of the two samples. If there are fewer than five successes or failures in either comparison group, then alternative procedures called exact methods must be used to estimate the difference in population proportions.[3,4]

Example 7.12. In Example 6.9, we analyzed data from $n = 3799$ participants who attended the fifth examination of the Offspring in the Framingham Heart Study. The outcome of interest was prevalent CVD and we compared prevalent CVD between participants who were and were not currently smoking cigarettes at the time of the fifth examination of the Framingham Offspring Study. The data are shown in Table 7–18. We will now use the data to test if the prevalence of CVD is significantly different in smokers as compared to nonsmokers.

The prevalence of CVD (or proportion of participants with prevalent CVD) among nonsmokers is $298 / 3055 = 0.0975$, and the prevalence of CVD among current smokers is $81 / 744 = 0.1089$. Here smoking status defines the comparison groups and we will call the current smokers Group 1 (exposed) and the nonsmokers (unexposed) Group 2. The test of hypothesis is conducted below using the five-step approach.

Step 1: Set up hypotheses and determine the level of significance.

$$H_0: p_1 = p_2,$$
$$H_1: p_1 \neq p_2,$$
$$\alpha = 0.05.$$

Step 2: Select the appropriate test statistic.

The formula for the test statistic is in Table 7–17. We must first check that the sample size is adequate. Specifically, we need to ensure that we have at least five successes and five failures in each comparison group. In this example, we have more than enough successes (cases of prevalent CVD) and failures (persons free of CVD) in each comparison group.

TABLE 7–17 Test Statistics for Testing $H_0: p_1 = p_2$

$\min[n_1\hat{p}_1, n_1(1-\hat{p}_1), n_2\hat{p}_2, n_2(1-\hat{p}_2)] \geq 5$	$z = \dfrac{\hat{p}_1 - \hat{p}_2}{\sqrt{\hat{p}(1-\hat{p})\left(1/n_1 + 1/n_2\right)}}$	Find critical value of z in Table 1B

TABLE 7–18 Prevalent CVD in Smokers and Nonsmokers

	Free of CVD	History of CVD	Total
Nonsmoker	2757	298	3055
Current smoker	663	81	744
Total	3420	379	3799

The sample size is more than adequate, so the following formula can be used:

$$z = \frac{\hat{p}_1 - \hat{p}_2}{\sqrt{\hat{p}(1-\hat{p})\left(1/n_1 + 1/n_2\right)}}.$$

Step 3: Set up the decision rule.
This is a two-tailed test, using a z statistic and a 5% level of significance. The appropriate critical value can be found in Table 1C in the Appendix and the decision rule is

Reject H_0 if $z \leq -1.960$ or if $z \geq 1.960$.

Step 4: Compute the test statistic.
We now substitute the sample data into the formula for the test statistic identified in Step 2. We first compute the overall proportion of successes:

$$\hat{p} = \frac{x_1 + x_2}{n_1 + n_2} = \frac{81 + 298}{744 + 3055} = \frac{379}{3799} = 0.0998.$$

We now substitute to compute the test statistic,

$$z = \frac{0.1089 - 0.0975}{\sqrt{0.0988(1-0.0988)\left(1/744 + 1/3055\right)}} =$$

$$\frac{0.0114}{0.0123} = 0.927.$$

Step 5: Conclusion.
We do not reject H_0 because $-1.960 < 0.927 < 1.960$. We do not have statistically significant evidence at $\alpha = 0.05$ to show that there is a difference in prevalent CVD between smokers and nonsmokers.

In Example 6.9, we estimated the 95% confidence interval for the difference in prevalent CVD (or risk difference) between smokers and nonsmokers as 0.0114 ± 0.0247, or between -0.0133 and 0.0361. Because the 95% confidence interval for the risk difference included 0, we could not conclude that there was a statistically significant difference in prevalent CVD

between smokers and nonsmokers. This is consistent with the test of hypothesis result.

In Example 6.11, we used the same data and estimated the relative risk along with a 95% confidence interval for the relative risk. We estimated that the prevalence of CVD was 1.12 times higher in smokers as compared to nonsmokers with a 95% confidence interval of 0.89 to 1.41. Because this confidence interval included the null value of 1, we could not conclude that there was a difference in prevalent CVD between smokers and nonsmokers.

In Example 6.13, we again used the same data and estimated the odds ratio along with a 95% confidence interval for the odds ratio. We estimated that the odds of CVD was 1.13 times higher in smokers as compared to nonsmokers with a 95% confidence interval estimate of 0.87 to 1.47. Because this confidence interval included the null value of 1, we could not conclude that there was a difference in prevalent CVD between smokers and nonsmokers.

Smoking has been shown to be a risk factor for cardiovascular disease. What might explain the fact that we did not observe a statistically significant difference using data from the Framingham Heart Study? (Hint: Here we consider prevalent CVD. Would the results have been different if we considered incident CVD?)

Example 7.13. In Example 6.10, we analyzed data from a randomized trial designed to evaluate the effectiveness of a newly developed pain reliever designed to reduce pain in patients following joint replacement surgery. The trial compared the new pain reliever to the pain reliever currently in use (called the standard of care). A total of 100 patients undergoing joint replacement surgery agreed to participate in the trial. Patients were randomly assigned to receive either the new pain reliever or the standard pain reliever following surgery and were blind to the treatment assignment. Before receiving the assigned treatment, patients were asked to rate their pain on a scale of 0 to 10, with higher scores indicative of more pain. Each patient was then given the assigned treatment and after 30 minutes was again asked to rate their pain on the same scale. The primary outcome was a reduction in pain of 3 or more scale points (defined by clinicians as a clinically meaningful reduction). The data shown in Table 7–19 were observed in the trial. We will now test whether there is a statistically significant difference in the proportions of patients reporting a meaningful reduction (i.e., a reduction of 3 or more scale points) using the five-stepapproach.

Step 1: Set up hypotheses and determine the level of significance.

$$H_0: p_1 = p_2,$$

TABLE 7–19 Pain Reduction by Treatment

| Treatment Group | n | Reduction of 3+ Points | |
		Number	Proportion
New pain reliever	50	23	0.46
Standard pain reliever	50	11	0.22

$$H_1: p_1 \neq p_2,$$

$$\alpha = 0.05.$$

Here the new pain reliever is represented as Group 1 and the standard pain reliever as Group 2.

Step 2: Select the appropriate test statistic.

The formula for the test statistic is in Table 7–17. We must first check that the sample size is adequate. Specifically, we need to ensure that we have at least five successes and five failures in each comparison group or that

$$\min[n_1 \hat{p}_1, n_1(1 - \hat{p}_1), n_2 \hat{p}_2, n_2(1 - \hat{p}_2)] \geq 5.$$

In this example, we have

$$\min[50(0.46), 50(1 - 0.46), 50(0.22), 50(1 - 0.22)] = \\ \min(23, 27, 11, 39) = 11.$$

The sample size is adequate, so the following formula can be used:

$$z = \frac{\hat{p}_1 - \hat{p}_2}{\sqrt{\hat{p}(1 - \hat{p})\left(\frac{1}{n_1} + \frac{1}{n_2}\right)}}.$$

Step 3: Set up the decision rule.

This is a two-tailed test, using a z statistic and a 5% level of significance. The appropriate critical value can be found in Table 1C in the Appendix and the decision rule is

Reject H_0 if $z \leq -1.960$ or if $z \geq 1.960$.

Step 4: Compute the test statistic.

We now substitute the sample data into the formula for the test statistic identified in Step 2. We first compute the overall proportion of successes:

$$\hat{p} = \frac{x_1 + x_2}{n_1 + n_2} = \frac{23 + 11}{50 + 50} = \frac{34}{100} = 0.34.$$

We now substitute to compute the test statistic,

$$z = \frac{0.46 - 0.22}{\sqrt{0.34(1 - 0.34)\left(\frac{1}{50} + \frac{1}{50}\right)}} = \frac{0.24}{0.095} = 2.526.$$

Step 5: Conclusion.

We reject H_0 because $2.526 \geq 1960$. We have statistically significant evidence at $\alpha = 0.05$ to show that there is a difference in the proportions of patients on the new pain reliever reporting a meaningful reduction (i.e., a reduction of 3 or more scale points) as compared to patients on the standard pain reliever.

In Example 6.10, we estimated a 95% confidence interval for the difference in proportions of patients on the new pain reliever reporting a meaningful reduction (i.e., a reduction of 3 or more scale points) as compared to patients on the standard pain reliever, and it was 0.24 ± 0.18, or between 0.06 and 0.42. Because the 95% confidence interval did not include 0, we concluded that there was a statistically significant difference in proportions, which is consistent with the test of hypothesis result.

In Example 6.12, we used the same data and estimated the relative risk along with a 95% confidence interval for the relative risk. We estimated that patients receiving the new pain reliever were 2.09 times more likely to report a meaningful reduction in pain as compared to patients receiving the standard pain reliever, with a 95% confidence interval of 1.14 to 3.82. Because this confidence interval did not include the null value of 1, we concluded that there was a significant difference in the relative risk of a meaningful reduction in pain in patients on the new and standard pain relievers.

In Example 6.12, we used the same data and estimated the odds ratio along with a 95% confidence interval for the odds ratio. We estimated that the odds that patients receiving the new pain reliever reported a meaningful reduction in pain was 3.02 times the odds that patients on standard pain reliever reported a meaningful reduction in pain, with a 95% confidence interval of 1.26 to 7.21. Because this confidence interval did not include the null value of 1, we concluded that there was a significant difference in the odds of a meaningful reduction in pain in patients on the new and standard pain relievers.

7.8 TESTS WITH MORE THAN TWO INDEPENDENT SAMPLES, CONTINUOUS OUTCOME

There are many applications where it is of interest to compare more than two independent groups with respect to their mean scores on a continuous outcome. For example, in some clinical trials there are more than two comparison groups. Suppose a clinical trial is designed to evaluate a new medication for asthma and investigators compare an experimental medication to a placebo and to a standard treatment (i.e., a medication currently being used). In an observational study such as the Framingham Heart Study, it might be of interest to compare mean blood pressures or mean cholesterol levels in persons who are underweight, normal weight, overweight, and obese.

The technique to test for a difference in more than two independent means is an extension of the two independent samples procedure discussed in Section 7.5 and is called *analysis of variance* (ANOVA). The ANOVA technique applies when there are more than two independent groups. The ANOVA procedure is used to compare the means of the comparison groups and is conducted using the same five-step approach used in the scenarios discussed in previous sections. However, because there are more than two groups the computation of the test statistic is more involved. The test statistic must take into account the sample sizes, sample means, and sample standard deviations in each of the comparison groups. Before illustrating the computation of the test statistic, we first present the logic of the procedure.

Consider an example with four independent groups and a continuous outcome measure. The independent groups might be defined by a particular characteristic of the participants, such as BMI (e.g., underweight, normal weight, overweight, or obese), or by the investigator (e.g., randomizing participants to one of four competing treatments, call them A, B, C, and D). Suppose that the outcome is systolic blood pressure and we wish to test whether there is a statistically significant difference in mean systolic blood pressures among the four groups. The sample data are organized as shown in Table 7–20.

The hypotheses of interest in an ANOVA are

$$H_0: \mu_1 = \mu_2 = ... = \mu_k,$$

$$H_1: \text{Means are not all equal,}$$

where k is the number of independent comparison groups. For the example just described, the hypotheses are

$$H_0: \mu_1 = \mu_2 = \mu_3 = \mu_4,$$

$$H_1: \text{Means are not all equal.}$$

TABLE 7–20 Summary Statistics for ANOVA

	Group 1	Group 2	Group 3	Group 4
Sample size	n_1	n_2	n_3	n_4
Sample mean	$\overline{X}_1$	$\overline{X}_2$	$\overline{X}_3$	$\overline{X}_4$
Sample standard deviation	s_1	s_2	s_3	s_4

The null hypothesis in ANOVA is always that there is no difference in the means. The research or alternative hypothesis is always that the means are not all equal and is usually written in words rather than in mathematical symbols. The research hypothesis captures any difference in means and includes the situation where all four means are unequal, where one is different from the other three, where two are different, and so on. The alternative hypothesis (as shown earlier) captures all possible situations other than equality of all means specified in the null hypothesis.

The test statistic for ANOVA is given in Table 7–21. The F statistic is computed by taking the ratio of what is called the "between treatment" variability to the "residual or error" variability. This is where the name of the procedure originates. In analysis of variance, we are testing for a difference in means (H_0: means are all equal versus H_1: means are not all equal) by evaluating variability in the data. The numerator captures between-treatment variability (i.e., differences among the sample means) and the denominator contains an estimate of the variability in the outcome. The test statistic is a measure that allows us to assess whether the differences among the sample

TABLE 7–21 Test Statistic for Testing $H_0: \mu_1 = \mu_2 = ... = \mu_k$

$F = \dfrac{\sum n_j(\overline{X}_j - \overline{X})^2/(k-1)}{\sum\sum(X - \overline{X}_j)^2/(N-k)}$	Find critical value in Table 4 ($df_1 = k - 1$, $df_2 = N - k$)

where nj = the sample size in the *j*th group (e.g., *j* = 1, 2, 3, and 4 when there are 4 comparision groups), $\overline{X}_j$ is the sample mean in the *j*th group, and $\overline{X}$ is the overall mean. *k* represents the number of independent groups ($k > 2$) and N represents the total number of observations in the analysis.

Note that N does not refer to a population size, but instead to the total sample size in the analysis (the sum of the sample sizes in the comparison groups, e.g., N = n1 + n2 + n3 + n4). The test statistic is complicated because it incorporates all of the sample data. While it is not easy to see the extension, the F statistic is a generalization of the test statistic shown in Table 7–11, which is appropriate for exactly two groups.

NOTE: The F statistic assumes equal variability in the k populations (i.e., the population variances are equal, or $\sigma_1^2 = \sigma_2^2 = ... = \sigma_k^2$). This means that the outcome is equally variable in each of the comparison populations. This assumption is the same as that assumed for appropriate use of the test statistics in Table 7–11 when there are two comparison groups. It is possible to assess the likelihood that the assumption of equal variances is true and the test can be conducted in most statistical computing packages.[7] If the variability in the k comparison groups is not similar, then alternative techniques must be used.[8]

means (numerator) are larger than would be expected by chance if the null hypothesis were true. Recall in the two independent samples test (see test statistics in Table 7–11), the test statistics (z or t) were computed by taking the ratio of the difference in sample means (numerator) to the variability in the outcome (estimated by $S_p\sqrt{\frac{1}{n_1}+\frac{1}{n_2}}$.

The decision rule for the F test in ANOVA is set up in a similar way to decision rules we established for z and t tests. The decision rule again depends on the level of significance and the degrees of freedom. The F statistic has two degrees of freedom. These are denoted df_1 and df_2, and called the numerator and denominator degrees of freedom, respectively. The degrees of freedom are defined as $df_1 = k - 1$ and $df_2 = N - k$, where k is the number of comparison groups and N is the total number of observations in the analysis. Similar to χ^2 tests, there is no upper-, lower-, or two-tailed distinction. If the null hypothesis is true, the between treatment variation (numerator) will be close in value to the residual or error variation (denominator) and the F statistic will be small. If the null hypothesis is false, then the F statistic will be large. The rejection region for the F test is always in the upper-tail (right) of the distribution, as shown in Figure 7–7.

Table 4 in the Appendix contains critical values for the F distribution for tests when $\alpha = 0.05$, indexed by df_1 and df_2. Figure 7–7 is an example for the situation with $\alpha = 0.05$, $df_1 = 3$, and $df_2 = 36$. The degrees of freedom are based on an application with four comparison groups ($k = 4$) and a sample size of 40 ($N = 40$). The appropriate critical value from Table 4 in the Appendix is 2.87, and the decision rule is

$$\text{Reject } H_0 \text{ if } F \geq 2.87.$$

We will next illustrate the ANOVA procedure using the five-step approach. Because the computation of the test statistic is involved, the computations are often organized in an ANOVA table. The ANOVA table breaks down the components of variation in the data into variation between treatments and error or residual variation. The ANOVA table is set up as shown in Table 7–22.

The ANOVA table is organized as follows. The first column is entitled *Source of Variation* and delineates the between-treatment and error or residual variation. The total variation is the sum of the between-treatment and error variation. The second column is entitled *Sums of Squares (SS)*. The between-treatment sums of squares is

$$\text{SSB} = \sum n_j(\overline{X}_j - \overline{X})^2,$$

and is computed by summing the squared differences between each treatment (or group) mean ($\overline{X}_j$) and the overall mean ($\overline{X}$). The squared differences are weighted by the sample sizes per group (n_j). The error sums of squares is

$$\text{SSE} = \sum\sum(X - \overline{X}_j)^2,$$

and is computed by summing the squared differences between each observation (X) and its group mean ($\overline{X}_j$) (i.e., the squared differences between each observation in Group 1 and the Group 1 mean, the squared differences between each observation in Group 2 and the Group 2 mean, and so on). The double summation ($\sum\sum$) indicates summation of the squared differences within each treatment and then summation of these totals across treatments to produce a single value. (This will be illustrated in the following examples.) The total sums of squares is

$$\text{SST} = \sum\sum(X - \overline{X})^2,$$

and is computed by summing the squared differences between each observation (X) and the overall sample mean ($\overline{X}$). In an

---

TABLE 7–22 ANOVA Table

Source of Variation	Sums of Squares (SS)	Degrees of Freedom (df)	Mean Squares (MS)	F
Between treatments	$\text{SSB} = \sum n_j(\overline{X}_j - \overline{X})^2$	$k - 1$	$\text{MSB} = \dfrac{\text{SSB}}{k - 1}$	$F = \dfrac{\text{MSB}}{\text{MSE}}$
Error or residual	$\text{SSE} = \sum\sum(X - \overline{X}_j)^2$	$N - k$	$\text{MSE} = \dfrac{\text{SSE}}{N - k}$	
Total	$\text{SST} = \sum\sum(X - \overline{X})^2$	$N - 1$		

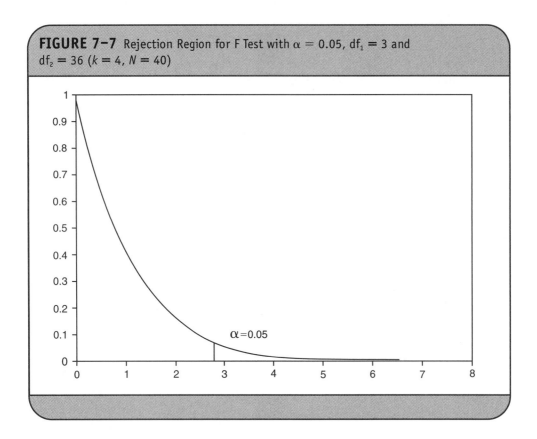

FIGURE 7-7 Rejection Region for F Test with $\alpha = 0.05$, $df_1 = 3$ and $df_2 = 36$ ($k = 4$, $N = 40$)

ANOVA, data are organized by comparison or treatment groups. If all of the data were pooled into a single sample, SST would reflect the numerator of the sample variance computed on the pooled or total sample. SST does not figure into the F statistic directly. However, SST = SSB + SSE, thus if two sums of squares are known, the third can be computed from the other two.

The third column contains degrees of freedom. The between treatment degrees of freedom is $df_1 = k - 1$. The error degrees of freedom is $df_2 = N - k$. The total degrees of freedom is $N - 1$, and it is also true that $(k - 1) + (N - k) = N - 1$. The fourth column contains *Mean Squares (MS)*, which are computed by dividing sums of squares (SS) by degrees of freedom (df), row by row. Specifically,

$$\text{MSB} = \frac{\text{SSB}}{k-1} \text{ and MSE} = \frac{\text{SSE}}{N-k}.$$

Dividing SST / $(N - 1)$ produces the variance of the total sample. The F statistic is in the right column of the ANOVA table and is computed by taking the ratio of MSB / MSE.

Example 7.14. A clinical trial is run to compare weight-loss programs, and participants are randomly assigned to one of the comparison programs and counseled on the details of the assigned program. Participants follow the assigned program

for 8 weeks. The outcome of interest is weight loss, defined as the difference in weight measured at the start of the study (baseline) and weight measured at the end of the study (8 weeks), measured in pounds.

Three popular weight-loss programs are considered. The first is a low-calorie diet. The second is a low-fat diet and the third is a low-carbohydrate diet. For comparison purposes, a fourth group is considered as a control group. Participants in the fourth group are told that they are participating in a study of healthy behaviors with weight loss being only one component of interest. The control group is included here to assess the placebo effect (i.e., weight loss due to simply participating in the study). A total of 20 patients agree to participate in the study and are randomly assigned to one of the four diet groups. Weights are measured at baseline and patients are counseled on the proper implementation of the assigned diet (with the exception of the control group). After 8 weeks, each patient's weight is again measured and the difference in weights is computed by subtracting the 8-week weight from the baseline weight. Positive differences indicate weight losses and negative differences indicate weight gains. For interpretation purposes, we refer to the differences in weights as weight losses and the observed weight losses are shown in Table 7–23. Is there a statistically

TABLE 7–23 Weight Loss in Each Treatment

Low-Calorie	Low-Fat	Low-Carbohydrate	Control
8	2	3	2
9	4	5	2
6	3	4	−1
7	5	2	0
3	1	3	3

TABLE 7–24 Summary Statistics on Weight Loss by Treatment

Low-Calorie	Low-Fat	Low-Carbohydrate	Control
$n_1 = 5$	$n_2 = 5$	$n_3 = 5$	$n_4 = 5$
$\overline{X}_1 = 6.6$	$\overline{X}_2 = 3.0$	$\overline{X}_3 = 3.4$	$\overline{X}_4 = 1.2$

significant difference in the mean weight loss among the four diets? We will run the ANOVA using the five-step approach.

Step 1: Set up hypotheses and determine the level of significance.

$$H_0: \mu_1 = \mu_2 = \mu_3 = \mu_4,$$

$$H_1: \text{Means are not all equal,}$$

$$\alpha = 0.05.$$

Step 2: Select the appropriate test statistic.

The test statistic is the F statistic for ANOVA,

$$F = \frac{\text{MSB}}{\text{MSE}}.$$

Step 3: Set up the decision rule.

The appropriate critical value can be found in Table 4 in the Appendix. To determine the critical value of F, we need degrees of freedom, $df_1 = k - 1$ and $df_2 = N - k$. In this example, $df_1 = k - 1 = 4 - 1 = 3$ and $df_2 = N - k = 20 - 4 = 16$. The critical value is 3.24, and the decision rule is

$$\text{Reject } H_0 \text{ if } F \geq 3.24.$$

Step 4: Compute the test statistic.

To organize our computations, we complete the ANOVA table. To compute the sums of squares, we first compute the sample means for each group (see Table 7–24). The overall mean based on the total sample ($n = 20$) is $\overline{X} = 3.6$. We can now compute SSB:

$$\text{SSB} = \overline{X} \sum n_j (\overline{X}_j - \overline{X})^2,$$

$$\text{SSB} = 5(6.6 - 3.6)^2 + 5(3.0 - 3.6)^2 +$$

$$5(3.4 - 3.6)^2 + 5(1.2 - 3.6)^2,$$

$$\text{SSB} = 45.0 + 0.2 + 28.8 + 1.8 = 75.8.$$

Next, we compute SSE. SSE requires computing the squared differences between each observation and its group mean. We will compute SSE in parts (see Tables 7–25, 7–26, 7–27, 7–28), and then sum.

$$\text{SSE} = \sum\sum(X - \overline{X}_j)^2 = 21.4 + 10.0 + 5.4 + 10.6 = 47.4.$$

We can now construct the ANOVA table (see Table 7–29).

Step 5: Conclusion.

We reject H_0 because $8.43 \geq 3.24$. We have statistically significant evidence at $\alpha = 0.05$ to show that there is a difference in mean weight loss among the four diets.

Note that Table 4 in the Appendix only provides critical values for the F test when $\alpha = 0.05$. Without tables for other levels of significance, we cannot approximate p-values for ANOVA. Because ANOVA is a tedious technique to implement by hand, it is usually performed with the use of a statistical computing package that produces, along with the ANOVA table, an exact p-value.

ANOVA is a test that provides a global assessment of a statistical difference in more than two independent means. In this example, we find that there is a statistically significant difference in mean weight loss among the four diets considered. In addition to reporting the results of the statistical test of hypothesis (i.e., that there is a statistically significant difference in mean weight loss at $\alpha = 0.05$), investigators should also report

TABLE 7–25 Deviations from Mean Weight Loss on Low-Calorie Diet

Low-Calorie	$(X - 6.6)$	$(X - 6.6)^2$
8	1.4	2.0
9	2.4	5.8
6	−0.6	0.4
7	0.4	0.2
3	−3.6	13.0
Total	0	21.4

TABLE 7-26 Deviations from Mean Weight Loss on Low-Fat Diet

Low-Fat	$(X - 3.0)$	$(X - 3.0)^2$
2	−1.0	1.0
4	1.0	1.0
3	0.0	0.0
5	2.0	4.0
1	−2.0	4.0
Total	0	10.0

TABLE 7-27 Deviations from Mean Weight Loss on Low-Carbohydrate Diet

Low-Carbohydrate	$(X - 3.4)$	$(X - 3.4)^2$
3	−0.4	0.2
5	1.6	2.6
4	0.6	0.4
2	−1.4	2.0
3	−0.4	0.2
Total	0	5.4

TABLE 7-28 Deviations from Mean Weight Loss in Control Group

Control	$(X - 1.2)$	$(X - 1.2)^2$
2	0.8	0.6
2	0.8	0.6
−1	−2.2	4.8
0	−1.2	1.4
3	1.8	3.2
Total	0	10.6

the observed sample means to facilitate interpretation of the results. In this example, participants in the low-calorie diet lost an average of 6.6 pounds over 8 weeks, as compared to 3.0 and 3.4 pounds in the low-fat and low-carbohydrate groups, respectively. Participants in the control group lost an average of 1.2 pounds, which could be called a placebo effect because these participants were not participating in an active arm of the trial specifically targeted for weight loss.

Example 7.15. Calcium is an essential mineral that regulates the heart, and is important for blood clotting and for building healthy bones. The National Osteoporosis Foundation recommends a daily calcium intake of 1000 to 1200 mg/day for adult men and women.[9] Whereas calcium is contained in some foods, most adults do not get enough calcium in their diets and take supplements. Unfortunately, some of the supplements have side effects such as gastric distress, making them difficult for some patients to take on a regular basis.

A study is designed to test whether there is a difference in mean daily calcium intake in adults with normal bone density, adults with osteopenia (a low bone density, which may lead to osteoporosis), and adults with osteoporosis. Adults 60 years of age with normal bone density, osteopenia, and osteoporosis are selected at random from hospital records and invited to participate in the study. Each participant's daily calcium intake is measured based on reported food intake and supplements. The data are shown in Table 7–30.

Is there a statistically significant difference in mean calcium intake in patients with normal bone density as compared to patients with osteopenia and osteoporosis? We will run the ANOVA using the five-step approach.

Step 1: Set up hypotheses and determine the level of significance.

$$H_0: \mu_1 = \mu_2 = \mu_3,$$

$$H_1: \text{Means are not all equal,}$$

$$\alpha = 0.05.$$

TABLE 7-29 ANOVA Table

Source of Variation	Sums of Squares (SS)	Degrees of Freedom (df)	Mean Squares (MS)	F
Between treatments	75.8	4 − 1 = 3	75.8 / 3 = 25.3	25.3 / 3.0 = 8.43
Error or residual	47.4	20 − 4 = 16	47.4 / 16 = 3.0	
Total	123.2	20 − 1 = 19		

TABLE 7–30 Calcium Intake in Each Treatment

Normal Bone Density	Osteopenia	Osteoporosis
1200	1000	890
1000	1100	650
980	700	1100
900	800	900
750	500	400
800	700	350

TABLE 7–31 Summary Statistics on Calcium Intake by Treatment

Normal Bone Density	Osteopenia	Osteoporosis
$n_1 = 6$	$n_2 = 6$	$n_3 = 6$
$\overline{X}_1 = 938.3$	$\overline{X}_2 = 715.0$	$\overline{X}_3 = 800.0$

TABLE 7–32 Deviations from Mean Calcium Intake in Patients with Normal Bone Density

Normal Bone Density	$(X - 938.3)$	$(X - 938.3)^2$
1200	261.7	68,486.9
1000	61.7	3806.9
980	41.7	1738.9
900	−38.3	1466.9
750	−188.3	35,456.9
800	−138.3	19,126.9
Total	0	130,083.4

TABLE 7–33 Deviations from Mean Calcium Intake in Patients with Osteopenia

Osteopenia	$(X - 715.0)$	$(X - 715.0)^2$
1000	285.0	81,225.0
1100	385.0	148,225.0
700	−15	225.0
800	85.0	7225.0
500	−215.0	46,225.0
700	−15	225.0
Total	0	283,350.0

Step 2: Select the appropriate test statistic.
The test statistic is the F statistic for ANOVA,

$$F = \frac{MSB}{MSE}.$$

Step 3: Set up the decision rule.
The appropriate critical value can be found in Table 4 in the Appendix. To determine the critical value of F, we need degrees of freedom, $df_1 = k - 1$ and $df_2 = N - k$. In this example, $df_1 = k - 1 = 3 - 1 = 2$ and $df_2 = N - k = 18 - 3 = 15$. The critical value is 3.68, and the decision rule is

Reject H_0 if $F \geq 3.68$.

Step 4: Compute the test statistic.
To organize our computations, we will complete the ANOVA table. To compute the sums of squares, we must first compute the sample means for each group (see Table 7–31). The overall mean is $\overline{X} = 817.7$. We can now compute SSB:

$$SSB = \sum n_j(\overline{X}_j - \overline{X})^2,$$

$$SSB = 6(938.3 - 817.7)^2 + 6(715.0 - 817.7)^2 + 6(800.0 - 817.7)^2,$$

$$SSB = 87,266.2 + 63,283.7 + 1879.7 = 152,429.6.$$

Next, we calculate SSE. SSE requires computing the squared differences between each observation and its group mean. We will compute SSE in parts (see Tables 7–32, 7–33, and 7–34), and then sum.

$$SSE = \sum\sum(X - \overline{X}_j)^2 = 130,083.4 + 283,350.0 + 493,100.0 = 906,533.4.$$

We can now construct the ANOVA table (see Table 7–35).

Step 5: Conclusion.
We do not reject H_0 because $1.26 < 3.68$. We do not have statistically significant evidence at $\alpha = 0.05$ to show that there is a difference in mean calcium intake in patients with normal bone density as compared to osteopenia and osteoporosis.

The ANOVA tests described here are called one-factor ANOVAs. There is one treatment or grouping factor with $k > 2$ levels and we wish to compare the means across the different categories of this factor. The factor might represent different diets, different classifications of risk for disease (e.g., osteoporosis), different medical treatments, different age groups, or different racial or ethic groups. There are situations

TABLE 7–34 Deviations from Mean Calcium Intake in Patients with Osteoporosis

Osteoporosis	$(X - 800.0)$	$(X - 800.0)^2$
890	90	8100.0
650	−150	22,500.0
1100	300	90,000.0
900	100	10,000.0
400	−400	160,000.0
350	−450	202,500.0
Total	0	493,100.0

where it may be of interest to compare means of a continuous outcome across two or more factors. For example, suppose a clinical trial is designed to compare five different treatments for joint pain in patients with osteoarthritis. Investigators might also hypothesize that there are differences in the outcome by gender. This is an example of a two-factor ANOVA where the factors are treatment (with five levels) and gender (with two levels). In the two-factor ANOVA, investigators can assess whether there are differences in means among treatments, by gender, or whether there is a difference in means by the combination or interaction of treatment and gender. Higher-order ANOVAs are conducted in the same way as one-factor ANOVAs presented here, and the computations are again organized in ANOVA tables with more rows to distinguish the different sources of variation (e.g., between treatments, between men and women). More details on higher-order ANOVA can be found in Snedecor and Cochran.[10]

7.9　TESTS FOR TWO OR MORE INDEPENDENT SAMPLES, DISCRETE OUTCOME

In Section 7.4, we presented the χ^2 goodness-of-fit test, which was used to test whether the distribution of responses to a discrete variable measured in a single sample followed a known distribution. Here we extend that application to the two or more independent samples case. Specifically, the outcome of interest is discrete with two or more responses, and the responses can be ordered or unordered (i.e., the outcome can be ordinal or categorical). We now consider the situation where there are two or more independent comparison groups, and the goal of the analysis is to compare the distribution of responses to the discrete outcome variable among several independent comparison groups.

The test is called the χ^2 *test of independence* and the null hypothesis is that there is no difference in the distribution of responses to the outcome across comparison groups. This is often stated as: The outcome variable and the grouping variable (e.g., the comparison treatments or comparison groups) are independent (hence the name of the test). Independence here implies homogeneity in the distribution of the outcome among comparison groups. The null hypothesis in the χ^2 test of independence is often stated in words as

H₀: The distribution of the outcome is independent of the groups.

The research hypothesis is that there is a difference in the distribution of the outcome variable among the comparison groups (i.e., that the distribution of responses "depends" on the group). To test the hypothesis, we measure the discrete outcome variable in each participant in each comparison group. The data of interest are the observed frequencies (or number of participants in each response category in each group). The formula for the test statistic for the χ^2 test of independence is given in Table 7–36.

The data for the χ^2 test of independence are organized in a two-way table. The outcome and grouping variable are shown in the rows and columns of the table. Table 7–37 illustrates the sample data layout. The table entries (blank) are the numbers of participants in each group responding to each response category of the outcome variable.

In Table 7–37, the grouping variable is shown in the rows of the table; *r* denotes the number of independent groups. The outcome variable is shown in the columns of

TABLE 7–35 ANOVA Table

Source of Variation	Sums of Squares (SS)	Degrees of Freedom (df)	Mean Squares (MS)	F
Between treatments	152,429.6	2	76,214.8	1.26
Error or residual	906,533.4	15	60,435.6	
Total	1,058,963.0	17		

<table>
<tr><td>

TABLE 7–36 Test Statistic for Testing
H_0: Distribution of Outcome Is Independent of Groups

$\chi^2 = \sum \dfrac{(O - E)^2}{E}$ Find critical value in Table 3,
df = (r − 1)(c − 1)

</td></tr>
</table>

the table; c denotes the number of response options in the outcome variable. Each combination of a row (group) and column (response) is called a cell of the table. The table has $r \times c$ cells and is sometimes called an $r \times c$ ("r by c") table. For example, if there are four groups and five categories in the outcome variable, the data are organized in a 4×5 table. The row and column totals are shown along the right margin and the bottom of the table, respectively. The total sample size, N, can be computed by summing the row totals or the column totals. Similar to ANOVA, N here does not refer to a population size but rather to the total sample size in the analysis. The sample data can be organized into a table like that shown. The numbers of participants within each group who select each response option are shown in the cells of the table, and these are the observed frequencies used in the test statistic.

The test statistic for the χ^2 test of independence involves comparing observed (sample data) and expected frequencies in each cell of the table. The expected frequencies are computed assuming that the null hypothesis is true. The null hypothesis states that the two variables (the grouping variable and the outcome) are independent. In Chapter 5, we introduced the concept of independence. The definition of independence is

Two events, A and B, are independent if P(A|B) = P(A),

or, equivalently,

Two events, A and B, are independent if P(A and B) = P(A) P(B).

The second statement indicates that if two events, A and B, are independent, then the probability of their intersection can be computed by multiplying the probability of each individual event. To conduct the χ^2 test of independence, we must compute expected frequencies in each cell of the table. Expected frequencies are computed by assuming that the grouping variable and outcome are independent (i.e., under the null hypothesis). Thus, if the null hypothesis is true, using the definition of independence:

P(Group 1 and Response Option 1) = P(Group 1)
P(Response Option 1).

The preceding states that the probability that an individual is in Group 1 and their outcome is Response Option 1 is computed by multiplying the probability that person is in Group 1 by the probability that a person gave Response Option 1. This is true if Group and Response are independent. To conduct the χ^2 test of independence, we need expected frequencies and not expected probabilities. To convert the probability to a frequency, we multiply by N. Consider the following example.

The data shown in Table 7–38 are measured in a sample of size $N = 150$. The frequencies in the cells of the table are the observed frequencies. If Group and Response are independent, then we can compute the probability that a person in the sample is in Group 1 and Response category 1 using

P(Group 1 and Response 1) = P(Group 1) P(Response 1),

P(Group 1 and Response 1) = (25 / 150)(62 / 150) = 0.069.

TABLE 7–37 Data Layout for Chi-Square Test of Independence

Grouping Variable	Response Option 1	Response Option 2	...	Response Option c	Row Totals
Group 1					
Group 2					
...					
Group r					
Column totals					N

TABLE 7–38 Observed Frequencies by Group

	Response 1	Response 2	Response 3	Total
Group 1	10	8	7	25
Group 2	22	15	13	50
Group 3	30	28	17	75
Total	62	51	37	150

Thus, if Group and Response are independent, we would expect 6.9% of the sample to be in the top-left cell of the table (Group 1 and Response 1). The expected frequency is $150(0.069) = 10.4$. We could do the same for Group 2 and Response 1:

$$P(\text{Group 2 and Response 1}) = P(\text{Group 2}) \, P(\text{Response 1}),$$

$$P(\text{Group 2 and Response 1}) = (50 / 150)(62 / 150) = 0.138.$$

The expected frequency in Group 2 and Response 1 is $150(0.138) = 20.7$.

The formula for determining the expected cell frequencies in the χ^2 test of independence is

$$\text{Expected cell frequency} = \frac{\text{Row total} \times \text{column total}}{N}.$$

The preceding equation computes the expected frequency in one step rather than computing the expected probability first and then converting to a frequency.

Example 7.16. In Example 7.6, we examined data from a survey of university graduates that assessed (among other things) how frequently they exercised. The survey was completed by 470 graduates. We used the χ^2 goodness-of-fit test to assess whether there was a shift in the distribution of responses to the exercise question following the implementation of a health promotion campaign on campus. We specifically considered one sample (all students) and compared the observed distribution to the distribution of responses the prior year (an historical control). Suppose we wish to assess whether there is a relationship between exercise on campus and students' living arrangements. As part of the same survey, graduates were asked where they lived their senior year. The response options were dormitory, on-campus apartment, off-campus apartment, and at home (i.e., commuted to and from the university). The data are shown in Table 7–39.

Based on the data, is there a relationship between exercise and a student's living arrangement? Here we have four independent comparison groups (living arrangements) and a discrete outcome variable with three response options. We specifically want to test whether living arrangement and exercise are independent. We will run the test using the five-step approach.

Step 1: Set up hypotheses and determine the level of significance.

H_0: Living arrangement and exercise are independent,

H_1: H_0 is false,

$\alpha = 0.05$.

The null and research hypotheses are written in words rather than in symbols. The research hypothesis is that the grouping variable (living arrangement) and the outcome variable (exercise) are dependent or related.

Step 2: Select the appropriate test statistic.
The formula for the test statistic is in Table 7–36 and is given as

$$\chi^2 = \sum \frac{(O-E)^2}{E}.$$

The condition for appropriate use of the preceding test statistic is that each expected frequency is at least five. In Step 4, we will compute the expected frequencies and ensure that the condition is met.

Step 3: Set up the decision rule.
The decision rule for the χ^2 test of independence is set up in a similar way to decision rules we established for z and t tests. The decision rule depends on the level of significance and the

TABLE 7–39 Exercise by Living Arrangement

	No Regular Exercise	Sporadic Exercise	Regular Exercise	Total
Dormitory	32	30	28	90
On-campus apartment	74	64	42	180
Off-campus apartment	110	25	15	150
At home	39	6	5	50
Total	255	125	90	470

degrees of freedom, defined as df $= (r - 1)(c - 1)$, where r and c are the numbers of rows and columns in the two-way data table. The row variable is the living arrangement, and there are four arrangements considered, thus $r = 4$. The column variable is exercise, and three responses are considered, thus $c = 3$. For this test, df $= (4 - 1)(3 - 1) = 3(2) = 6$. Again, with χ^2 tests there are no upper-, lower-, or two-tailed tests. If the null hypothesis is true, the observed and expected frequencies will be close in value and the χ^2 statistic will be close to 0. If the null hypothesis is false, then the χ^2 statistic will be large. The rejection region for the χ^2 test of independence is always in the upper tail (right) of the distribution, as shown in Figure 7–6.

Table 3 in the Appendix contains critical values for the χ^2 test indexed by degrees of freedom and the desired level of significance. For df $= 6$ and a 5% level of significance, the appropriate critical value from Table 3 is 12.59, and the decision rule is

$$\text{Reject } H_0 \text{ if } \chi^2 \geq 12.59.$$

Step 4: Compute the test statistic.

We now compute the expected frequencies using the formula,

$$\text{Expected cell frequency} = \frac{\text{Row total} \times \text{column total}}{N}.$$

The computations can be organized in a two-way table. The expected frequencies are taken to one decimal place and the sums of the observed frequencies are equal to the sums of the expected frequencies in each row and column of the table (see Table 7–40).

Recall in Step 2 that a condition for the appropriate use of the test statistic was that each expected frequency is at least five. This is true for this sample (the smallest expected

TABLE 7-40 Expected Frequencies

	No Regular Exercise	Sporadic Exercise	Regular Exercise	Total
Dormitory	48.8	23.9	17.2	90
On-campus apartment	97.7	47.9	34.5	180
Off-campus apartment	81.4	39.9	28.7	150
At home	27.1	13.3	9.6	50
Total	255	125	90	470

frequency is 9.6) and therefore it is appropriate to use the test statistic. The test statistic is computed as follows:

$$\chi^2 = \frac{(32 - 48.8)^2}{48.8} + \frac{(30 - 23.9)^2}{23.9} + \frac{(28 - 17.2)^2}{17.2} +$$

$$\frac{(74 - 97.7)^2}{97.7} + \frac{(64 - 47.9)^2}{47.9} + \frac{(42 - 34.5)^2}{34.5} +$$

$$\frac{(110 - 81.4)^2}{81.4} + \frac{(25 - 39.9)^2}{39.9} + \frac{(15 - 28.7)^2}{28.7} +$$

$$\frac{(39 - 27.1)^2}{27.1} + \frac{(6 - 13.3)^2}{13.3} + \frac{(5 - 9.6)^2}{9.6},$$

$$\chi^2 = 5.78 + 1.56 + 6.78 + 5.75 + 5.41 + 1.63 + 10.05 + 5.56 + 6.54 + 5.23 + 4.01 + 2.20 = 60.5.$$

Step 5: Conclusion.

We reject H_0 because $60.5 \geq 12.59$. We have statistically significant evidence at $\alpha = 0.05$ to show that H_0 is false or that living arrangement and exercise are not independent (i.e., they are dependent or related). Using Table 3 in the Appendix, we can approximate the p-value. We need to look at critical values for smaller levels of significance with df $= 6$. Using Table 3, the p-value is $p, 0.005$.

The χ^2 test of independence is used to test whether the distribution of the outcome variable is different across the comparison groups. In Example 7.16, we rejected H_0 and concluded that the distribution of exercise is not independent of living arrangement, or that there is a relationship between living arrangement and exercise. The test provides an overall assessment of statistical significance. When the null hypothesis is rejected, it is important to review the sample data to understand the nature of the relationship. Consider again the data in Example 7.16.

Because there are different numbers of students in each living situation, it makes the comparisons of exercise patterns difficult on the basis of the frequencies alone. Table 7–41 displays the percentages of students in each exercise category by living arrangement. The percentages sum to 100% in each row of the table. For comparison purposes, percentages are also shown for the total sample along the bottom row of the table. From Table 7–41, it is clear that higher percentages of students living in dormitories and in on-campus apartments reported regular exercise (31% and 23%) as compared to students living in off-campus apartments and at home (10% each).

Example 7.17. In Example 7.13, we analyzed data from a randomized trial designed to evaluate the effectiveness of a

TABLE 7–41 Percentages of Students Exercising by Living Arrangement

	No Regular Exercise	Sporadic Exercise	Regular Exercise
Dormitory	36	33	31
On-campus apartment	41	36	23
Off-campus apartment	73	17	10
At home	78	12	10
Total	54	27	19

TABLE 7–42 Pain Reduction by Treatment

	Meaningful Reduction (3 + Points)	No Meaningful Reduction (< 3 Points)	Total
New pain reliever	23	27	50
Higher dose of new pain reliever	30	20	50
Standard pain reliever	11	39	50
Total	64	86	150

newly developed pain reliever to reduce pain in patients following joint replacement surgery. The trial compared a new pain reliever to the pain reliever currently in use (called the standard of care). Suppose there was a third arm of the trial and patients assigned to the third arm received a higher dose of the newly developed pain reliever. Suppose that $N = 150$ patients agreed to participate in the trial and were randomly assigned to one of the three treatments. Before receiving the assigned treatment, patients were asked to rate their pain on a scale of 0 to 10, with higher scores indicative of more pain. Each patient was then given the assigned treatment and after 30 minutes was again asked to rate their pain on the same scale. The primary outcome was a reduction in pain of 3 or more scale points (defined by clinicians as a clinically meaningful reduction). The data shown in Table 7–42 were observed in the trial.

Here we have three independent comparison groups and a discrete (dichotomous) outcome variable. We want to test whether there is a difference in the proportions of patients reporting a meaningful reduction in pain among the three treatments, and we will run the test using the five-step approach.

Step 1: Set up hypotheses and determine the level of significance.

H_0: Treatment and reduction in pain are independent,

H_1: H_0 is false,

$\alpha = 0.05$.

Step 2: Select the appropriate test statistic.
The formula for the test statistic is in Table 7–36 and is given as

$$\chi^2 = \sum \frac{(O - E)^2}{E}.$$

The condition for appropriate use of the preceding test statistic is that each expected frequency is at least five. In Step 4, we will compute the expected frequencies and we will ensure that the condition is met.

Step 3: Set up the decision rule.
The row variable is the treatment and there are three considered here ($r = 3$). The column variable is the outcome and two responses are considered ($c = 2$). For this test, df $= (3 - 1)(2 - 1) = 2(1) = 2$. For df $= 2$ and a 5% level of significance, the appropriate critical value from Table 3 in the Appendix is 5.99, and the decision rule is

$$\text{Reject } H_0 \text{ if } \chi^2 \geq 5.99.$$

Step 4: Compute the test statistic.
We now compute the expected frequencies using the formula,

$$\text{Expected cell frequency} = \frac{\text{Row total} \times \text{column total}}{N}.$$

The expected frequencies are shown in Table 7–43.

The test statistic is computed as

$$\chi^2 = \frac{(23 - 21.3)^2}{21.3} + \frac{(27 - 28.7)^2}{28.7} + \frac{(30 - 21.3)^2}{21.3} +$$
$$\frac{(20 - 28.7)^2}{28.7} + \frac{(11 - 21.3)^2}{21.3} + \frac{(39 - 28.7)^2}{28.7},$$

$$\chi^2 = 0.14 + 0.10 + 3 + 2.64 + 4.98 + 3.70 = 15.11.$$

Step 5: Conclusion.
We reject H_0 because $15.11 \geq 5.99$. We have statistically significant evidence at $\alpha = 0.05$ to show that H_0 is false, or that there is a difference in the proportions of patients reporting a

TABLE 7–43 Expected Frequencies

	Meaningful Reduction (3+ Points)	No Meaningful Reduction (< 3 Points)	Total
New pain reliever	21.3	28.7	50
Higher dose of new pain reliever	21.3	28.7	50
Standard pain reliever	21.3	28.7	50
Total	64	86	150

meaningful reduction in pain among the three treatments. Using Table 3 in the Appendix, we can approximate the p-value. We need to look at critical values for smaller levels of significance for df = 2. Using Table 3 in the Appendix, the *p*-value is $p < 0.005$.

What is the nature of the observed differences in treatments?

7.10 SUMMARY

In this chapter, we presented hypothesis testing techniques. Tests of hypothesis involve several steps, including specifying the null and alternative or research hypothesis, selecting and computing an appropriate test statistic, setting up a decision rule, and drawing a conclusion. There are many details to consider in hypothesis testing. The first is to determine the appropriate test. We discussed z, t, χ^2, and F tests here for different applications. The appropriate test depends on the distribution of the outcome variable (continuous, dichotomous, or discrete), the number of comparison groups (one, two, or more than two), and whether the comparison groups are independent or dependent. Table 7–44 summarizes the different tests of hypothesis discussed here.

Once the type of test is determined, the details of the test must be specified. Specifically, the null and research hypotheses must be clearly stated. The null hypothesis always reflects the "no change" or "no difference" situation. The alternative or research hypothesis reflects the investigator's belief. The investigator might hypothesize that a parameter (e.g., a mean, proportion, difference in means or proportions) will increase, will decrease, or will be different under specific conditions (sometimes the conditions are different experimental conditions and other times the conditions are defined by participant attributes). Once the hypotheses are specified, data are collected and summarized. The appropriate test is then conducted according to the five-step

approach. If the test leads to rejection of the null hypothesis, an approximate *p*-value is computed to summarize the significance of the findings. When tests of hypothesis are conducted using statistical computing packages, exact *p*-values are computed. Because the statistical tables in this textbook are limited, we can only approximate *p*-values. If the test fails to reject the null hypothesis, then a weaker concluding statement is made.

In hypothesis testing, there are two types of errors that can be committed. A Type I error occurs when a test incorrectly rejects the null hypothesis. This is referred to as a false positive result, and the probability that this occurs is equal to the level of significance, α. The investigator chooses the level of significance and purposely chooses a small value, such as $\alpha = 0.05$, to control the probability of committing a Type I error. A Type II error occurs when a test fails to reject the null hypothesis when, in fact, it is false. The probability that this occurs is equal to β. Unfortunately, the investigator cannot specify β because it depends on several factors, including the sample size (smaller samples have higher β), the level of significance and the difference in the parameter under the null and alternative hypothesis. (For more details, see D'Agostino, Sullivan, and Beiser.[5])

We noted in several examples the relationship between confidence intervals and tests of hypothesis. While the approaches are somewhat different, they are clearly related. It is possible to draw a conclusion about statistical significance by examining a confidence interval. For example, if a 95% confidence interval does not contain the null value (e.g., 0 when analyzing a mean difference or risk difference, 1 when analyzing relative risks or odds ratios), then we can conclude that a two-sided test of hypothesis would reject the null hypothesis at $\alpha = 0.05$. It is important to note that the correspondence between a confidence interval and a test of hypothesis relates to a two-sided test, and that the confidence level corresponds to a specific two-sided level of significance (e.g., 95% to $\alpha = 0.05$, 90% to $\alpha = 0.10$, and so on). The exact significance of the test, the *p*-value, can only be determined using the hypothesis testing approach.

7.11 PRACTICE PROBLEMS

1. A clinical trial evaluated a new compound designed to improve wound healing in trauma patients. The new compound was compared against a placebo. After treatment for 5 days with the new compound or placebo, the extent of wound healing was measured and the data are shown in Table 7–45. Is there a difference in the extent of wound healing by

TABLE 7-44 Summary of Key Formulas

Outcome Variable, Number of Groups: Null Hypothesis	Test Statistic*
Continuous outcome, one sample: $H_0: \mu = \mu_0$	$z = \dfrac{\overline{X} - \mu_0}{s/\sqrt{n}}$
Continuous outcome, two independent samples: $H_0: \mu_1 = \mu_2$	$z = \dfrac{\overline{X}_1 - \overline{X}_2}{S_p\sqrt{1/n_1 + 1/n_2}}$
Continuous outcome, two matched samples: $H_0: \mu_d = 0$	$z = \dfrac{\overline{X}_d - \mu_d}{s_d/\sqrt{n}}$
Continuous outcome, more than two independent samples: $H_0: \mu_1 = \mu_2 = \ldots = \mu_k$	$F = \dfrac{\sum n_j (\overline{X}_j - \overline{X})^2/(k-1)}{\sum\sum(X - \overline{X}_j)^2/(N-k)} = \dfrac{MSB}{MSE}$
Dichotomous outcome, one sample: $H_0: p = p_0$	$Z = \dfrac{\hat{p}_1 - p_0}{\sqrt{\dfrac{p_0(1-p_0)}{n}}}$
Dichotomous outcome, two independent samples: $H_0: p_1 = p_2$ RD = 0, RR = 1, OR = 1	$z = \dfrac{\hat{p}_1 - \hat{p}_2}{\sqrt{\hat{p}(1-\hat{p})\left(1/n_1 + 1/n_2\right)}}$
Discrete outcome, one sample: $H_0: p_1 = p_{10}, p_2 = p_{20}, \ldots, p_k = p_{k0}$	$\chi^2 = \sum \dfrac{(O-E)^2}{E}$, df = $k - 1$
Discrete outcome, two or more independent samples: H_0: Outcome and groups are independent	$\chi^2 = \sum \dfrac{(O-E)^2}{E}$, df = $(r-1)(c-1)$

*See Table 7–4, 7–11, and 7–14 for alternative formulas that are appropriate for small samples.

treatment? Run the appropriate test at a 5% level of significance. (Hint: Are treatment and the percent of wound healing independent?)

2. Use the data in Problem 1 and pool the data across the treatments into one sample of size $n = 250$. Use the pooled data to test whether the distribution of the percent of wound healing is approximately normal. Specifically, use the following distribution: 30%, 40%, 20%, and 10%, and $\alpha = 0.05$ to run the appropriate test.

3. Table 7–46 displays descriptive statistics on the subjects involved in the study described in Problem 1. Are any of the characteristics significantly different between groups? Justify briefly. (Hint: No calculations, just an interpretation.)

4. An investigator hypothesizes that cholesterol levels in children might be affected by educating their parents on proper nutrition and exercise. A sample of 40 families with a child between the ages of 10 to 15 who has been diagnosed with high cholesterol

TABLE 7-45 Wound Healing by Treatment

	Percent Wound Healing			
Treatment	0–25	26–50	51–75	76–100
New compound ($n = 125$)	15	37	32	41
Placebo ($n = 125$)	36	45	34	10

TABLE 7–46 Descriptive Statistics by Treatment

	New Compound	Placebo	*p*-value
Mean age (years)	47.2	46.1	0.7564
Men (%)	44	59	0.0215
Mean educational level (years)	13.1	14.2	0.6898
Mean annual income	$36,560	$37,470	0.3546
Mean body mass index (BMI)	24.7	25.1	0.0851

TABLE 7–47 Fetal Heart Rate by Position

Back	Side	Sitting	Standing
20	21	24	26
24	23	25	25
26	25	27	28
21	24	28	29
19	16	24	25
Mean = 22.0	Mean = 21.8	Mean = 25.6	Mean = 26.6

agree to participate in the study. All parents are provided educational information on nutrition and exercise. After following the prescribed program, their child's total cholesterol level is measured. The childrens' mean cholesterol level is 175 with a standard deviation of 19.5. Is there significant evidence of a reduction in total cholesterol in the children? Run the appropriate test at the 5% level of significance and assume that the null value for total cholesterol is 191.

5. An experiment is designed to investigate the impact of different positions of the mother on fetal heart rate. Fetal heart rate is measured by ultrasound in beats per minute. The study included 20 women who were assigned to one position and had the fetal heart rate measured in that position. Each woman was between 28 and 32 weeks gestation. The data are shown in Table 7–47. Is there a significant difference in mean fetal heart rates by position? Run the test at a 5% level of significance.

6. A clinical trial is conducted comparing a new pain reliever for arthritis to a placebo. Participants are randomly assigned to receive the new treatment or

a placebo and the outcome is pain relief within 30 minutes. The data are shown in Table 7–48 Is there a significant difference in the proportions of patients reporting pain relief? Run the test at a 5% level of significance.

7. A clinical trial is planned to compare an experimental medication designed to lower blood pressure to a placebo. Before starting the trial, a pilot study is conducted involving seven participants. The objective of the study is to assess how systolic blood pressures change over time if left untreated. Systolic blood pressures are measured at baseline and again 4 weeks later. Is there a statistically

TABLE 7–48 Pain Relief by Treatment

	Pain Relief	No Pain Relief
New medication	44	76
Placebo	21	99

TABLE 7–49 Outcomes by Treatment

	Experimental (n = 100)	Placebo (n = 100)
Mean (SD) systolic blood pressure	120.2 (15.4)	131.4 (18.9)
Hypertensive (%)	14	22
Side effects (%)	6	8

TABLE 7–50 Hypertensive Status by Treatment

	Site 1	Site 2	Site 3
Hypertensive	10	14	12
Not hypertensive	68	56	40

significant difference in blood pressures over time? Run the test at a 5% level of significance.

Baseline: 120 145 130 160 152 143 126

4 Weeks: 122 142 135 158 155 140 130

8. The main trial in Problem 7 is conducted and involves a total of 200 patients. Patients are enrolled and randomized to receive either the experimental medication or the placebo. The data shown in Table 7–49 are collected at the end of the study after 6 weeks on the assigned treatment.
   a. Test if there is a significant difference in mean systolic blood pressures between groups using $\alpha = 0.05$.
   b. Test if there is a significant difference in the proportions of hypertensive patients between groups using $\alpha = 0.05$.

9. Suppose in the trial described in Problem 8 that patients were recruited from three different clinical sites. Use the data in Table 7–50 to test if there is a difference in the proportions of hypertensive patients across clinical sites. Run the test at a 5% level of significance.

10. A clinical trial is conducted to compare an experimental medication to a placebo to reduce the symptoms of asthma. Two hundred participants are enrolled in the study and randomized to receive either the experimental medication or a placebo. The primary outcome is self-reported reduction of symptoms. Among 100 participants who received the experimental medication, 38 reported a reduction of symptoms as compared to 21 participants of 100 assigned to placebo. Test if there is a significant difference in the proportions of participants reporting a reduction of symptoms between the experimental and placebo groups. Use $\alpha = 0.05$.

11. Suppose more detail was recorded in the primary outcome in the clinical trial described in Problem 10. The data are shown in Table 7–51. Is there a difference in the change in symptoms by the treatment group? Run the appropriate test at a 5% level of significance.

12. Suppose a secondary outcome was recorded in the trial described in Problem 10 reflecting asthma symptom severity measured on a scale of 0 to 100, with higher scores indicating more severe symptoms. In the participants who received the experimental medication, the mean symptom score was 74 with a standard deviation of 5.6, and in the placebo group, the mean symptom score was 85 with a standard deviation of 6.0. Is there a significant difference in mean symptom scores between groups? Run the appropriate test at a 5% level of significance.

13. Recent recommendations suggest 60 minutes of physical activity per day. A sample of 50 adults in a study of cardiovascular risk factors report exercising a mean

TABLE 7–51 Change in Symptoms by Treatment

Treatment	Change in Symptoms				
	Much Worse	Worse	No Change	Better	Much Better
Experimental	10	17	35	28	10
Placebo	12	25	42	12	9

TABLE 7–52 Systolic Blood Pressure by Treatment

Standard Treatment	Placebo	New Treatment
124	134	114
111	143	117
133	148	121
125	142	124
128	150	122
115	160	128

TABLE 7–53 Cholesterol Levels by Treatment

Diet Program	Sample Size	Mean Cholesterol	Std Dev Cholesterol
Low-carbohydrate	50	225.4	24.5
Conventional	75	203.8	21.6

of 38 minutes per day with a standard deviation of 19 minutes. Based on the sample data, is the physical activity significantly less than recommended? Run the appropriate test at a 5% level of significance.

14. Suppose a hypertension trial is mounted and 18 participants are randomly assigned to one of three comparison treatments. Each participant takes the assigned medication and their systolic blood pressure is recorded after 6 months on the assigned treatment. The data are shown in Table 7–52. Is there a difference in mean systolic blood pressure among treatments? Run the appropriate test at $\alpha = 0.05$.

15. A study is conducted to compare mean cholesterol levels for individuals following a low-carbohydrate diet for at least 6 months to individuals following a conventional (low-fat, low-calorie) diet for at least 6 months. The data are summarized in Table 7–53. Test if there is a significant difference in mean cholesterol levels between the diet programs using a 5% level of significance.

16. Another outcome variable in the study described in Problem 15 is hypercholesterolemia, defined as total cholesterol over 220. Among the individuals who followed the low-carbohydrate diet, 56% were

hypercholesterolemic, and among the individuals who followed the conventional diet, 40% were hypercholesterolemic. Test if there is a significant difference in the proportions using a 5% level of significance.

17. Table 7–54 compares background characteristics of the participants involved in the study described in Problem 15. Are there any statistically significant differences in patient characteristics between the different diet programs? Justify briefly.

18. Suppose the results of the analyses in Problem 15 through Problem 17 are reported and criticized because the participants were not randomized to different diets, and that there may be other factors associated with changes in cholesterol. A third study is run to attempt to estimate the effect of the low-carbohydrate diet on cholesterol levels. In the third study, participants' cholesterol levels are measured before starting the program and then again after 6 months on the program. The data are shown below:

Before Program	210	230	190	215	260	200

After 6 Months	215	240	190	200	280	210

Is there a significant increase in cholesterol after 6 months on the low-carbohydrate program? Run the appropriate test at a 5% level of significance.

TABLE 7–54 Background Characteristics by Treatment

	Low Carbohydrate (n = 50)	Conventional (n = 75)	p-value
Mean age (years)	52.1	53.4	0.7564
Men (%)	42	34	0.0145
Mean educational level (years)	15.3	12.9	0.0237
Mean family income	$39,540	$47,980	0.0576

TABLE 7–55 Weight Reduction by Treatment

	A	B	C	Placebo
Mean (SD) weight reduction	6.4 (4.1)	8.9 (4.0)	2.2 (3.9)	2.5 (4.3)

19. Suppose a new study is conducted to compare three new appetite suppressants (A, B, and C) to a placebo in terms of their effects on weight reduction. A total of 80 participants are involved and they are randomly assigned to the comparison groups in equal numbers. The outcome of interest is weight reduction, measured in pounds. The data shown in Table 7–55 are observed after 3 months on treatment. Is there a significant difference in mean weight reduction among the four treatments? Use a 5% level of significance. (Hint: SST = 4520.)

20. The mean lifetime for cardiac stents is 8.9 years. A medical device company has implemented some improvements in the manufacturing process and hypothesizes that the lifetime is now longer. A study of 40 new devices reveals a mean lifetime of 9.7 years with a standard deviation of 3.4 years. Is there statistical evidence of a prolonged lifetime of the stents? Run the test at a 5% level of significance.

REFERENCES

1. Ogden, C.L., Fryar, C.D., Carroll, M.D., and Flegal, K.M. "Mean body weight, height, and body mass index, United States 1960–2002." *Advance Data from Vital and Health Statistics* 2004; 347.

2. National Center for Health Statistics. *Health, United States, 2005 with Chartbook on Trends in the Health of Americans.* Hyattsville, MD: U.S. Government Printing Office, 2005.

3. Agresti, A. *Categorical Data Analysis* (2nd ed.). New York: John Wiley & Sons, 2002.

4. StatXact Version 7© 2006 by Cytel, Inc., Cambridge, MA.

5. D'Agostino, R.B., Sullivan, L.M., and Beiser, A. *Introductory Applied Biostatistics.* Belmont, CA: Duxbury-Brooks/Cole, 2004.

6. Rosner, B. *Fundamentals of Biostatistics.* Belmont, CA: Duxbury-Brooks/Cole, 2006.

7. SAS version 9.1© 2002–2003 by SAS Insitute, Inc., Cary, NC.

8. Glantz, S.A. and Slinker, B.K. *Primer of Applied Regression and Analysis of Variance.* New York: McGraw-Hill, 2001.

9. National Osteoporosis Foundation. Available at: http://www.nof.org.

10. Snedecor, G.W. and Cochran, W.G. *Statistical Methods.* Ames, IA: Iowa State University Press, 1980.

CHAPTER 8

Power and Sample Size Determination

In Chapter 6 and Chapter 7, we presented techniques for estimation and hypothesis testing, respectively. In Chapter 6, we saw that confidence interval estimates based on larger samples had smaller margins of error. In Chapter 7, we saw that tests of hypothesis based on larger samples were more likely to detect small increases, decreases, or differences in the parameter of interest. Larger samples produce more precise analyses. However, there is a point at which a larger sample size does not substantially improve the precision in the analysis.

Studies should be designed to include a sufficient number of participants to adequately address the research question. Realizing at the end of a study that the sample was simply too small to answer the research question is wasteful in terms of participant and investigator time, resources to conduct the assessments, analytic efforts, and so on. It can also be viewed as unethical as participants may have been put at risk as part of a study that was unable to answer an important question. Alternatively, studies should not be too large because again resources can be wasted and some participants may be unnecessarily placed at risk.

A critically important aspect of study design is determining the appropriate sample size to answer the research question. There are formulas that can be used to estimate the sample size needed to produce a confidence interval estimate with a specified margin of error, or to ensure that a test of hypothesis has a high probability of detecting a meaningful difference in the parameter. Ideally, these formulas are used to generate estimates of the sample size needed to answer the study question before any data are collected.

The formulas we present here generate the sample sizes required to satisfy statistical criteria. In many studies, the sample size is determined by financial or logistical constraints. For example, suppose a study is proposed to evaluate a new screening test for Down Syndrome. Suppose that the screening test is based on the analysis of a blood sample taken from women early in pregnancy. To evaluate the properties of the screening test (e.g., the sensitivity and specificity), each pregnant woman will be asked to provide a blood sample and in addition to undergo an amniocentesis. The amniocentesis is included as the gold standard, and the plan is to compare the results of the screening test to the results of the amniocentesis. Suppose that the collection and processing of the blood sample costs $250 per participant and that the amniocentesis costs $900 per participant. These financial constraints alone might substantially limit the number of women who can be enrolled. Just as it is important to consider both statistical and practical issues in interpreting the results of a statistical analysis, it is also important to weigh both statistical and logistical issues in determining the sample size for an analysis. Our focus here is on statistical considerations. Investigators must evaluate whether the sample size determined to be sufficient from a statistical standpoint is realistic and feasible.

8.1 ISSUES IN ESTIMATING SAMPLE SIZE FOR CONFIDENCE INTERVALS ESTIMATES

In Chapter 6, we presented confidence intervals for various parameters—e.g., μ, p, $(\mu_1 - \mu_2)$, μ_d, $(p_1 - p_2)$. Confidence intervals for every parameter take the following general form:

$$\text{Point estimate} \pm \text{Margin of error.}$$

In Chapter 6, when we introduced the concept of confidence intervals, we derived the expression for the confidence interval for μ as

$$\overline{X} \pm z \frac{\sigma}{\sqrt{n}}.$$

The point estimate for the population mean is the sample mean and the margin of error is $z \sigma / \sqrt{n}$. In planning studies, we want to determine the sample size needed to ensure that the margin of error is sufficiently small to be informative. For example, suppose we want to estimate the mean weight of female college students. We conduct a study and generate a 95% confidence interval as 125 ± 40 lbs, or 85 to 165 lbs. The margin of error is so wide that the confidence interval is uninformative. To be informative, an investigator might want the margin of error to be no more than 5 or 10 lbs (meaning that the 95% confidence interval would have a width—lower limit to upper limit—of 10 or 20 lbs). To determine the sample size needed, the investigator must specify the desired margin of error. It is important to note that this is not a statistical issue but a clinical or a practical one. The sample size needed also depends on the outcome variable under consideration. For example, suppose we want to estimate the mean birth weight of infants born to mothers who smoke cigarettes during pregnancy. Birth weights in infants clearly have a much more restricted range than weights of female college students. Therefore, we would probably want to generate a confidence interval for the mean birth weight that has a margin of error not exceeding 1 or 2 lbs.

The margin of error in the one sample confidence interval for μ can be written as

$$E = z \frac{\sigma}{\sqrt{n}}.$$

We want to determine the sample size, n, that ensures that the margin of error, E, does not exceed a specified value. We can take the preceding formula and, with some algebra, solve for n:

$$n = \left(\frac{z\sigma}{E} \right)^2.$$

This formula generates the sample size, n, required to ensure that the margin of error, E, does not exceed a specified value. To solve for n, we must input z, σ, and E. z is the value from Table 1B in the Appendix for the desired confidence level (e.g., $z = 1.96$ for 95% confidence) and E is the margin of error that the investigator specifies as important from a practical standpoint. The last input is σ, the standard deviation of the outcome of interest. Sometimes it is difficult to estimate σ. When we use the prior sample size formula (or one of the

other formulas that we will present in the sections that follow), we are planning a study to estimate the unknown mean of a particular outcome variable in a population. It is unlikely that we would know the standard deviation of that variable. In sample size computations, investigators often use a value for the standard deviation from a previous study or a study done in a different but comparable population.

The sample size computation is not an application of statistical inference and therefore it is reasonable to use an appropriate estimate for the standard deviation. The estimate can be derived from a different study that was reported in the literature; some investigators perform a small pilot study to estimate the standard deviation. A pilot study usually involves a small number of participants (e.g., $n = 10$) who are selected by convenience as opposed to random sampling. Data from the participants in the pilot study can be used to compute sample standard deviation, s, which serves as a good estimate for σ in the sample size formula. Regardless of how the estimate of the variability of the outcome is derived, it should always be conservative (i.e., as large as is reasonable), so that the resultant sample size is not too small.

The formula for n produces the minimum sample size to ensure that the margin of error in a confidence interval will not exceed E. In planning studies, investigators should also consider attrition or loss to follow-up. Sample size formulas for confidence intervals give the number of participants needed with complete data to ensure that the margin of error in the confidence interval does not exceed E. We will illustrate how attrition is addressed in planning studies through examples in the following sections.

8.1.1 Sample Size for One Sample, Continuous Outcome

In studies where the plan is to estimate the mean of a continuous outcome variable in a single population, the formula for determining sample size is

$$n = \left(\frac{z\sigma}{E} \right)^2$$

where z is the value from the standard normal distribution reflecting the confidence level that will be used (e.g., $z = 1.96$ for 95%), σ is the standard deviation of the outcome variable, and E is the desired margin of error. The preceding formula generates the minimum number of subjects required to ensure that the margin of error in the confidence interval for μ does not exceed E.

Example 8.1. An investigator wants to estimate the mean systolic blood pressure in children with congenital heart disease who are between the ages of 3 and 5 years old. How many children should be enrolled in the study?

To determine the requisite sample size, the investigator must provide the necessary inputs for the sample size formula,

$$n = \left(\frac{z\sigma}{E}\right)^2.$$

Suppose that a 95% confidence interval is planned; thus, $z = 1.96$. The investigator must then specify the margin of error. Suppose the investigator decides that a margin of error of 5 units will be sufficiently precise. The final input is the standard deviation of systolic blood pressure in children with congenital heart disease. A suitable estimate might be found in the literature. There are certainly data on systolic blood pressure in the Framingham Heart Study but those data might not be sufficiently comparable as they are based on adults, most of whom are probably free of congenital heart disease.

Suppose the investigators conduct a literature search and find that the standard deviation of systolic blood pressures in children with other cardiac defects is between 15 and 20. To estimate the sample size, we consider the larger standard deviation. This will produce the most conservative (largest) sample size,

$$n = \left(\frac{z\sigma}{E}\right)^2 = \left(\frac{1.96 \times 20}{5}\right)^2 = 61.5.$$

To ensure that the 95% confidence interval estimate of the mean systolic blood pressure in children between the ages of 3 and 5 with congenital heart disease is within 5 units of the true mean, a sample of size 62 is needed. Note that we always round up, as the sample size formulas always generate the minimum number of subjects needed to ensure the specified precision.

Had we assumed a standard deviation of 15, the sample size would have been $n = 35$. Because the estimates of the standard deviation were derived from studies of children with other cardiac defects, it would be advisable to use the larger standard deviation and plan for a study with 62 children. Selecting the smaller sample size could potentially produce a confidence interval estimate with a much larger margin of error.

Example 8.2. An investigator wants to estimate the mean birth weight of infants born full term (approximately 40 weeks gestation) to mothers who are 19 years of age and under. The mean birth weight of infants born full term to mothers 20 years of age and older is 3510 g with a standard deviation of 385 g.[1] How many women 19 years of age or younger must be enrolled in the study to ensure that a 95% confidence interval estimate of the mean birth weight of their infants has a margin of error not exceeding 100 g?

$$n = \left(\frac{z\sigma}{E}\right)^2 = \left(\frac{1.96 \times 385}{100}\right)^2 = 56.9.$$

To ensure that the 95% confidence interval estimate of the mean birth weight is within 100 g of the true mean, a sample of size 57 is needed. In planning the study, the investigator must consider the fact that some women may deliver prematurely. If women are enrolled into the study during pregnancy, then more than 57 women will need to be enrolled so that after excluding those who deliver prematurely, 57 with complete outcome information will be available for analysis. For example, if 5% of the women are expected to delivery prematurely (i.e., 95% will deliver full term), then 60 women must be enrolled to ensure that 57 deliver full term. The number of women who must be enrolled, N, is computed as

$$N \text{ (number to enroll)} \times (\% \text{ retained}) = \text{Desired sample size},$$

$$N \times 0.95 = 57,$$

$$N = \frac{57}{0.95} = 60.$$

8.1.2 Sample Size for One Sample, Dichotomous Outcome

In studies where the plan is to estimate the proportion of successes in a dichotomous outcome variable in a single population, the formula for determining sample size is

$$n = p(1-p)\left(\frac{z}{E}\right)^2.$$

where z is the value from the standard normal distribution reflecting the confidence level that will be used (e.g., $z = 1.96$ for 95%), E is the desired margin of error, and p is the proportion of successes in the population. Here we are planning a study to generate a 95% confidence interval for the unknown population proportion, p, and the formula to estimate the sample size needed requires p! Obviously, this is a circular problem—if we knew the proportion of successes in the population, then a study would not be necessary. To estimate the sample size, we need an approximate value of p. The range of p is 0 to 1 and therefore the range of $p(1 - p)$ is 0 to 1. The value of p that maximizes $p(1 - p)$ is $p = 0.5$. Thus, if there is no information available to approximate p, then $p = 0.5$ can be used to generate the most conservative, or largest, sample size.

Example 8.3. An investigator wants to estimate the proportion of freshmen at his university who currently smoke cigarettes (i.e., the prevalence of smoking). How many freshmen should be involved in the study to ensure that a 95% confidence interval estimate of the proportion of freshmen who smoke is within 5% of the true proportion?

If we have no information on the proportion of freshmen who smoke, we use the following to estimate the sample size:

$$n = p(1-p)\left(\frac{z}{E}\right)^2 = 0.5(1-0.5)\left(\frac{1.96}{0.05}\right)^2 = 384.2.$$

To ensure that the 95% confidence interval estimate of the proportion of freshmen who smoke is within 5% of the true proportion, a sample of size 385 is needed.

Suppose that a similar study was conducted two years ago and found that the prevalence of smoking was 27% among freshmen. If the investigator believes that this is a reasonable estimate of prevalence two years later, it can be used to plan the study:

$$n = p(1-p)\left(\frac{z}{E}\right)^2 = 0.27(1-0.27)\left(\frac{1.96}{0.05}\right)^2 = 302.9.$$

To ensure that the 95% confidence interval estimate of the proportion of freshmen who smoke is within 5% of the true proportion, a sample of size 303 is needed. Notice that this sample size is substantially smaller than the one estimated previously. Having some information on the magnitude of the proportion in the population will always produce a sample size that is less than or equal to the one based on a population proportion of 0.5. However, the estimate must be realistic.

Example 8.4. An investigator wants to estimate the prevalence of breast cancer among women who are between 40 and 45 years of age living in Boston. How many women must be involved in the study to ensure that the estimate is precise? National data suggest that 1 in 235 women are diagnosed with breast cancer by age 40.[2] This translates to a proportion of 0.0043 (0.43%), or a prevalence of 43 per 10,000 women. Suppose the investigator wants the estimate to be within 10 per 10,000 women with 95% confidence. The sample size is computed as

$$n = p(1-p)\left(\frac{z}{E}\right)^2 =$$

$$0.0043(1-0.0043)\left(\frac{1.96}{0.0010}\right)^2 = 16,447.8.$$

A sample of size $n = 16,448$ will ensure that a 95% confidence interval estimate of the prevalence of breast cancer is within 0.0010 (or within 10 women per 10,000) of its true value.

This is a situation where investigators might decide that a sample of this size is not feasible. Suppose that the investigators thought a sample of size 5000 would be reasonable from a practical point of view. How precisely can we estimate the prevalence with a sample of size $n = 5000$? Recall from Chapter 6 that the confidence interval formula to estimate prevalence is

$$\hat{p} \pm z\sqrt{\frac{\hat{p}(1-\hat{p})}{n}}.$$

Assuming that the prevalence of breast cancer in the sample will be close to that based on national data, we would expect the margin of error to be approximately equal to

$$z\sqrt{\frac{\hat{p}(1-\hat{p})}{n}} = 1.96\sqrt{\frac{0.0043(1-0.0043)}{5000}} = 0.0018.$$

With $n = 5000$ women, a 95% confidence interval would be expected to have a margin of error of 0.0018 (or 18 per 10,000). The investigators must decide if this would be sufficiently precise to answer the research question. Note that this calculation is based on the assumption that the prevalence of breast cancer in Boston is similar to that reported nationally. This may or may not be a reasonable assumption. In fact, it is the objective of the current study to estimate the prevalence in Boston. With input from clinical investigators and biostatisticians, the research team must carefully evaluate the implications of selecting a sample of size $n = 5000$, $n = 16,448$, or any size in between.

8.1.3 Sample Sizes for Two Independent Samples, Continuous Outcome

In studies where the plan is to estimate the difference in means between two independent populations, the formula for determining the sample sizes required in each comparison group is

$$n_i = 2\left(\frac{z\sigma}{E}\right)^2$$

where n_i is the sample size required in each group ($i = 1, 2$), z is the value from the standard normal distribution reflecting the confidence level that will be used (e.g., $z = 1.96$ for 95%), and E is the desired margin of error. σ again reflects the standard deviation of the outcome variable. Recall from Chapter 6 that when we generated a confidence interval estimate for the difference in means, we used S_p (the pooled estimate of the common standard deviation) as a measure of variability in the outcome, where S_p is computed as

$$S_p = \sqrt{\frac{(n_1-1)s_1^2 + (n_2-1)s_2^2}{n_1 + n_2 - 2}}.$$

If data are available on the variability of the outcome in each comparison group, then S_p can be computed and used in the sample size formula. However, it is more often the case that data on the variability of the outcome are available from only one group, often the untreated (e.g., placebo control) or unexposed group. When planning a clinical trial to investigate a new drug or procedure, data are often available from other trials that involved a placebo or an active control group (i.e., a standard medication or treatment given for the condition under study). The standard deviation of the outcome variable measured in patients assigned to the placebo, control, or un-exposed group can be used to plan a future trial. This situation is illustrated below.

Note that the formula shown here generates sample size estimates for samples of equal size. If a study is planned where different numbers of patients will be assigned or different numbers of patients will comprise the comparison groups, then alternative formulas can be used. Interested readers can see Howell for more details.[3]

Example 8.5. An investigator wants to plan a clinical trial to evaluate the efficacy of a new drug designed to increase HDL cholesterol (the "good" cholesterol). The plan is to enroll participants and to randomly assign them to receive either the new drug or a placebo. HDL cholesterol will be measured in each participant after 12 weeks on the assigned treatment. Based on prior experience with similar trials, the investigator expects that 10% of all participants will be lost to follow up or will drop out of the study. A 95% confidence interval will be estimated to quantify the difference in mean HDL levels between patients taking the new drug as compared to the placebo. The investigator would like the margin of error to be no more than 3 units. How many patients should be recruited into the study?

The sample sizes (i.e., the number of participants who must receive the new drug and the number who must receive a placebo) are computed as

$$n_i = 2\left(\frac{z\sigma}{E}\right)^2.$$

A major issue is determining the variability in the outcome of interest (σ), here the standard deviation of HDL cholesterol. To plan this study, we can use data from the Framingham Heart Study. In participants who attended the seventh examination of the Offspring Study and were not on treatment for high cholesterol, the standard deviation of HDL cholesterol is 17.1. We will use this value and the other inputs to compute the sample sizes:

$$n_i = 2\left(\frac{z\sigma}{E}\right)^2 = 2\left(\frac{1.96 \times 17.1}{3}\right)^2 = 249.6.$$

Samples of size $n_1 = 250$ and $n_2 = 250$ will ensure that the 95% confidence interval for the difference in mean HDL levels will have a margin of error of no more than 3 units. Again, these sample sizes refer to the numbers of participants with complete data. The investigators hypothesized a 10% attrition (or drop-out) rate in both groups. To ensure that a total

sample size of 500 is available at 12 weeks, the investigator needs to recruit more participants to allow for attrition.

N (number to enroll) $\times$ (% retained) = Desired sample size.

$$N \times 0.90 = 500.$$

$$N = \frac{500}{0.90} = 556.$$

The investigator must enroll 556 participants. Each patient will be randomly assigned to receive either the new drug or a placebo; assuming that 10% are lost to follow up, 500 will be available for analysis.

Example 8.6. An investigator wants to compare two diet programs in children who are obese. One diet is a low-fat diet and the other is a low-carbohydrate diet. The plan is to enroll children and weigh them at the start of the study. Each child will then be randomly assigned to either the low-fat or the low-carbohydrate diet. Each child will follow the assigned diet for 8 weeks, at which time they will again be weighed. The number of pounds lost will be computed for each child. Based on data reported from diet trials in adults, the investigator expects that 20% of all children will not complete the study. A 95% confidence interval will be estimated to quantify the difference in weight lost between the two diets, and the investigator would like the margin of error to be no more than 3 lbs. How many children should be recruited into the study?

The sample sizes (i.e., the number of children who must follow the low-fat diet and the number of children who must follow the low-carbohydrate diet) are computed as

$$n_i = 2\left(\frac{z\sigma}{E}\right)^2.$$

Again, the issue is determining the variability in the outcome of interest (σ), here the standard deviation in pounds lost over 8 weeks. To plan this study, investigators use data from adult studies. Suppose one such study compared the same diets in adults and involved 100 participants in each diet group. The study reported a standard deviation in weight lost over 8 weeks on a low-fat diet of 8.4 lbs and a standard deviation in weight lost over 8 weeks on a low-carbohydrate diet of 7.7 lbs. These data can be used to estimate the common standard deviation in weight lost as

$$S_p = \sqrt{\frac{(n_1-1)s_1^2 + (n_2-1)s_2^2}{n_1 + n_2 - 2}} =$$

$$\sqrt{\frac{(100-1)(8.4)^2 + (100-1)(7.7)^2}{100 + 100 - 2}} = 8.1.$$

We will now use this value and the other inputs to compute the sample sizes:

$$n_i = 2\left(\frac{z\sigma}{E}\right)^2 = 2\left(\frac{1.96 \times 8.1}{3}\right)^2 = 56.0.$$

Samples of size $n_1 = 56$ and $n_2 = 56$ will ensure that the 95% confidence interval for the difference in weight lost between diets will have a margin of error of no more than 3 lbs. Again, these sample sizes refer to the numbers of children with complete data. The investigators hypothesized a 20% attrition rate. To ensure that the total sample size of 112 is available at 8 weeks, the investigator needs to recruit more participants to allow for attrition.

$$N \text{ (number to enroll)} \times (\% \text{ retained}) = \text{Desired sample size.}$$

$$N \times 0.80 = 112.$$

$$N = \frac{112}{0.80} = 140.$$

The investigator must enroll 140 children. Each child will be randomly assigned to either the low-fat or low-carbohydrate diet; assuming that 20% are lost to follow up, 112 will be available for analysis.

8.1.4 Sample Size for Matched Samples, Continuous Outcome

In studies where the plan is to estimate the mean difference of a continuous outcome based on matched data, the formula for determining sample size is

$$n = \left(\frac{z\sigma_d}{E}\right)^2$$

where z is the value from the standard normal distribution reflecting the confidence level that will be used (e.g., $z = 1.96$ for 95%), E is the desired margin of error, and σ_d is the standard deviation of the difference scores. It is extremely important that the standard deviation of the difference scores (e.g., the differences based on measurements over time, or the differences between matched pairs) is used here to appropriately estimate the sample size.

Example 8.7. Consider again the diet study proposed in Example 8.6. Suppose the investigator is considering an alternative design—a crossover trial. In the crossover trial, each child follows each diet for 8 weeks. At the end of each 8-week period, the weight lost during that period is measured. Children will be randomly assigned to the first diet (i.e., some will follow the low-fat diet first while others will follow the low-carbohydrate diet first). The investigators expect to lose 30% of the participants over the course of the 16 week study. The difference in weight lost on the low-fat diet and the low-carbohydrate diet will be computed for each child, and a confidence interval for the mean difference in weight lost will be computed. How many children are required to ensure that a 95% confidence interval estimate for the mean difference in weight lost has a margin of error of no more than 3 lbs?

To compute the sample size, we need an estimate of the variability in the difference in weight lost between diets as opposed to the variability in weight loss in either diet program, as was required in Example 8.6. Suppose that the standard deviation of the difference in weight loss between a low-fat diet and a low-carbohydrate diet is approximately 9.1 lbs based on a crossover trial conducted in adults. The sample size is computed as

$$n = \left(\frac{z\sigma_d}{E}\right)^2 = \left(\frac{1.96 \times 9.1}{3}\right)^2 = 35.3.$$

To ensure that the 95% confidence interval estimate of the mean difference in weight lost between diets is within 3 lbs of the true mean, a sample of size 36 children with complete data is needed. The investigators hypothesized a 30% attrition rate. To ensure that the total sample size of 36 is available at 16 weeks, the investigator needs to recruit 52 participants to allow for attrition:

$$N \text{ (number to enroll)} \times (\% \text{ retained}) = \text{Desired sample size.}$$

$$N \times 0.70 = 36.$$

$$N = \frac{36}{0.70} = 52.$$

Notice that fewer patients are needed in the crossover trial as compared to the trial with two concurrent or parallel comparison groups considered in Example 8.6. In the crossover trial, each child is given each treatment (diet). Crossover trials can be efficient in terms of sample size. However, the crossover can be challenging in other respects. The crossover trial is problematic when there is loss to follow up. Because each participant contributes data on each treatment, when a participant is lost after completing the first treatment, their data is unusable without information on the second treatment. Diet studies are particularly problematic in terms of participant loss to follow up. Sometimes participants start to lose weight and feel they no longer need the study, and so they drop out. Other participants do not lose weight and become frustrated and drop out. These and other issues must be considered carefully in determining the most appropriate design for any study.

8.1.5 Sample Sizes for Two Independent Samples, Dichotomous Outcome

In studies where the plan is to estimate the difference in proportions between two independent populations (i.e., to estimate the risk difference), the formula for determining the sample sizes required in each comparison group is given as

$$n_i = \left[p_1(1-p_1) + p_2(1-p_2) \right] \left(\frac{z}{E} \right)^2$$

where n_i is the sample size required in each group ($i = 1, 2$), z is the value from the standard normal distribution reflecting the confidence level that will be used (e.g., $z = 1.96$ for 95%), E is the desired margin of error, and p_1 and p_2 are the proportions of successes in each comparison group. Again, here we are planning a study to generate a 95% confidence interval for the difference in unknown proportions, and the formula to estimate the sample sizes needed requires p_1 and p_2. To estimate the sample size, we need approximate values of p_1 and p_2. The values of p_1 and p_2 that maximize the sample sizes are $p_1 = p_2 = 0.5$. Thus, if there is no information available to approximate p_1 and p_2, 0.5 can be used to generate the most conservative, or largest, sample sizes.

Similar to the situation we presented in Section 8.1.3 for two independent samples and a continuous outcome, it may be the case that data are available on the proportion of successes in one group, usually the untreated (e.g., placebo control) or unexposed group. If so, that known proportion can be used for both p_1 and p_2 in the formula shown here.

This formula generates sample size estimates for samples of equal size. If a study is planned where different numbers of patients will be assigned or different numbers of patients will comprise the comparison groups, then alternative formulas can be used. Interested readers can see Fleiss for more details.[4]

Example 8.8. An investigator wants to estimate the impact of smoking during pregnancy on premature delivery. Normal pregnancies last approximately 40 weeks and premature deliveries are those that occur before 37 weeks. The 2005 National Vital Statistics report indicates that approximately 12% of infants are born prematurely in the United States.[5] The investigator plans to collect data through medical record review and generate a 95% confidence interval for the difference in proportions of infants born prematurely to women who smoked during pregnancy as compared to those who did not. How many women should be enrolled in the study to ensure that the 95% confidence interval for the difference in proportions has a margin of error of no more than 4%?

The sample sizes (i.e., numbers of women who smoked and did not smoke during pregnancy) can be computed using the previous formula. National data suggest that 12% of infants are born prematurely. We will use that estimate for both groups in the sample size computation:

$$n_i = \left[p_1(1-p_1) + p_2(1-p_2) \right] \left(\frac{z}{E} \right)^2 =$$

$$\left[0.12(1-0.12) + 0.12(1-0.12) \right] \left(\frac{1.96}{0.04} \right)^2 = 507.1.$$

Samples of size $n_1 = 508$ women who smoked during pregnancy and $n_2 = 508$ women who did not smoke during pregnancy will ensure that the 95% confidence interval for the difference in proportions who deliver prematurely will have a margin of error of no more than 4%. Is attrition an issue here?

Example 8.9. An investigator wants to estimate the impact of smoking on the incidence of prostate cancer. The incidence of prostate cancer by age 70 is approximately 1 in 6 men (17%). A United States study reported that heavy smokers (defined as men smoking more than a pack a day for 40 years) had twice the risk of developing prostate cancer as compared to nonsmokers.[6] An investigator plans to replicate the study in England using a cohort study design. Men who are free of prostate cancer will be enrolled at age 50 and followed for 30 years. The plan is to enroll approximately equal numbers of smokers and nonsmokers in the study and follow them prospectively for the outcome of interest—a diagnosis of prostate cancer. The plan is to generate a 95% confidence interval for the difference in proportions of smoking and nonsmoking men who develop prostate cancer. The study will follow men for 30 years and investigators expect to lose approximately 20% of the participants over the course of the follow-up period. How many men should be enrolled in the study to ensure that the 95% confidence interval for the difference in proportions has a margin of error of no more than 5%?

The sample sizes (i.e., numbers of men who smoke and do not smoke) can be computed using the previous formula. The estimates of the incidence of prostate cancer from the United States study will be used to design the study planned for England (i.e., $p_1 = 0.34$ and $p_2 = 0.17$ are the estimates of prostate cancer in smokers versus nonsmokers, respectively):

$$n_i = \left[p_1(1-p_1) + p_2(1-p_2) \right] \left(\frac{z}{E} \right)^2 =$$

$$\left[0.34(1-0.34) + 0.17(1-0.17) \right] \left(\frac{1.96}{0.05} \right)^2 = 561.6.$$

Samples of size $n_1 = 562$ men who smoke and $n_2 = 562$ men who do not smoke will ensure that the 95% confidence interval for the difference in the incidence of prostate cancer will have a margin of error of no more than 5%.

The sample sizes here refer to the numbers of men with complete data. The investigators hypothesized a 20% attrition rate (in both groups). To ensure that the total sample size of 1124 is available for analysis, the investigator needs to recruit more participants to allow for attrition:

$$N \text{ (number to enroll)} \times (\% \text{ retained}) = \text{Desired sample size}.$$

$$N \times 0.80 = 1,124.$$

$$N = \frac{1124}{0.80} = 1405.$$

The investigator must enroll 1405 men. Because enrollment will be on the basis of smoking status at baseline, the investigator will enroll approximately 703 men who smoke and 703 men who do not.

8.2   ISSUES IN ESTIMATING SAMPLE SIZE FOR HYPOTHESIS TESTING

In Chapter 7, we introduced hypothesis testing techniques for means, proportions, differences in means, and differences in proportions. Whereas each test involved details that were specific to the outcome of interest (continuous, dichotomous, or discrete) and to the number of comparison groups (one, two, or more than two), there were common elements to each test.

For example, in each test of hypothesis there are two errors that can be committed. The first is called a Type I error and refers to the situation where we incorrectly reject H_0 when, in fact, it is true. In the first step of any test of hypothesis, we select a level of significance, α, and

$$\alpha = P(\text{Type I error}) = P(\text{Reject } H_0 \mid H_0 \text{ is true}).$$

Because we purposely select a small value for α, we control the probability of committing a Type I error. The second type of error is called a Type II error and it is defined as the probability we do not reject H_0 when it is false. The probability of a Type II error is denoted β, and

$$\beta = P(\text{Type II error}) = P(\text{Do not reject } H_0 \mid H_0 \text{ is false}).$$

In hypothesis testing, we usually focus on *power*, which is defined as the probability that we reject H_0 when it is false,

$$\text{Power} = 1 - \beta = P(\text{Reject } H_0 \mid H_0 \text{ is false}).$$

Power is the probability that a test correctly rejects a false null hypothesis. A good test is one with low probability of committing a Type I error (i.e., small α) and high power (i.e., small β, high power).

In the following sections, we present formulas to determine the sample size required to ensure that a test has high power. The sample size computations depend on the level of significance, α, the desired power of the test (equivalent to $1 - \beta$), the variability of the outcome, and the effect size. The effect size is the difference in the parameter of interest that represents a clinically meaningful difference. Similar to the margin of error in confidence interval applications, the effect size is determined based on clinical or practical criteria and not statistical criteria. The concept of statistical power can be difficult to grasp. Before presenting the formulas to determine the sample size required to ensure high power in a test, we will first discuss power from a conceptual point of view.

Suppose we want to test the following hypotheses at $\alpha = 0.05$,

$$H_0: \mu = 90,$$

$$H_1: \mu \neq 90.$$

To test the hypotheses, suppose we select a sample of size $n = 100$. For this example, assume that the standard deviation of the outcome is $\sigma = 20$. We compute the sample mean and then must decide whether the sample mean provides evidence to support the research hypothesis or not. This is done by computing a test statistic and comparing the test statistic to an appropriate critical value.

If the null hypothesis is true ($\mu = 90$), then we are likely to select a sample whose mean is close in value to 90. However, it is also possible to select a sample whose mean is much larger or much smaller than 90. Recall from the Central Limit Theorem (see Chapter 5), that for large n (here $n = 100$ is sufficiently large), the distribution of the sample means is approximately normal with a mean of $\mu_{\overline{X}} = \mu = 90$ and a standard deviation of $\sigma_{\overline{X}} = \sigma/\sqrt{n} = 20/\sqrt{100} = 2.0$ If the null hypothesis is true, it is possible to observe any sample mean shown in Figure 8–1, as all are possible under H_0: $\mu = 90$.

When we set up the decision rule for our test of hypotheses, we determine critical values based on $\alpha = 0.05$ and a two-sided test. When we run tests of hypotheses, we usually standardize the data (e.g., convert to z or t) and the critical values are appropriate values from the probability distribution used in the test. To facilitate interpretation, we continue this discussion with $\overline{X}$ as opposed to z. The critical values of $\overline{X}$ for a two-sided test with $\alpha = 0.05$ are 86.08 and 93.92 (these values correspond to -1.96 and 1.96, respectively, on the z scale), so the decision rule is

$$\text{Reject } H_0 \text{ if } \overline{X} \leq 86.08 \text{ or if } \overline{X} \geq 93.92.$$

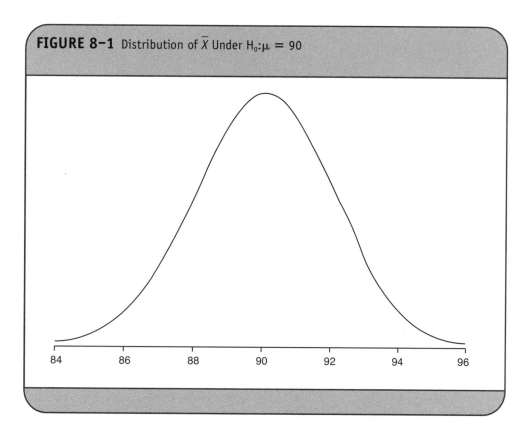

FIGURE 8–1 Distribution of $\bar{X}$ Under $H_0 : \mu = 90$

The rejection region is shown in the tails of Figure 8–2. The areas in the two tails of the curve represent the probability of a Type I error, $\alpha = 0.05$. This concept was discussed in some detail in Chapter 7.

Now suppose that the alternative hypothesis, H_1, is true ($\mu \neq 90$) and that the true mean is actually 94. Figure 8–3 shows the distributions of the sample mean under the null and alternative hypotheses. The values of the sample mean are shown along the horizontal axis.

If the true mean is 94, then the alternative hypothesis is true. In our test, we selected $\alpha = 0.05$ and will reject H_0 if the observed sample mean exceeds 93.92 (focusing on the upper tail of the rejection region for now). The critical value (93.92) is indicated by the vertical line. The probability of a Type II error is denoted β, and

$$\beta = P(\text{Do not reject } H_0 \mid H_0 \text{ is false}).$$

β is shown in Figure 8.3 as the area under the rightmost curve (H_1) to the left of the vertical line (where we do not reject H_0). Power is defined as

$$1 - \beta = P(\text{Reject } H_0 \mid H_0 \text{ is false})$$

and is shown in Figure 8.3 as the area under the rightmost curve (H_1) to the right of the vertical line (where we reject H_0).

We previously noted that β and power were related to α, the variability of the outcome and the effect size. From Figure 8–3 we can see what happens to β and power if we increase α. For example, suppose we increase α to $\alpha = 0.10$. The upper critical value would be 92.56 instead of 93.92. The vertical line would shift to the left, increasing α, decreasing β, and increasing power. Whereas a better test is one with higher power, it is not advisable to increase α as a means to increase power. Nonetheless, there is a direct relationship between α and power (as α increases, so does power).

β and power are also related to the variability of the outcome and to the effect size. The effect size is the difference in the parameter of interest (e.g., μ) that represents a clinically meaningful difference. Figure 8–3 graphically displays α, β, and power when the difference in the mean under the null as compared to the alternative hypothesis is 4 units (i.e., 90 versus 94). Figure 8–4 shows the same components for the situation where the mean under the alternative hypothesis is 98.

Notice that there is much higher power when there is a larger difference between the mean under H_0 as compared to H_1 (i.e., 90 versus 98). A statistical test is much more likely to reject the null hypothesis in favor of the alternative if the true mean is 98 than if the true mean is 94. Notice in Figure 8–4 that there is little overlap in the distributions under the null and alternative hypotheses. If a sample mean of 97 or higher is observed, it is very unlikely that it came from a distribution whose

FIGURE 8–2 Rejection Region for Test $H_0: \mu = 90$ Versus $H_1: \mu \neq 90$ at $\alpha = 0.05$

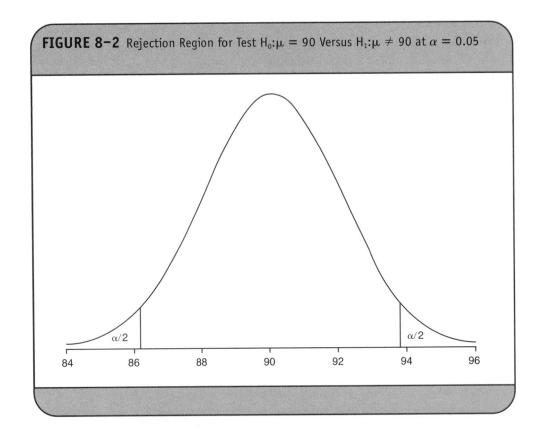

FIGURE 8–3 Distribution of $\bar{X}$ Under $H_0: \mu = 90$ Under $H_1: \mu = 94$

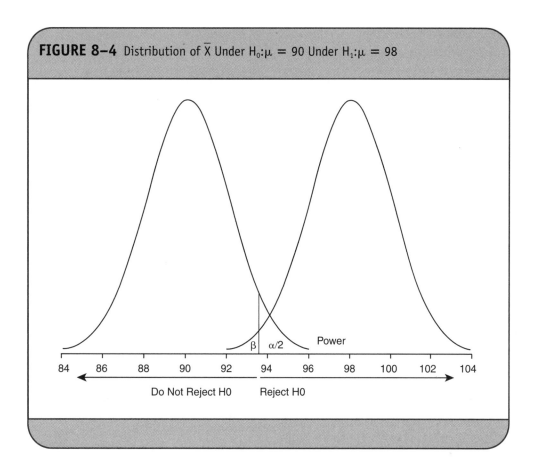

FIGURE 8-4 Distribution of $\overline{X}$ Under $H_0:\mu = 90$ Under $H_1:\mu = 98$

Do Not Reject H0   Reject H0

---

mean is 90. In Figure 8.3, if we observed a sample mean of 93, it would not be as clear as to whether it came from a distribution whose mean is 90 or one whose mean is 94.

In the following sections, we provide formulas to determine the sample size needed to ensure that a test has high power. In designing studies, most people consider power of 80% or 90% (just as we generally use 95% as the confidence level for confidence interval estimates). The inputs for the sample size formulas include the desired power, the level of significance, and the effect size. The effect size is selected to represent a clinically meaningful or practically important difference in the parameter of interest. This will be illustrated in examples that follow.

The formulas we present produce the minimum sample size to ensure that the test of hypothesis will have a specified probability of rejecting the null hypothesis when it is false (i.e., a specified power). In planning studies, investigators again must account for attrition or loss to follow up. The formulas shown produce the number of participants needed with complete data. In the examples, we also illustrate how attrition is addressed in planning studies.

8.2.1 Sample Size for One Sample, Continuous Outcome

In studies where the plan is to perform a test of hypothesis comparing the mean of a continuous outcome variable in a single population to a known mean, the hypotheses of interest are

$$H_0: \mu = \mu_0,$$

$$H_1: \mu \neq \mu_0$$

where μ_0 is the known mean (e.g., a historical control). The formula for determining sample size to ensure that the test has a specified power is

$$n = \left(\frac{z_{1-\alpha/2} + z_{1-\beta}}{\text{ES}}\right)^2$$

where α is the selected level of significance and $z_{1-\alpha/2}$ is the value from the standard normal distribution holding $1-\alpha/2$ below it. For example, if $\alpha = 0.05$, then $1-\alpha/2 = 0.975$ and $z = 1.960$. $1-\beta$ is the selected power and $z_{1-\beta}$ is the value from the standard normal distribution holding $1-\beta$ below it. Sample size estimates for hypothesis testing are often based on achieving 80% or 90% power. The $z_{1-\beta}$ values for these popular scenarios are

$$80\% \text{ power} \qquad z_{0.8} = 0.84$$

$$90\% \text{ power} \qquad z_{0.9} = 1.282$$

ES is the effect size, defined as

$$\text{ES} = \frac{|\mu_1 - \mu_0|}{\sigma},$$

where μ_0 is the mean under H_0, μ_1 is the mean under H_1, and σ is the standard deviation of the outcome of interest. The numerator of the effect size, the absolute value of the difference in means $|\mu_1 - \mu_0|$, represents what is considered a clinically meaningful or practically important difference in means. Similar to the issue we faced when planning studies to estimate confidence intervals, it can sometimes be difficult to estimate the standard deviation. In sample size computations, investigators often use a value for the standard deviation from a previous study or a study performed in a different population. Regardless of how the estimate of the variability of the outcome is derived, it should always be conservative (i.e., as large as is reasonable) so that the resultant sample size will not be too small.

Example 8.10. An investigator hypothesizes that in people free of diabetes, fasting blood glucose—a risk factor for coronary heart disease—is higher in those who drink at least two cups of coffee per day. A cross-sectional study is planned to assess the mean fasting blood glucose levels in people who drink at least two cups of coffee per day. The mean fasting blood glucose level in people free of diabetes is reported as 95.0 mg/dl with a standard deviation of 9.8 mg/dl.[7] If the mean blood glucose level in people who drink at least two cups of coffee per day is 100 mg/dl, this would be important clinically. How many patients should be enrolled in the study to ensure that the power of the test is 80% to detect this difference? A two-sided test will be used with a 5% level of significance.

We first compute the effect size,

$$\text{ES} = \frac{|\mu_1 - \mu_0|}{\sigma} = \frac{|100 - 95|}{9.8} = 0.51.$$

We now substitute the effect size and the appropriate z values for the selected α and power to compute the sample size.

$$n = \left(\frac{z_{1-\alpha/2} + z_{1-\beta}}{\text{ES}}\right)^2 = \left(\frac{1.96 + 0.84}{0.51}\right)^2 = 30.1.$$

A sample of size $n = 31$ will ensure that a two-sided test with $\alpha = 0.05$ has 80% power to detect a 5-mg/dl difference in mean fasting blood glucose levels.

In the planned study, participants will be asked to fast overnight and to provide a blood sample for the analysis of glucose levels. Based on prior experience, the investigators hypothesize that 10% of the participants will fail to fast or will refuse to submit the blood sample (i.e., they will fail to follow the study protocol). Therefore, a total of 35 participants will be enrolled in the study to ensure that 31 are available for analysis:

$$N \text{ (number to enroll)} \times (\% \text{ following protocol}) = \\ \text{Desired sample size}$$

$$N \times 0.90 = 31$$

$$N = \frac{31}{0.90} = 35.$$

Example 8.11. In Example 7.1, we conducted a test of hypothesis to assess whether there was a reduction in expenditures on health care and prescription drugs in 2006 as compared to 2002. In 2002, Americans paid an average of \$3302 per year on health care and prescription drugs.[8] An investigator sampled 100 Americans and found that they spent a mean of \$3190 on health care and prescription drugs with a standard deviation of \$890. The test failed to reject the null hypothesis and the investigator is concerned that the sample size was too small. How many participants are needed to ensure that the test has 80% power to detect a difference of \$150 in expenditures (a difference the investigator feels is meaningful)? A two-sided test will be used with a 5% level of significance.

We first compute the effect size,

$$\text{ES} = \frac{|\mu_1 - \mu_0|}{\sigma} = \frac{150}{890} = 0.17.$$

Notice that the numerator is 150, the difference specified by the investigator. We also use the standard deviation measured in the previous study ($s = 890$) to inform the design of the next study.

We now substitute the effect size and the appropriate z values for the selected α and power to compute the sample size,

$$n = \left(\frac{z_{1-\alpha/2} + z_{1-\beta}}{\text{ES}}\right)^2 = \left(\frac{1.96 + 0.84}{0.17}\right)^2 = 271.3.$$

A sample of size $n = 272$ will ensure that a two-sided test with $\alpha = 0.05$ has 80% power to detect a \$150 difference in expenditures. Thus, the study with $n = 100$ participants had lower power to detect a difference of \$150 in expenditures.

8.2.2 Sample Size for One Sample, Dichotomous Outcome

In studies where the plan is to perform a test of hypothesis comparing the proportion of successes in a dichotomous outcome variable in a single population to a known proportion, the hypotheses of interest are

$$H_0: p = p_0,$$

$$H_1: p \neq p_0$$

where p_0 is the known proportion (e.g., an historical control). The formula for determining the sample size to ensure that the test has a specified power is

$$n = \left(\frac{z_{1-\alpha/2} + z_{1-\beta}}{ES} \right)^2$$

where α is the selected level of significance and $z_{1-\alpha/2}$ is the value from the standard normal distribution holding $1-\alpha/2$ below it. $1-\beta$ is the selected power, $z_{1-\beta}$ is the value from the standard normal distribution holding $1-\beta$ below it, and ES is the effect size, defined as

$$ES = \frac{|p_1 - p_0|}{\sqrt{p_0(1-p_0)}},$$

where p_0 is the proportion under H_0 and p_1 is the proportion under H_1. The numerator of the effect size, the absolute value of the difference in proportions $|p_1 - p_0|$, again represents what is considered a clinically meaningful or practically important difference in proportions.

Example 8.12. A recent report from the Framingham Heart Study indicated that 26% of people free of cardiovascular disease had elevated LDL cholesterol levels, defined as LDL of more than 159 mg/dl.[9] An investigator hypothesizes that a higher proportion of patients with a history of cardiovascular disease will have elevated LDL cholesterol. How many patients should be studied to ensure that the power of the test is 90% to detect a 5% difference in the proportion with elevated LDL cholesterol? A two-sided test will be used with a 5% level of significance.

We first compute the effect size,

$$ES = \frac{|p_1 - p_0|}{\sqrt{p_0(1-p_0)}} = \frac{0.05}{\sqrt{0.26(1-0.26)}} = 0.11.$$

We now substitute the effect size and the appropriate z values for the selected α and power to compute the sample size,

$$n = \left(\frac{z_{1-\alpha/2} + z_{1-\beta}}{ES} \right)^2 = \left(\frac{1.96 + 1.282}{0.11} \right)^2 = 868.6.$$

A sample of size $n = 869$ will ensure that a two-sided test with $\alpha = 0.05$ has 90% power to detect a 5% difference in the proportion of patients with a history of cardiovascular disease who have an elevated LDL cholesterol level.

Example 8.13. A medical device manufacturer produces implantable stents. During the manufacturing process, approximately 10% of the stents are deemed to be defective. The manufacturer wants to test whether the proportion of defective stents is more than 10%. If the process produces more than 15% defective stents, then corrective action must be taken. Therefore, the manufacturer wants the test to have 90% power to detect a difference in proportions of this magnitude. How many stents must be evaluated? A two-sided test will be used with a 5% level of significance.

We first compute the effect size,

$$ES = \frac{|p_1 - p_0|}{\sqrt{p_0(1-p_0)}} = \frac{|0.15 - 0.10|}{\sqrt{0.10(1-0.10)}} = 0.17.$$

We now substitute the effect size and the appropriate z values for the selected α and power to compute the sample size,

$$n = \left(\frac{z_{1-\alpha/2} + z_{1-\beta}}{ES} \right)^2 = \left(\frac{1.96 + 1.282}{0.17} \right)^2 = 363.7.$$

A sample of size $n = 364$ stents will ensure that a two-sided test with $\alpha = 0.05$ has 90% power to detect a 5% difference in the proportion of defective stents produced.

8.2.3 Sample Sizes for Two Independent Samples, Continuous Outcome

In studies where the plan is to perform a test of hypothesis comparing the means of a continuous outcome variable in two independent populations, the hypotheses of interest are:

$$H_0: \mu_1 = \mu_2,$$

$$H_1: \mu_1 \neq \mu_2$$

where μ_1 and μ_2 are the means in the two comparison populations. The formula for determining the sample sizes to ensure that the test has a specified power is

$$n_i = 2\left(\frac{z_{1-\alpha/2} + z_{1-\beta}}{ES} \right)^2$$

where n_i is the sample size required in each group ($i = 1, 2$), α is the selected level of significance, $z_{1-\alpha/2}$ is the value from the standard normal distribution holding $1-\alpha/2$ below it, $1-\beta$ is the selected power, and $z_{1-\beta}$ is the value from the standard normal distribution holding $1-\beta$ below it. ES is the effect size, defined as

$$ES = \frac{|\mu_1 - \mu_2|}{\sigma},$$

where $|\mu_1 - \mu_2|$ is the absolute value of the difference in means between the two groups expected under the alternative hypothesis, H_1. σ is the standard deviation of the outcome of interest.

Recall from Chapter 6 when we performed tests of hypothesis comparing the means of two independent groups, we used S_p (the pooled estimate of the common standard deviation) as a measure of variability in the outcome. If data are available on variability of the outcome in each comparison group, then S_p can be computed and used to generate the sample sizes. However, it is more often the case that data on the variability of the outcome are available from only one group, usually the untreated (e.g., placebo control) or unexposed group. When planning a clinical trial to investigate a new drug or procedure, data are often available from other trials that may have involved a placebo or an active control group (i.e., a standard medication or treatment given for the condition under study). The standard deviation of the outcome variable measured in patients assigned to the placebo, control, or unexposed group can be used to plan a future trial. This situation is illustrated in the following examples.

Note that the formula shown previously generates sample size estimates for samples of equal size. If a study is planned where different numbers of patients will be assigned or different numbers of patients will comprise the comparison groups, then alternative formulas can be used. Interested readers can see Howell for more details.[3]

Example 8.14. An investigator is planning a clinical trial to evaluate the efficacy of a new drug designed to reduce systolic blood pressure. The plan is to enroll participants and to randomly assign them to receive either the new drug or a placebo. Systolic blood pressures will be measured in each participant after 12 weeks on the assigned treatment. Based on prior experience with similar trials, the investigator expects that 10% of all participants will be lost to follow up or will drop from the study. If the new drug shows a 5 unit reduction in mean systolic blood pressure, this would represent a clinically meaningful reduction. How many patients should be enrolled in the trial to ensure that the power of the test is 80% to detect this difference? A two-sided test will be used with a 5% level of significance.

To compute the effect size, an estimate of the variability in systolic blood pressures is needed. Analysis of data from the Framingham Heart Study (see Table 4.20), showed that the standard deviation of systolic blood pressure was $s = 19.0$. This value can be used to plan the trial.

The effect size is

$$ES = \frac{|\mu_1 - \mu_2|}{\sigma} = \frac{5}{19.0} = 0.26.$$

We now substitute the effect size and the appropriate z values for the selected α and power to compute the sample size,

$$n_i = 2\left(\frac{z_{1-\alpha/2} + z_{1-\beta}}{ES}\right)^2 = 2\left(\frac{1.96 + 0.84}{0.26}\right)^2 = 232.0.$$

Samples of size $n_1 = 232$ and $n_2 = 232$ will ensure that the test of hypotheses will have 80% power to detect a 5 unit difference in mean systolic blood pressures in patients receiving the new drug as compared to patients receiving the placebo. These sample sizes refer to the numbers of participants required with complete data. The investigators hypothesized a 10% attrition rate in both groups. To ensure that the total sample size of 464 is available at 12 weeks, the investigator needs to recruit more participants to allow for attrition:

N (number to enroll) $\times$ (% retained) = Desired sample size

$$N \times 0.90 = 464$$

$$N = \frac{464}{0.90} = 516$$

The investigator must enroll 516 participants. Each patient will be randomly assigned to receive either the new drug or placebo; assuming that 10% are lost to follow up, 464 will be available for analysis.

Example 8.15. An investigator is planning a study to assess the association between alcohol consumption and grade point average among college seniors. The plan is to categorize students as heavy drinkers or not using five or more drinks on a typical drinking day as the criterion for heavy drinking. Mean grade point averages will be compared between students classified as heavy drinkers versus not using a two independent samples test of means. The standard deviation in grade point averages is assumed to be 0.42 and a meaningful difference in grade point averages (relative to drinking status) is 0.25 units.

How many college seniors should be enrolled in the study to ensure that the power of the test is 80% to detect a 0.25 unit difference in mean grade point averages? A two-sided test will be used with a 5% level of significance.

We first compute the effect size,

$$ES = \frac{|\mu_1 - \mu_2|}{\sigma} = \frac{0.25}{0.42} = 0.60.$$

We now substitute the effect size and the appropriate z values for the selected α and power to compute the sample size,

$$n_i = 2\left(\frac{z_{1-\alpha/2} + z_{1-\beta}}{ES}\right)^2 = 2\left(\frac{1.96 + 0.84}{0.60}\right)^2 = 43.6.$$

Samples of size $n_1 = 44$ heavy drinkers and $n_2 = 44$ who drink fewer than five drinks per typical drinking day will ensure that the test of hypothesis will have 80% power to detect a 0.25 unit difference in mean grade point averages.

This computation assumes that approximately equal numbers of students will be classified as heavy drinkers versus not. A study by Wechsler et al. showed that approximately 44% of college students were binge drinkers (defined as drinking five or more drinks per occasion for men and four or more per occasion for women).[9] To ensure that this study has at least 44 heavy drinkers, a total of $N = 100$ college students should be selected. This will ensure that approximately 44 (44% of 100) are heavy drinkers and 56 (56% of 100) are not.

8.2.4   Sample Size for Matched Samples, Continuous Outcome

In studies where the plan is to perform a test of hypothesis on the mean difference in a continuous outcome variable based on matched data, the hypotheses of interest are

$$H_0: \mu_d = 0$$

$$H_1: \mu_d \neq 0$$

where μ_d is the mean difference in the population. The formula for determining the sample size to ensure that the test has a specified power is

$$n = \left(\frac{z_{1-\alpha/2} + z_{1-\beta}}{ES} \right)^2,$$

where α is the selected level of significance and $z_{1-\alpha/2}$ is the value from the standard normal distribution holding $1 - \alpha/2$ below it. $1 - \beta$ is the selected power, $z_{1-\beta}$ is the value from the standard normal distribution holding $1 - \beta$ below it and ES is the effect size, defined as

$$ES = \frac{\mu_d}{\sigma_d},$$

where μ_d is the mean difference expected under the alternative hypothesis, H_1, and σ_d is the standard deviation of the difference in the outcome (e.g., the difference based on measurements over time or the difference between matched pairs).

Example 8.16. In Example 8.7, we generated sample size requirements for a crossover trial to compare two diet programs for their effectiveness in promoting weight loss. The planned analysis was a confidence interval estimate for the mean difference in weight lost on the low-fat as compared to the low-carbohydrate diet. Suppose we design the same study with a test of hypothesis as the primary analysis. The proposed study will have each child follow each diet for 8 weeks. At the end of each 8-week period, the weight lost during that period will be measured. Children will be randomly assigned to the

first diet (i.e., some will follow the low-fat diet first while others will follow the low-carbohydrate diet first). The investigators expect to lose 30% of the participants over the course of the 16-week study. The difference in weight lost on the low-fat diet and the low-carbohydrate diet will be computed for each child; here we will test if there is a statistically significant difference in weight lost between the diets. How many children are required to ensure that a two-sided test with a 5% level of significance has 80% power to detect a mean difference in weight lost between the two diets of 3 lbs?

To compute the sample size, we again need an estimate of the variability of the difference in weight lost between diets. In Example 8.7, we used a value from a previous study of 9.1 lbs (this was based on a similar trial conducted in adults).

We first compute the effect size,

$$ES = \frac{\mu_d}{\sigma_d} = \frac{3}{9.1} = 0.33.$$

We now substitute the effect size and the appropriate z values for the selected α and power to compute the sample size,

$$n = \left(\frac{z_{1-\alpha/2} + z_{1-\beta}}{ES} \right)^2 = \left(\frac{1.96 + 0.84}{0.33} \right)^2 = 72.0.$$

A sample of size $n = 72$ children will ensure that a two-sided test with $\alpha = 0.05$ has 80% power to detect a mean difference of 3 lbs between diets using a crossover trial. The investigators hypothesized a 30% attrition rate. To ensure that the total sample size of 72 is available at 16 weeks, the investigator needs to recruit 103 participants:

$$N \text{ (number to enroll)} \times (\% \text{ retained}) = \text{Desired sample size}$$

$$N \times 0.70 = 72$$

$$N = \frac{72}{0.70} = 103$$

Notice that different numbers of children are needed depending on the analysis plan. In Example 8.7, we determined that 36 children would be needed to ensure that a 95% confidence interval for the mean difference has a margin of error of no more than 3 lbs. With a test of hypothesis, to ensure 80% power in detecting a mean difference of 3 lbs between diets we need 72 children. The analysis plan is key in the design of the study as it clearly affects the sample size.

Example 8.17. An investigator wants to evaluate the efficacy of an acupuncture treatment for reducing pain in patients with chronic migraine headaches. The plan is to enroll patients who suffer from migraine headaches. Each will be asked to rate the severity of the pain they experience with their next migraine before any treatment is administered. Pain will be recorded on a scale of 1 to 100 with higher scores indicative of more severe pain. Each patient will then undergo the acupuncture treatment. On their next migraine (post-treatment), each patient will again be asked to rate the severity of the pain. The difference in pain will be computed for each patient. A two-sided test of hypothesis will be conducted at $\alpha = 0.05$ to assess whether there is a statistically significant difference in pain scores before and after treatment. How many patients should be involved in the study to ensure that the test has 80% power to detect a difference of 10 units on the pain scale? Assume that the standard deviation in the difference scores is approximately 20 units.

We first compute the effect size,

$$ES = \frac{\mu_d}{\sigma_d} = \frac{10}{20} = 0.50.$$

We now substitute the effect size and the appropriate z values for the selected α and power to compute the sample size,

$$n = \left(\frac{z_{1-\alpha/2} + z_{1-\beta}}{ES}\right)^2 = \left(\frac{1.96 + 0.84}{0.50}\right)^2 = 31.4.$$

A sample of size $n = 32$ patients with migraines will ensure that a two-sided test with $\alpha = 0.05$ has 80% power to detect a mean difference of 10 points in pain before and after treatment. (Note that this assumes that all 32 patients complete the treatment and have available pain measurements before and after treatment.)

8.2.5 Sample Sizes for Two Independent Samples, Dichotomous Outcome

In studies where the plan is to perform a test of hypothesis comparing the proportions of successes in two independent populations, the hypotheses of interest are

$$H_0: p_1 = p_2$$

$$H_1: p_1 \neq p_2$$

where p_1 and p_2 are the proportions in the two comparison populations. The formula for determining the sample sizes to ensure that the test has a specified power is

$$n_i = 2\left(\frac{z_{1-\alpha/2} + z_{1-\beta}}{ES}\right)^2$$

where n_i is the sample size required in each group ($i = 1, 2$), α is the selected level of significance, and $z_{1-\alpha/2}$ is the value from the standard normal distribution holding $1-\alpha/2$ below it, $1-\beta$ is the selected power, and $z_{1-\beta}$ is the value from the standard

normal distribution holding $1-\beta$ below it. ES is the effect size, defined as

$$ES = \frac{|p_1 - p_2|}{\sqrt{p(1-p)}},$$

where $|p_1 - p_2|$ is the absolute value of the difference in proportions between the two groups expected under the alternative hypothesis, H_1, and p is the overall proportion, based on pooling the data from the two comparison groups.

Example 8.18. In Example 8.14, we determined the sample size needed for a clinical trial proposed to evaluate the efficacy of a new drug designed to reduce systolic blood pressure. The primary outcome was systolic blood pressure measured after 12 weeks on the assigned treatment, and the proposed analysis was a comparison of mean systolic blood pressures between treatments. We now consider a similar trial with a different primary outcome. Suppose we consider a diagnosis of hypertension (yes/no) as the primary outcome. Hypertension will be defined as a systolic blood pressure above 140 or a diastolic blood pressure above 90. Suppose we expect that 30% of the participants will meet the criteria for hypertension in the placebo group. The new drug will be considered efficacious if there is a 20% reduction in the proportion of patients receiving the new drug who meet the criteria for hypertension (i.e., if the proportion is 24% among patients receiving the new drug). How many patients should be enrolled in the trial to ensure that the power of the test is 80% to detect this difference in the proportions of patients with hypertension? A two-sided test will be used with a 5% level of significance.

We first compute the effect size by substituting the proportions of hypertensive patients expected in each group, $p_1 = 0.24$ and $p_2 = 0.30$, and the overall proportion, $p = 0.27$,

$$ES = \frac{|p_1 - p_2|}{\sqrt{p(1-p)}} = \frac{|0.24 - 0.30|}{\sqrt{0.27(1 - 0.27)}} = 0.135.$$

We now substitute the effect size and the appropriate z values for the selected α and power to compute the sample size,

$$n_i = 2\left(\frac{z_{1-\alpha/2} + z_{1-\beta}}{ES}\right)^2 = 2\left(\frac{1.96 + 0.84}{0.135}\right)^2 = 860.4.$$

Samples of size $n_1 = 861$ patients on the new drug and $n_2 = 861$ patients on placebo will ensure that the test of hypothesis will have 80% power to detect a 20% difference in the proportions of patients who meet the criteria for hypertension. In the trial proposed in Example 8.14, the investigators hypothesized a 10% attrition rate in both groups. To ensure that the total sample size of 1722 is available at 12 weeks, the investigator needs to recruit more participants to allow for attrition:

$$N \text{ (number to enroll)} \times (\% \text{ retained}) = \text{Desired sample size}$$

$$N \times 0.90 = 1722$$

$$N = \frac{1722}{0.90} = 1914$$

The investigator must enroll 1914 participants. Each patient will be randomly assigned to receive either the new medication or a placebo. Assuming that 10% are lost to follow up, 1722 will be available for analysis.

Example 8.19. An investigator hypothesizes that there is a higher incidence of flu among students who use their athletic facility regularly than their counterparts who do not. The study will be conducted in the spring. Each student will be asked if they used the athletic facility regularly over the past 6 months and whether or not they had the flu. A test of hypothesis will be conducted to compare the proportion of students who used the athletic facility regularly and got flu with the proportion of students who did not and got flu. During a typical year, approximately 35% of the students experience flu. The investigators feel that a 30% increase in flu among those who used the athletic facility regularly would be clinically meaningful. How many students should be enrolled in the study to ensure that the power of the test is 80% to detect this difference in the proportions? A two-sided test will be used with a 5% level of significance.

We first compute the effect size by substituting the proportions of students in each group who are expected to develop flu, $p_1 = 0.46$ and $p_2 = 0.35$, and the overall proportion, $p = 0.41$,

$$\text{ES} = \frac{|p_1 - p_2|}{\sqrt{p(1-p)}} = \frac{|0.46 - 0.35|}{\sqrt{0.41(1-0.41)}} = 0.22.$$

We now substitute the effect size and the appropriate z values for the selected α and power to compute the sample size,

$$n_i = 2\left(\frac{z_{1-\alpha/2} + z_{1-\beta}}{\text{ES}}\right)^2 = 2\left(\frac{1.96 + 0.84}{0.22}\right)^2 = 324.0.$$

Samples of size $n_1 = 324$ and $n_2 = 324$ will ensure that the test of hypothesis will have 80% power to detect a 30% difference in the proportions of students who develop flu between those who do and do not use the athletic facilities regularly.

8.3   SUMMARY

Determining the appropriate design of a study is more important than the statistical analysis. A poorly designed study can never be salvaged, whereas a poorly analyzed study can always be re-analyzed. A critical component in study design is the determination of the appropriate sample size. The sample size must be large enough to adequately answer the research question yet not too large so as to involve too many patients when fewer would have sufficed. The determination of the appropriate sample size involves statistical criteria as well as clinical or practical considerations. Sample size determination involves teamwork; biostatisticians must work closely with clinical investigators to determine the sample size that will address the research question of interest with adequate precision or power to produce results that are clinically meaningful.

Table 8–1 summarizes the sample size formulas for each scenario described here. The formulas are organized by the proposed analysis, a confidence interval estimate, or a test of hypothesis.

8.4   PRACTICE PROBLEMS

1. Suppose we want to design a new placebo-controlled trial to evaluate an experimental medication to increase lung capacity. The primary outcome is peak expiratory flow rate, a continuous variable measured in liters per minute. The primary outcome will be measured after 6 months on treatment. The expected peak expiratory flow rate in adults is 300 with a standard deviation of 50. How many subjects should be enrolled to ensure 80% power to detect a difference of 15 l/min with a two-sided test and $\alpha = 0.05$? The investigators expect to lose 10% of the participants over the course of follow up.

2. An investigator wants to estimate caffeine consumption in high school students. How many students would be required to ensure that a 95% confidence interval estimate for the mean caffeine intake (measured in mg) is within 15 units of the true mean? Assume that the standard deviation in caffeine intake is 68 mg.

3. Consider the study proposed in Problem 2. How many students would be required to estimate the proportion of students who consume coffee? Suppose we want the estimate to be within 5% of the true proportion with 95% confidence.

4. A clinical trial was conducted comparing a new compound designed to improve wound healing in trauma patients to a placebo. After treatment for five days, 58% of the patients taking the new compound had a substantial reduction in the size of their wound as compared to 44% in the placebo group. The trial failed to show significance. How many subjects would

TABLE 8-1 Sample Size Formulas

Outcome Variable, Number of Groups: Planned Analysis	Sample Size to Estimate Confidence Interval (CI)	Sample Size for Test of Hypothesis
Continuous outcome, one sample: CI for μ, H_0: $\mu = \mu_0$	$n = \left(\dfrac{Z\sigma}{E}\right)^2$	$n = \left(\dfrac{Z_{1-\alpha/2} + Z_{1-\beta}}{ES}\right)^2$ $ES = \dfrac{\lvert \mu_1 - \mu_0 \rvert}{\sigma}$
Continuous outcome, two independent samples: CI for $(\mu_1 - \mu_2)$, H_0: $\mu_1 = \mu_2$	$n_i = 2\left(\dfrac{Z\sigma}{E}\right)^2$	$n_i = 2\left(\dfrac{Z_{1-\alpha/2} + Z_{1-\beta}}{ES}\right)^2$ $ES = \dfrac{\lvert \mu_1 - \mu_2 \rvert}{\sigma}$
Continuous outcome, two matched samples: CI for μ_d, H_0: $\mu_d = 0$	$n = \left(\dfrac{Z\sigma_d}{E}\right)^2$	$n = \left(\dfrac{Z_{1-\alpha/2} + Z_{1-\beta}}{ES}\right)^2$ $ES = \dfrac{\mu_d}{\sigma_d}$
Dichotomous outcome, one sample: CI for p, H_0: $p = p_0$	$n = p(1-p)\left(\dfrac{Z}{E}\right)^2$	$n = \left(\dfrac{Z_{1-\alpha/2} + Z_{1-\beta}}{ES}\right)^2$ $ES = \dfrac{\lvert p_1 - p_0 \rvert}{\sqrt{p_0(1-p_0)}}$
Dichotomous outcome, two independent samples: CI for $(p_1 - p_2)$, H_0: $p_1 = p_2$	$n_i = \left[p_1(1-p_1) + p_2(1-p_2)\right]\left(\dfrac{Z}{E}\right)^2$	$n_i = 2\left(\dfrac{Z_{1-\alpha/2} + Z_{1-\beta}}{ES}\right)^2$ $ES = \dfrac{\lvert p_1 - p_2 \rvert}{\sqrt{p(1-p)}}$

be required to detect the difference in proportions observed in the trial with 80% power? A two-sided test is planned at $\alpha = 0.05$.

5. A crossover trial is planned to evaluate the impact of an educational intervention program to reduce alcohol consumption in patients determined to be at risk for alcohol problems. The plan is to measure alcohol consumption (the number of drinks on a typical drinking day) before the intervention and then again after participants complete the educational intervention program. How many participants would be required to ensure that a 95% confidence interval for the mean difference in the number of drinks is within 2 drinks of the true mean? Assume that the standard deviation of the difference in the mean number of drinks is 6.7 drinks and that 20% of the participants will drop out over the course of follow up.

6. An investigator wants to design a study to estimate the difference in the proportions of men and women

who develop early onset cardiovascular disease (defined as cardiovascular disease before age 50). A study conducted 10 years ago found that 15% and 8% of men and women, respectively, developed early onset cardiovascular disease. How many men and women are needed to generate a 95% confidence interval estimate for the difference in proportions with a margin of error not exceeding 4%?

7. The mean body mass index (BMI) for boys age 12 years old is 23.6. An investigator wants to test if the BMI is higher in 12-year-old boys living in New York City. How many boys are needed to ensure that a two-sided test of hypothesis has 80% power to detect an increase in BMI of 2 units? Assume that the standard deviation in BMI is 5.7.

8. An investigator wants to design a study to estimate the difference in the mean BMI between boys and girls 12 years old living in New York City. How many boys and girls are needed to ensure that a 95% confidence interval estimate for the difference in mean BMI between boys and girls has a margin of error not exceeding 2 units? Use the estimate of the variability in BMI from Problem 7.

REFERENCES

1. Buschman, N.A., Foster, G., and Vickers, P. "Adolescent girls and their babies: Achieving optimal birth weight. Gestational weight gain and pregnancy outcome in terms of gestation at delivery and infant birth weight: A comparison between adolescents under 16 and adult women." *Child: Care, Health and Development*. 2001; 27(2): 163–171.

2. Feuer, E.J. and Wun, L.M. DEVCAN: Probability of Developing or Dying of Cancer, Version 4.0. Bethesda, MD: National Cancer Institute, 1999.

3. Howell, D.C. *Statistical Methods for Psychology*. Boston: Duxbury Press, 1982.

4. Fleiss, J.L. *Statistical Methods for Rates and Proportions*. New York: John Wiley & Sons, 1981.

5. National Center for Health Statistics. *Health, United States, 2005 with Chartbook on Trends in the Health of Americans*. Hyattsville, MD: US Government Printing Office, 2005.

6. Plaskon, L.A., Penson, D.F., Vaughan, T.L., and Stanford, J.L. "Cigarette smoking and risk of prostate cancer in middle-aged men." *Cancer Epidemiology Biomarkers & Prevention*. 2003; 12: 604–609.

7. Rutter, M.K., Meigs, J.B., Sullivan, L.M., D'Agostino, R.B., and Wilson, P.W. "C-reactive protein, the metabolic syndrome, and prediction of cardiovascular events in the Framingham Offspring Study." *Circulation*. 2004; 110: 380–385.

8. Vasan, R.S., Sullivan, L.M., Wilson, P.W., Sempos, C.T., Sundstrom, J., Kannel, W.B., Levy, D., and D'Agostino, R.B. "Relative importance of borderline and elevated levels of coronary heart disease risk factors." *Annals of Internal Medicine*. 2005; 142: 393–402.

9. Wechsler, H., Lee, J.E., Kuo, M., and Lee, H. "College binge drinking in the 1990s: A continuing problem. Results of the Harvard School of Public Health, 1999 College Alcohol Study." *Journal of American College Health*, 2000; 48: 199–210.

CHAPTER 9

Multivariable Methods

In Chapter 6 and Chapter 7, we presented statistical inference procedures for estimation and hypothesis testing. We discussed many scenarios that differed in terms of the nature of the outcome variable (continuous, dichotomous, or discrete), the number of comparison groups (one, two, or more than two) and whether the groups were independent or dependent (physically separate or matched). In each scenario, we considered one outcome variable and we investigated whether there were differences in that outcome variable among the comparison groups or whether there was an association between an exposure or risk factor and that outcome. What we have not considered up to this point is the possibility that observed differences or associations might be due to other characteristics or variables. Multivariable statistical methods are used to assess the interrelationships among several risk factors or exposure variables and a single outcome. The topic of multivariable analysis is extensive. We will describe only general principles and concepts here. Interested readers should see Kleinbaum, Kupper, and Muller, Jewell, and Hosmer and Lemeshow for more in-depth discussion.[1–3]

We will specifically discuss the use of multivariable modeling techniques to address confounding and effect modification. In Chapter 2, we defined *confounding* as a distortion of the effect of an exposure or risk factor on an outcome by another characteristic or variable. *Effect modification* occurs when there is a different relationship between the exposure or risk factor and the outcome depending on the level of another characteristic or variable. In both situations, the third variable can exaggerate or mask the association between the risk factor and the outcome.

Analytically, confounding and effect modification are handled differently. When there is confounding, multivariable methods can be used to generate an estimate of the association between an exposure or risk factor and an outcome adjusting for or taking into account the impact of the confounder. In contrast, with effect modification there is a different relationship between the risk factor and outcome depending on the level of a third variable, and therefore an overall estimate of association does not accurately convey the information in the data. In the presence of effect modification, results are generally presented separately for each level of the third variable (using the techniques presented in Chapter 6 and Chapter 7). To formalize these concepts, we first present some examples and then move into the methods.

Suppose we want to assess the association between smoking and cardiovascular disease in a cohort study. We may find that smokers in the cohort are much more likely to develop cardiovascular disease. Suppose that we estimate a relative risk of $\hat{R}R = 2.6$ with a 95% confidence interval of $(1.5, 4.1)$. In our study, smokers are 2.6 times more likely to develop cardiovascular disease than nonsmokers. However, it may also be the case that the smokers are less likely to exercise and have higher cholesterol levels. Without examining these other characteristics, we could incorrectly infer that there is a strong association between smoking and cardiovascular disease when the relationship may be due, in part, to lack of exercise or to high cholesterol. Multivariable methods can be used to address these complex relationships and to tease out what proportion of the association might be due to smoking, as opposed to other risk factors. In other words, we use these methods to adjust the magnitude of association for the impact of other variables (e.g., the association between smoking and cardiovascular disease adjusted for exercise and cholesterol). Methods will also be discussed that allow us to assess whether an association remains statistically significant after adjusting for the impact of other variables.

Multivariable methods can also be used to assess effect modification—specifically, the situation in which the relationship between a risk factor and the outcome of interest varies by a third variable. For example, suppose we are interested in the efficacy of a new drug designed to lower total cholesterol. A clinical trial is conducted and the drug is shown to be effective with a statistically significant reduction in total cholesterol in patients who receive the new drug as compared to patients who receive a placebo. Suppose that the investigators look more closely at the data and find that the reduction (or effect of the drug) is only present in participants with a specific genetic marker and that there is no reduction in persons who do not possess the marker. This is an example of effect modification, or statistical interaction. The effect of the treatment is different depending on the presence or absence of the genetic marker. Multivariable methods can be used to identify effect modification. When effect modification is present, the strategy is to present separate results according to the third variable (i.e., to report the effect of the treatment separately in persons with and without the marker).

Other uses of multivariable methods include the consideration of several risk factors simultaneously, where the goal is to assess the relative importance of each with regard to a single outcome variable. For example, the Framingham Heart Study has a long history of developing multivariable risk functions.[4,5] These risk functions are used to predict the likelihood that a person will develop cardiovascular disease over a fixed period (e.g., the next 10 years) as a function of their risk factors. The risk factors include age, gender, systolic blood pressure, total and HDL cholesterol levels, current smoking, and diabetes status. Multivariable techniques are used in this setting to account for all of the risk factors simultaneously. This application is similar to the first, except that rather than focusing on the association between one risk factor and the outcome (adjusting for others) we are interested in the relationships between each of the risk factors and the outcome.

There are many other uses of multivariable methods. We will focus here on only a few specific applications. Because the computations are intensive, our presentation is more general with particular emphasis on interpretation rather than computation. In practice, the computations would be performed using a statistical computing package.[6]

It is important to note that the statistical analysis of any study should begin with a complete description of the study data using the methods described in Chapter 4. The primary analyses should proceed as planned to either generate estimates of unknown parameters or to perform tests of hypothesis using the techniques described in Chapter 6 and Chapter 7, respectively. The analyses we presented in Chapter 6 and Chapter 7 are called *unadjusted* or *crude analyses*. Multivariable methods are used after the study data are described and after unadjusted analyses are performed. In the clinical trials setting, the unadjusted analyses are generally the final analyses due primarily to the randomization component that (in theory) eliminates the possibility of confounding. While the multivariable methods we describe are a means to account for confounding, they should not be relied on to "correct" problems in a study.

Multivariable models are used for the statistical adjustment of confounding, whereas careful study design can provide much more in the way of minimizing confounding. Randomization is a very effective means of minimizing confounding. Unfortunately, not all studies are suitable for randomization. There are other options to minimize confounding (e.g., matching), but in all cases it is important to recognize that multivariable models can only adjust or account for differences in confounding variables that are measured in the study. Therefore, investigators must carefully plan studies not only with an eye toward minimizing confounding whenever possible but also with forethought to measure variables that might be potential confounders.

9.1   CONFOUNDING AND EFFECT MODIFICATION

Confounding is present when the relationship between a risk factor and an outcome is modified by a third variable, called the confounding variable. A *confounding variable* or the *confounder* is one that is related to the exposure or risk factor of interest and also to the outcome. Identification of confounding variables requires a strong working knowledge of the substantive area under investigation. (An additional consideration in determining whether the third variable is a confounder is assessing whether or not the third variable is part of a causal chain. A confounder is not in the causal chain from exposure to outcome. This is a complex issue; for more details, see Aschengrau and Seage.[7])

Confounding can be assessed in a number of different ways. Some investigators use formal statistical tests and others use clinical or practical judgment. We will discuss both approaches. Effect modification, also called statistical interaction, occurs when there is a different association between the risk factor and outcome depending on a third variable. Effect modification is generally assessed by statistical significance using regression techniques (discussed in Section 9.4 and Section 9.5). We will illustrate confounding and effect modification in Example 9.1 and Example 9.2, respectively.

Example 9.1. Consider a study designed to assess the association between obesity—defined as a body mass index (BMI) of 30 or more—and the incidence of cardiovascular disease. Data are collected in a cohort study in which participants between the ages of 35 and 65 who are free of cardiovascular disease (CVD) are enrolled and followed over 10 years. Each participant's BMI is assessed at baseline and participants are followed for 10 years for incident cardiovascular disease. A summary of the data are contained in Table 9–1.

The proportion of obese persons at baseline who develop CVD (or the incidence of CVD among obese persons) is

TABLE 9–1 Baseline Obesity and Incident CVD Over 10-Year Follow-Up

	Incident CVD	No CVD	Total
Obese	46	254	300
Not obese	60	640	700
Total	106	894	1000

46 / 300 = 0.153, and the proportion of non-obese persons who develop CVD (or the incidence of CVD among non-obese persons) is 60 / 700 = 0.086. The 10-year incidence rates are shown graphically in Figure 9–1. The estimate of the relative risk of CVD in obese as compared to non-obese persons is

$$\hat{RR} = \frac{\hat{p}_1}{\hat{p}_2} = \frac{0.153}{0.086} = 1.78.$$

Obese persons are 1.78 times more likely to develop CVD than non-obese persons in this study.

Many studies have shown an increase in the risk of CVD with advancing age. Could age be a confounder in this analysis? Could any of the observed association between obesity and incident CVD be attributable to age? A confounder is a variable that is associated with the risk factor and with the outcome. Is age associated with obesity? Is age associated with incident CVD?

In this study, age is measured as a continuous variable (in years). For interpretation purposes, suppose we dichotomize age at 50 years (less than 50 years of age versus 50 years and older). In this study, $n = 600$ (60%) participants are less than

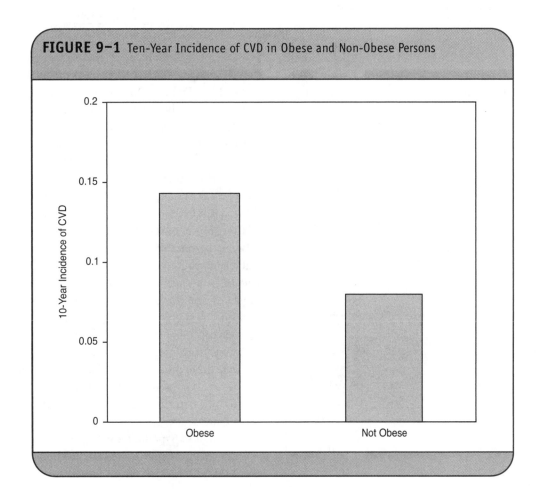

FIGURE 9–1 Ten-Year Incidence of CVD in Obese and Non-Obese Persons

50 years of age and $n = 400$ (40%) are 50 years of age and older. Table 9–2 shows the relationship between age and obesity.

Age is related to obesity. A higher proportion of persons 50 years of age and older are obese ($200 / 400 = 0.500$) as compared to persons less than 50 years of age ($100 / 600 = 0.167$). Looking at the data another way, a much higher proportion of obese persons are 50 years of age and older ($200 / 300 = 0.667$) as compared to non-obese persons ($200 / 700 = 0.286$). Could the fact that the majority of the obese persons are older explain the association between obesity and incident CVD? Is age driving the association?

Table 9–3 shows the relationship between age and incident CVD. Age is related to incident CVD. A much higher proportion of persons 50 years of age and older developed CVD ($61 / 400 = 0.153$) as compared to persons less than 50 years of age ($45 / 600 = 0.075$).

A higher proportion of the obese persons are older, and age is related to incident CVD. Thus, age meets the definition of a confounder (i.e., it is associated with the risk factor, obesity, and the outcome, incident CVD). We will now examine the relationship between obesity and incident CVD in persons less than 50 years of age and in persons 50 years of age and older separately (see Table 9–4).

Among people less than 50 years of age, the proportion of obese persons who develop CVD is $10 / 100 = 0.100$, and the proportion of non-obese persons who develop CVD is $35 / 500 = 0.070$. The relative risk of CVD in persons less than 50 years of age who are obese as compared to non-obese is

$$\hat{RR} = \frac{\hat{p}_1}{\hat{p}_2} = \frac{0.100}{0.070} = 1.43.$$

TABLE 9–2 Baseline Age and Baseline Obesity

Age	Obese	Not Obese	Total
< 50	100	500	600
50+	200	200	400
Total	300	700	1000

TABLE 9–3 Baseline Age and Incident CVD Over 10-Year Follow-Up

Age	Incident CVD	No CVD	Total
< 50	45	555	600
50+	61	339	400
Total	110	890	1000

TABLE 9–4 Baseline Obesity and Incident CVD by Age Group

	Age < 50		
	Incident CVD	No CVD	Total
Obese	10	90	100
Not obese	35	465	500
Total	45	555	600

	Age 50+		
	Incident CVD	No CVD	Total
Obese	36	164	200
Not obese	25	175	200
Total	65	335	400

Among people 50 years of age and older, the proportion of obese persons who develop CVD is $36 / 200 = 0.180$, and the proportion of non-obese persons who develop CVD is $25 / 200 = 0.125$. The relative risk of CVD in persons 50 years of age and older who are obese as compared to non-obese is

$$\hat{RR} = \frac{\hat{p}_1}{\hat{p}_2} = \frac{0.180}{0.125} = 1.44.$$

The relative risk based on the combined sample suggests a much stronger association between obesity and incident CVD ($\hat{RR} = 1.78$). Figure 9–2 shows the 10-year incidence rates for obese and non-obese persons in each age group.

There are different methods to determine whether a variable is a confounder or not. Some investigators perform formal tests of hypothesis to assess whether the variable is associated with the risk factor and with the outcome; other investigators do not conduct statistical tests but instead inspect the data and if there is a practically important or clinically meaningful relationship between the variable and the risk factor and between the variable and the outcome (regardless of whether that relationship reaches statistical significance), the variable is said to be a confounder. The data in Table 9–2 through Table 9–5 would suggest that age is a confounder by the latter method. (In Section 9.3, we will provide yet another method to assess confounding that again is based on evaluation of associations from a practical or clinical point of view.) We now illustrate the approach to assessing confounding using tests of hypothesis. We specifically test whether there is a statistically significant association between age and obesity and between age and incident CVD.

The tests of hypothesis can be performed using the χ^2 test of independence. In the first test, we determine whether age and obesity are related. The data for the test are shown in Table 9–2.

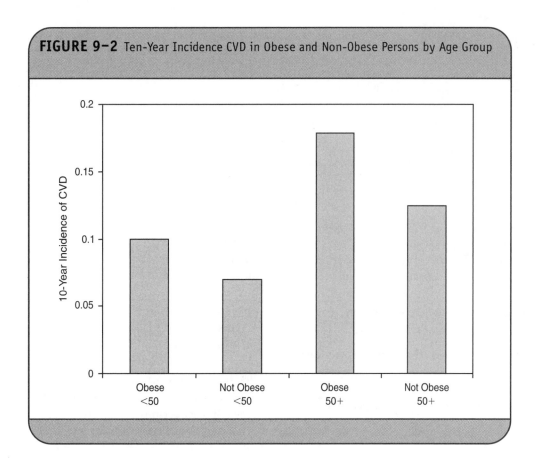

FIGURE 9-2 Ten-Year Incidence CVD in Obese and Non-Obese Persons by Age Group

Step 1. Set up hypotheses and determine the level of significance.

H_0: Age and obesity are independent

H_1: H_0 is false

$\alpha = 0.05$

Step 2. Select the appropriate test statistic.

The formula for the test statistic is in Table 7–44 and is given as

$$\chi^2 = \sum \frac{(O-E)^2}{E}.$$

The condition for appropriate use of the preceding test statistic is that each expected frequency in each cell of the table is five or more. In Step 4, we will compute the expected frequencies and ensure that the condition is met.

Step 3. Set up the decision rule.

The row variable is age ($r = 2$) and the column variable is obesity ($c = 2$), so for this test, df $= (2 - 1)(2 - 1) = 1(1) = 1$. For df $= 1$ and a 5% level of significance, the appropriate

critical value from Table 3 in the Appendix is 3.84, and the decision rule is

Reject H_0 if $\chi^2 \geq 3.84$.

Step 4. Compute the test statistic.

We now compute the expected frequencies using the formula,

$$\text{Expected frequency} = \frac{\text{Row total} \times \text{column total}}{N}.$$

The numbers in each cell of the table are the observed frequencies and the expected frequencies, shown in parentheses (see Table 9–5). The test statistic is computed as

$$\chi^2 = \frac{(100-180)^2}{180} + \frac{(500-420)^2}{420} +$$

$$\frac{(200-120)^2}{120} + \frac{(200-280)^2}{280},$$

$$\chi^2 = 35.56 + 15.23 + 53.33 + 22.86 = 126.98.$$

TABLE 9–5 Age and Obesity Frequencies

Age	Obese	Not Obese	Total
< 50	100 (180)	500 (420)	600
50+	200 (120)	200 (280)	400
Total	300	700	1000

Step 5. Conclusion.

We reject H_0 because $126.98 \geq 3.84$. We have statistically significant evidence at $\alpha = 0.05$ to show that H_0 is false; age and obesity are not independent (i.e., they are related). Using Table 3 in the Appendix, the *p*-value is $p < 0.005$.

The second test is to assess whether age is associated with incident CVD. We will again use the χ^2 test of independence, and the data for the test are shown in Table 9–3.

Step 1. Set up hypotheses and determine the level of significance.

$$H_0: \text{Age and incident CVD are independent}$$

$$H_1: H_0 \text{ is false}$$

$$\alpha = 0.05$$

Step 2. Select the appropriate test statistic.

The formula for the test statistic is in Table 7–44 and is given below:

$$\chi^2 = \sum \frac{(O-E)^2}{E}.$$

The condition for appropriate use of the preceding test statistic is that each expected frequency is five or more. In Step 4, we will compute the expected frequencies and ensure that the condition is met.

Step 3. Set up the decision rule.

The row variable is age ($r = 2$) and the column variable is incident CVD ($c = 2$), so for this test, df $= (2 - 1)(2 - 1) = 1(1) = 1$. For df $= 1$ and a 5% level of significance, the decision rule is

$$\text{Reject } H_0 \text{ if } \chi^2 \geq 3.84.$$

Step 4. Compute the test statistic.

We now compute the expected frequencies using the formula,

$$\text{Expected frequency} = \frac{\text{Row total} \times \text{column total}}{N}.$$

The numbers in each cell of the table are the observed frequencies and the expected frequencies, shown in parentheses (see Table 9–6). The test statistic is computed as

$$\chi^2 = \frac{(45-63.6)^2}{63.6} + \frac{(555-536.4)^2}{536.4} +$$

$$\frac{(65-42.4)^2}{42.4} + \frac{(335-357.6)^2}{357.6},$$

$$\chi^2 = 5.44 + 0.64 + 8.16 + 0.97 = 15.21.$$

Step 5. Conclusion.

We reject H_0 because $15.21 \geq 3.84$. We have statistically significant evidence at $\alpha = 0.05$ to show that H_0 is false; age and incident CVD are not independent. Using Table 3 in the Appendix, the *p*-value is $p < 0.005$.

Because age is related to obesity (17% of younger persons are obese as compared to 50% of older persons, and 67% of obese persons are 50 years of age and older as compared to 29% of non-obese persons) and age is related to incident CVD (7.5% of younger persons developed CVD as compared to 15.3% of older persons), age is a confounder. Therefore, some of the association between obesity and incident CVD can be attributed to age. In Section 9.2 to Section 9.5, we will discuss multivariable methods that can be used to estimate the magnitude of the association between obesity and incident CVD adjusting for age.

Example 9.2. A clinical trial is conducted to evaluate the efficacy of a new drug to increase HDL cholesterol (the "good" cholesterol). One hundred patients are enrolled in the trial and randomized to receive either the new drug or a placebo. Background characteristics (e.g., age, gender, educational level, income) and clinical characteristics (e.g., height, weight, blood pressure, total and HDL cholesterol levels) are measured at baseline. Suppose that the background and clinical characteristics (including baseline HDL levels) are comparable between groups (data not shown). Each patient is instructed to take the assigned medication for

TABLE 9–6 Age and CVD Frequencies

Age	Incident CVD	No CVD	Total
< 50	45 (63.6)	555 (536.4)	600
50+	65 (42.4)	335 (357.6)	400
Total	110	890	1000

8 weeks, at which time their HDL cholesterol is measured. Summary statistics on the primary outcome, HDL cholesterol, are shown in Table 9–7.

On average, the mean HDL levels are 0.95 units higher in patients treated with the new drug. A two-sample test to compare mean HDL levels between treatments (i.e., H$_0$: $\mu_1 = \mu_2$ versus H$_1$: $\mu_1 \neq \mu_2$) has a test statistic of $z = -1.13$, which is not statistically significant at $\alpha = 0.05$. Figure 9–3 shows the mean HDL levels in each group. The error bars represent the standard errors (SE) in each group.

Suppose that the lack of effect concerns investigators as they had expected a significant result on the basis of

preliminary studies. They wonder whether other variables might be masking the effect of the treatment. Suppose other studies had shown differential effectiveness of a similar drug in men and women. In this study, there are 19 men and 81 women. Table 9–8 shows the number and percentage of men assigned to each treatment.

There does not appear to be a difference in the proportions of men assigned to the treatments. A two-sample test of independent proportions or an χ^2 test of independence can be used to compare the proportions of men between treatments (i.e., H$_0$: $p_1 = p_2$ versus H$_1$: $p_1 \neq p_2$, or H$_0$: Gender and treatment are independent versus H$_1$: H$_0$ is false). The test of proportions has a test statistic of $z = 0.25$ (and the χ^2 test has $\chi^2 = 0.06$), which is not statistically significant at $\alpha = 0.05$.

Thus, gender is not a confounder as it is not related to the treatment. There is no meaningful difference in the proportions of men assigned to receive the new drug or the placebo; the difference in proportions is also not statistically significant. (Recall that a confounder is related to both the risk factor—the treatment variable in this case—and the outcome.) The investigators then wonder whether there might be effect modification by gender. Effect modification is a difference in

TABLE 9–7 HDL By Treatment

	Sample Size	Mean HDL	Standard Deviation of HDL
New drug	50	40.16	4.46
Placebo	50	39.21	3.91

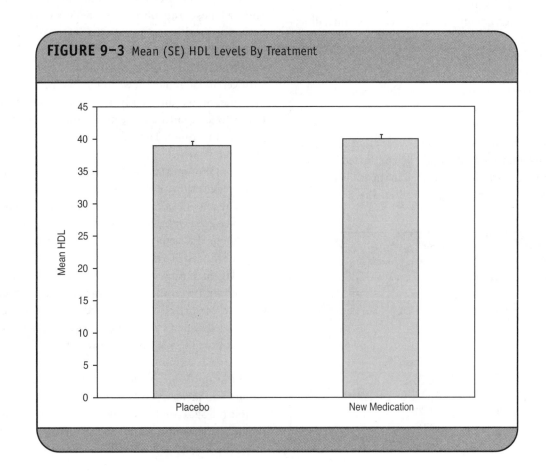

FIGURE 9–3 Mean (SE) HDL Levels By Treatment

TABLE 9-8 Number (%) of Men in Each Treatment Group

	Sample Size	Number	Percentage
New drug	50	10	20
Placebo	50	9	18

the effect of treatment depending on the participant's gender. The mean HDL levels for men and women assigned to the new drug and placebo are shown in Table 9–9.

On average, the mean HDL levels are 0.36 units lower in women treated with the new drug as compared to a placebo. On average, the mean HDL levels are 6.19 units higher in men treated with the new drug. This is an example of effect modification by gender. There is a different relationship between treatment and outcome depending on the gender of the participant. There is very little, if any, effect of treatment among women and a large effect among men.

Figure 9–4 shows the mean HDL levels in each treatment group, stratified (or presented separately) by gender. Among women, there is almost no difference in mean HDL levels by treatment. However, among men there is a substantial difference in mean HDL, with men assigned to the new drug having a much higher mean HDL than men assigned to the placebo. It is important to note that there are very few men in the analysis. Thus, the comparison of the mean HDL levels among men assigned to the new drug versus the placebo should be interpreted carefully.

It is also important to note that in the clinical trials setting, the only analyses that should be conducted are those that are planned *a priori* and specified in the study protocol. In contrast, in epidemiologic studies there are often

TABLE 9-9 HDL by Treatment and Gender

	Women		
	Sample Size	Mean HDL	Std Dev of HDL
New drug	40	38.88	3.97
Placebo	41	39.24	4.21
	Men		
	Sample Size	Mean HDL	Std Dev of HDL
New drug	10	45.25	1.89
Placebo	9	39.06	2.22

exploratory analyses that are conducted to fully understand associations (or lack thereof). However, these analyses should also be restricted to those that are biologically sensible.

When there is effect modification, analysis of the pooled data can be misleading. In this example, the pooled data (men and women combined) show no effect of the treatment. Because there is effect modification by gender, it is important to look at the differences in HDL levels among men and women, considered separately (or stratified by gender). However, in stratified analyses investigators must be careful to ensure that the sample size is adequate to provide a meaningful analysis. In Section 9.3 to Section 9.5, we will discuss methods to formally assess effect modification.

9.2 THE COCHRAN-MANTEL-HAENSZEL METHOD

In Example 9.1 and Example 9.2, we illustrated the concepts of confounding and effect modification, respectively. Confounding occurs when a third variable, the confounder, affects the relationship between the risk factor or exposure and the outcome. In Example 9.1, age was the confounder. Age was related to obesity and to incident CVD. Stated differently, there was an imbalance in the age distribution among obese and non-obese persons. The association between obesity and incident CVD was similar among younger and older persons (in stratified analysis). When the data were pooled (all ages combined), the effect looked stronger. In Example 9.2, we found that gender was an effect modifier. Stated differently, there was a statistical interaction between gender and treatment on mean HDL levels (the primary outcome). The effect of treatment was different in men and women.

The *Cochran-Mantel-Haenszel method* is a technique that generates an estimate of an association between a risk factor or exposure and an outcome accounting for confounding. The method is used with a dichotomous outcome variable and a dichotomous risk factor and essentially computes a weighted average of the relative risks (or odds ratios, whichever measure is used to quantify association) across the stratum (or groups) defined by the confounding variable. To implement the Cochran-Mantel-Haenszel method, the confounder must be categorized so that a series of two-by-two tables can be generated showing the association between the risk factor and outcome in each stratum.

In Example 9.1, we found that the association between obesity and incident CVD was much stronger in the pooled sample (all ages combined) than in either age group. The estimate based on the pooled sample is sometimes called an unadjusted or crude estimate. We generated a crude estimate

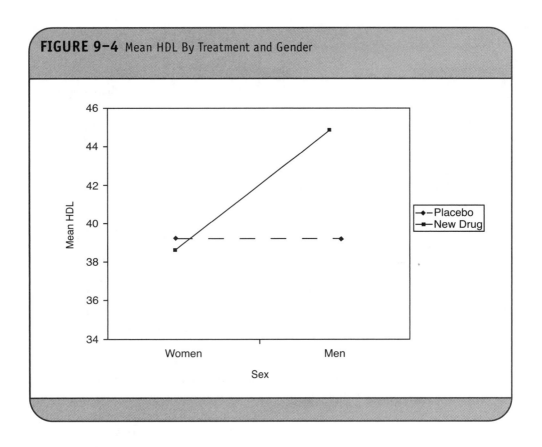

FIGURE 9–4 Mean HDL By Treatment and Gender

of the relative risk of 1.78. The crude or unadjusted odds ratio is 1.93. We now want to estimate the association between obesity and incident CVD that accounts for confounding by age.

Table 9–10 is a two-by-two table summarizing the association between a dichotomous risk factor and a dichotomous outcome. In previous chapters, we estimated the relative risk and the odds ratios as

$$\hat{RR} = \frac{\hat{p}_1}{\hat{p}_2} \text{ and } \hat{OR} = \frac{\hat{p}_1/(1-\hat{p}_1)}{\hat{p}_2/(1-\hat{p}_2)}.$$

TABLE 9–10 Data Layout for Cochran-Mantel-Haenszel Estimates

	Outcome Present	Outcome Absent	Total
Risk factor present (exposed)	a	b	$a + b$
Risk factor absent (unexposed)	c	d	$c + d$
Total	$a + c$	$b + d$	n

Using the notation in Table 9–10, the relative risk and odds ratio are equivalent to

$$\hat{RR} = \frac{a/(a + b)}{c/(c + d)} \text{ and } \hat{OR} = \frac{a/b}{c/d} = \frac{ad}{bc}.$$

When there is a confounding variable, we set up a series of two-by-two tables, one for each stratum (category) of the confounding variable. For example, in Example 9.1 we considered two age groups and thus we set up two tables showing the association between obesity and incident CVD in each of the two age strata.

The Cochran-Mantel-Haenszel estimates of the relative risk and odds ratio adjusted for confounding are

$$\hat{RR}_{CMH} = \frac{\sum a_i(c_i + d_i)/n_i}{\sum c_i(a_i + b_i)/n_i} \text{ and } \hat{OR}_{CMH} = \frac{\sum a_i d_i/n_i}{\sum b_i c_i/n_i},$$

where a_i, b_i, c_i, and d_i are the numbers of participants in the cells of the two-by-two table in the ith stratum of the confounding variable (see Table 9–10). n_i represents the number of participants in the ith stratum. We will illustrate the use of the Cochran-Mantel-Haenszel method in Example 9.3.

Example 9.3. Consider again the data in Example 9.1. We will use those data to estimate the relative risk and odds ratio describing the association between obesity and incident CVD

TABLE 9–11 Obesity and Incident CVD by Age Group

	Age < 50		
	Incident CVD	**No CVD**	**Total**
Obese	10	90	100
Not obese	35	465	500
Total	45	555	600
	Age 50+		
	Incident CVD	**No CVD**	**Total**
Obese	36	164	200
Not obese	25	175	200
Total	61	339	400

TABLE 9–12 Estimates of Association Between Obesity and CVD

	Relative Risk	**Odds Ratio**
Crude, unadjusted	1.78	1.93
Age < 50	1.43	1.48
Age 50+	1.44	1.52
Adjusted for age	1.44	1.52

adjusting for age. We will again consider two age groups or stratum, less than 50 years of age and 50 years of age and older. The data are shown in Table 9–11 for each age stratum.

The Cochran-Mantel-Haenszel method produces a single, summary measure of association that accounts for the fact that there is a different association in each age stratum. The adjusted relative risk and adjusted odds ratio are

$$\hat{RR}_{CMH} = \frac{\sum a_i(c_i + d_i)/n_i}{\sum c_i(a_i + b_i)/n_i} =$$

$$\frac{10(35 + 465)/600 + 36(25 + 175)/400}{35(10 + 90)/600 + 25(36 + 164)/400} = 1.44$$

and

$$\hat{OR}_{CMH} = \frac{\sum a_i d_i/n_i}{\sum b_i c_i/n_i} =$$

$$\frac{10(465)/600 + 36(175)/400}{90(35)/600 + 164(25)/400} = 1.52.$$

Table 9–12 summarizes the relative risks and odds ratios we have computed thus far to summarize the association between obesity and incident CVD.

Notice that the adjusted relative risk and adjusted odds ratio, 1.44 and 1.52, are not equal to the unadjusted or crude relative risk and odds ratio, 1.78 and 1.93. The adjustment for age produces estimates of the relative risk and odds ratio that are much closer to the stratum-specific estimates (the adjusted estimates are weighted averages of the stratum-specific estimates).

9.3 INTRODUCTION TO REGRESSION ANALYSIS

Regression analysis is a technique to assess the relationship between an outcome variable and one or more risk factors or confounding variables. The outcome variable is also called the *response* or *dependent variable* and the risk factors and confounders are called the *predictors, explanatory,* or *independent variables.* There is one potentially misleading aspect to this nomenclature. The term *predictor* can be interpreted as the ability to predict even beyond the limits of the data. The term *explanatory* might give an impression of an effect (when inferences should be limited to associations). The terms *independent* and *dependent* variable are less subject to these interpretations as they do not strongly imply cause and effect.

Regression analysis is a very general and widely applied technique. We will again focus on the general conceptual framework and somewhat specifically on the application of regression analysis to assess and account for confounding and to assess effect modification. Interested readers should see Kleinbaum, Kupper, and Muller for more details on regression analysis and its many applications.[1]

We first present a simple scenario to establish notation and general principles and then revisit the previous examples. Suppose we want to assess the association between total cholesterol and body mass index (BMI). In this application, total cholesterol is the dependent variable and BMI is the independent variable. In regression analysis, the dependent variable is denoted y and the independent variable is denoted x. We could expand this analysis and consider other potential predictors or independent variables associated with total cholesterol such as age, gender, and smoking. When there are more independent variables, they are denoted x_1, x_2, ... x_p. Considering only BMI, y = total cholesterol and x = BMI.

When there is a single continuous dependent variable and a single independent variable, the analysis is called a *simple linear regression analysis.* This analysis assumes that there is a linear association between the two variables. (If a different relationship is hypothesized, such as a curvilinear or exponential relationship, alternative regression analyses are performed.) Figure 9–5 displays data on BMI and total cholesterol measured in a sample of $n = 20$ participants. The data are displayed in a scatter diagram, where each point represents the (x, y) pair (in this case, BMI and total cholesterol) measured in each participant. Scatter diagrams display the independent variable on the horizontal axis and the dependent variable on the vertical axis.

Figure 9.5 shows a positive or direct association between BMI and total cholesterol. Participants with lower BMI are more likely to have lower total cholesterol levels and participants with higher BMI are more likely to have higher total cholesterol levels. In contrast, suppose we examine the association between BMI and HDL cholesterol. Figure 9–6 is a scatter diagram of BMI and HDL cholesterol measured in the same sample of $n = 20$ participants.

Figure 9–6 shows a negative or inverse association between BMI and HDL cholesterol. Participants with lower BMI are more likely to have higher HDL cholesterol levels and participants with higher BMI are more likely to have lower HDL cholesterol levels.

In simple linear regression analysis, we estimate the equation of the line that best describes the association between the independent variable and the dependent variable. The simple linear regression equation is

$$\hat{y} = b_0 + b_1 x,$$

where $\hat{y}$ is the predicted or expected value of the outcome, x is the predictor, b_0 is the estimated y-intercept, and b_1 is the estimated slope. The y-intercept and slope are estimated from the sample data and minimize the sum of the squared differences between the observed (y) and the predicted ($\hat{y}$) values of the outcome—i.e., the estimates minimize $\Sigma(\hat{y} - y)^2$. These differences are called *residuals.* The estimates of the y-intercept and slope minimize the sum of the squared residuals, and are called the *least squares estimates.*[1] The y-intercept is the value of the dependent variable (y) when the independent variable (x) is 0. The slope is the change in the dependent variable (y) relative to a one-unit change in the independent variable (x).

The least squares estimates of the regression coefficients, b_0 and b_1, describing the relationship between BMI and total

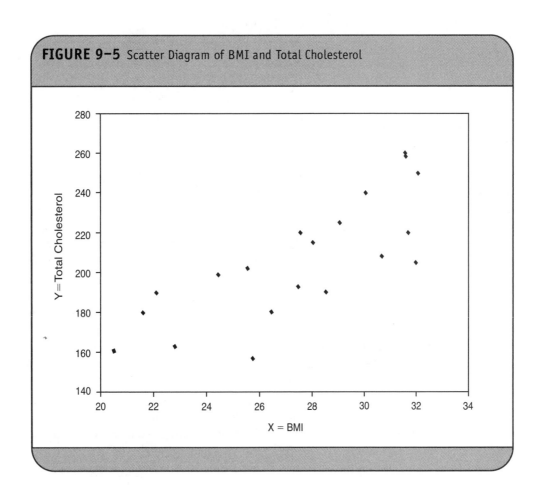

FIGURE 9–5 Scatter Diagram of BMI and Total Cholesterol

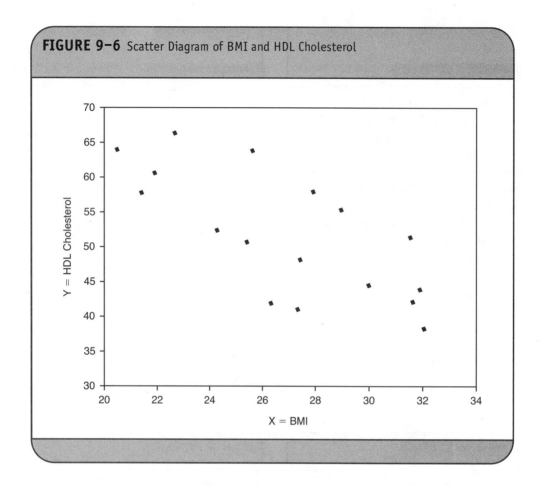

FIGURE 9-6 Scatter Diagram of BMI and HDL Cholesterol

cholesterol are $b_0 = 27.96$ and $b_1 = 6.49$. The estimate of the y-intercept ($b_0 = 27.96$) represents the estimated total cholesterol level when BMI is 0. Because a BMI of 0 is meaningless, the y-intercept is not informative. The estimate of the slope ($b_1 = 6.49$) represents the change in total cholesterol relative to a one-unit change in BMI. For example, if we compare two participants whose BMIs differ by one unit, we would expect their total cholesterols to differ by approximately 6.49 units (with the person with the higher BMI having the higher total cholesterol). The equation of the regression line is

$$\hat{y} = 27.96 + 6.49 \text{ BMI}.$$

The regression equation can be used to estimate a participant's total cholesterol as a function of their BMI. For example, suppose a participant has a BMI of 25. We would estimate their total cholesterol to be $27.96 + 6.49(25) = 190.21$. The equation can also be used to estimate total cholesterol for other values of BMI. However, the equation should only be used to estimate cholesterol levels for persons whose BMIs are in the range of the data used to generate the regression equation. In our sample, BMI ranges from 20 to 32, thus the equation

should only be used to generate estimates of total cholesterol for persons with BMI in that range.

There are statistical tests that can be performed to assess whether the estimated regression coefficients (b_0 and b_1) provide evidence that the respective coefficients in the population are statistically significantly different from 0. The test of most interest is usually H_0: $\beta_1 = 0$ versus H_1: $\beta_1 \neq 0$, where β_1 is the population slope. If the population slope is significantly different from 0, we conclude that there is a statistically significant association between the independent and dependent variables. These tests are conducted in most statistical computing packages (we omit the details here). Figure 9–7 shows the estimated regression line superimposed on the scatter diagram of BMI and total cholesterol.

The least squares estimates of the regression coefficients, b_0 and b_1, describing the relationship between BMI and HDL cholesterol are $b_0 = 111.77$ and $b_1 = -2.35$. Again, the y-intercept is uninformative because a BMI of 0 is meaningless. The estimate of the slope ($b_1 = -2.35$) represents the change in HDL cholesterol relative to a one-unit change in BMI. If we compare two participants whose BMIs differ by one unit, we would expect their HDL cholesterols to differ by approximately 2.35 units

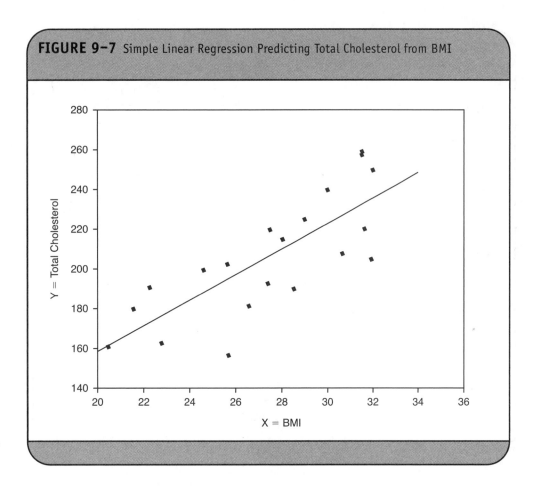

FIGURE 9–7 Simple Linear Regression Predicting Total Cholesterol from BMI

(with the person with the higher BMI having the lower HDL cholesterol). Figure 9–8 shows the regression line superimposed on the scatter diagram of BMI and HDL cholesterol.

In linear regression analysis, the dependent variable is continuous. There is an assumption that the distribution of the dependent variable (y) at each value of the independent variable (x) is approximately normally distributed. The independent variable can be continuous (e.g., BMI) or can be dichotomous.

In Example 9.2, we considered data from a clinical trial designed to evaluate the efficacy of a new drug to increase HDL cholesterol. One hundred patients enrolled in the study and were randomized to receive either the new drug or a placebo. Summary statistics on the primary outcome, HDL cholesterol, were shown in Table 9–7. We compared the mean HDL levels between treatment groups using a two independent samples t test. Regression analysis can also be used to compare mean HDL levels between treatments. HDL cholesterol is the continuous dependent variable and treatment (new drug versus placebo) is the independent variable. A simple linear regression equation is estimated as

$$\hat{y} = 39.21 + 0.95x,$$

where $\hat{y}$ is the estimated HDL level and x is a dichotomous (also called an indicator) variable reflecting the assigned treatment. In this example, x is coded as 1 for participants who received the new drug and as 0 for participants who received the placebo. The estimate of the y-intercept is $b_0 = 39.21$. The y-intercept is the value of y (HDL cholesterol) when x is 0. In this example, $x = 0$ indicates the placebo group. Thus, the y-intercept is exactly equal to the mean HDL level in the placebo group. The slope is $b_1 = 0.95$. The slope represents the change in y (HDL cholesterol) relative to a one-unit change in x. A one-unit change in x represents a difference in treatment assignment (placebo versus new drug). The slope represents the difference in mean HDL levels between the treatment groups (see Table 9–7; the mean HDL in the placebo group is 39.21 and the difference in means is 0.95 units).

In Section 9.4 and Section 9.5, we will extend the simple regression concept to include additional independent variables. In Section 9.4, we will present multiple linear regression analysis, which applies in situations where the outcome is

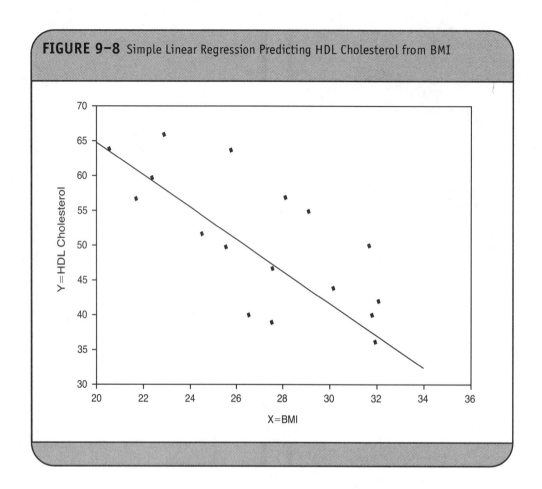

FIGURE 9–8 Simple Linear Regression Predicting HDL Cholesterol from BMI

continuous and there is more than one independent variable. The independent variables can be continuous or dichotomous (indicators). In Section 9.5, we will present multiple logistic regression analysis, which applies in situations where the outcome is dichotomous (e.g., incident CVD).

9.4   MULTIPLE LINEAR REGRESSION ANALYSIS

Multiple linear regression analysis is an extension of simple linear regression analysis and is used to assess the association between two or more independent variables and a single continuous dependent variable. The multiple linear regression equation is

$$\hat{y} = b_0 + b_1 x_1 + b_2 x_2 + \ldots + b_p x_p,$$

where $\hat{y}$ is the predicted or expected value of the dependent variable, x_1 through x_p are p distinct independent or predictor variables, b_0 is the value of y when all of the independent variables (x_1 through x_p) are equal to 0, and b_1 through b_p are the estimated regression coefficients. Each regression coefficient represents the change in y relative to a one-unit change in the respective independent variable holding the remaining

independent variables constant. For example, in the multiple regression situation, b_1 is the change in y relative to a one-unit change in x_1, holding all other independent variables constant (i.e., when the remaining independent variables are held at the same value or are fixed). Again, statistical tests can be performed to assess whether each regression coefficient is significantly different from 0.

Multiple regression analysis can be used to assess whether confounding exists. In Section 9.1, we mentioned that confounding can be assessed by formal statistical testing (i.e., testing whether the potential confounder is significantly associated with the risk factor and significantly associated with the outcome). We also mentioned that confounding can be assessed by examining the association between the potential confounder and the risk factor and between the potential confounder and the outcome (e.g., we used Table 9.2 through Table 9.5 to make that assessment in Example 9.1). Multiple regression analysis can be used to identify confounding as follows: Suppose we have a risk factor or an exposure variable, which we denote x_1 (e.g., obesity or treatment) and an outcome or dependent variable which we denote y. We can estimate a simple linear regression equation relating the risk factor (the independent variable) to the dependent variable as

$$\hat{y} = b_0 + b_1 x_1,$$

where b_1 is the estimated regression coefficient that quantifies the association between the risk factor and the outcome.

Suppose we now want to assess whether a third variable (e.g., age) is a confounder. We denote the potential confounder x_2 and then estimate a multiple linear regression equation as

$$\hat{y} = b_0 + b_1 x_1 + b_2 x_2.$$

In the multiple linear regression equation, b_1 is the estimated regression coefficient that quantifies the association between the risk factor x_1 and the outcome, adjusted for x_2 (b_2 is the estimated regression coefficient that quantifies the association between the potential confounder and the outcome). Some investigators assess confounding by assessing the extent to which the regression coefficient associated with the risk factor changes after adjusting for the potential confounder. In this case, we compare b_1 from the simple linear regression model to b_1 from the multiple linear regression model. As an informal rule, if the regression coefficient from the simple linear regression model changes by more than 10%, then x_2 is said to be a confounder. We will illustrate this approach in the following examples.

Once a variable is identified as a potential confounder, we can then use multiple linear regression analysis to estimate the association between the risk factor and the outcome adjusting for that confounder. The test of significance of the regression coefficient associated with the risk factor can be used to assess whether the association between the risk factor is statistically significant after accounting for one or more confounding variables. This is also illustrated in Example 9.4.

Example 9.4. Suppose we want to assess the association between BMI and systolic blood pressure using data collected in the seventh examination of the Framingham Offspring Study. A total of $n = 3539$ participants attended the exam and their mean systolic blood pressure is 127.3 with a standard deviation of 19.0. The mean BMI in the sample is 28.2 with a standard deviation of 5.3. A simple linear regression analysis reveals the following:

$$\hat{y} = 108.28 + 0.81(\text{BMI}),$$

where $\hat{y}$ is the predicted or expected systolic blood pressure. Suppose we now want to assess whether current smoking status (yes/no) and gender are potential confounders and if so,

appropriately account for these using multiple regression analysis. For analytic purposes, current smoking is coded as $1 =$ yes and $0 =$ no. Gender is coded as $1 =$ male and $0 =$ female. A multiple regression analysis reveals the following:

$$\hat{y} = 108.28 + 0.64(\text{BMI}) - 4.24(\text{Current smoking status}) + 1.36(\text{Gender}).$$

Notice that the association between BMI and systolic blood pressure is smaller (0.64 versus 0.81) after accounting for current smoking status and gender. The regression coefficient decreased by 21%. Using the informal rule (i.e., a change in the coefficient in either direction by 10% or more), we meet the criteria for confounding. Thus, part of the association between BMI and systolic blood pressure can be explained by current smoking status and gender.

As noted previously, most statistical computing packages produce p-values for each of the regression coefficients that can be used to assess the statistical significance of BMI after adjusting for current smoking status and gender. The p-values can also be used to assess the significance of current smoking status and gender as independent variables. It might be the case that after adjustment, BMI is no longer statistically significant. In that case, we might investigate explicitly the associations between current smoking and systolic blood pressure, between gender and systolic blood pressure, between current smoking status and BMI and between gender and BMI. Supposing that the association between BMI and systolic blood pressure remained significant after adjustment, we might then look specifically at the significance of the associations between current smoking and systolic blood pressure and between gender and systolic blood pressure. Some investigators would argue that regardless of whether current smoking and gender reach statistical significance, they should be retained in the model as they meet the criteria for confounding. Others would only retain variables that were statistically significant. This is yet another example of the complexity involved in multivariable modeling.

The multiple regression model produces an estimate of the association between BMI and systolic blood pressure that accounts for differences due to smoking and gender. A one-unit increase in BMI is associated with a 0.64-unit increase in systolic blood pressure, holding smoking and gender constant. Current smokers have lower systolic blood pressures—on average—by about 4.24 units, holding BMI and gender constant, and men have higher systolic blood pressures by about 1.36 units, holding BMI and current smoking status constant.

The multiple regression equation can be used to estimate systolic blood pressures as a function of a participant's

BMI, current smoking status, and gender. For example, we can estimate the blood pressure of a nonsmoking man with a BMI of 25 as

$$\hat{y} = 108.28 + 0.64(25) - 4.24(0) + 1.36(1) = 125.64.$$

We can estimate the blood pressure of a nonsmoking woman with a BMI of 28 as

$$\hat{y} = 108.28 + 0.64(28) - 4.24(0) + 1.36(0) = 126.20.$$

Example 9.5. In Example 9.2, we considered data from a clinical trial designed to evaluate the efficacy of a new drug to increase HDL cholesterol. One hundred patients enrolled in the study and were randomized to receive either the new drug or a placebo, and summary statistics on the primary outcome, HDL cholesterol, are shown in Table 9.7. In Section 9.3, we compared mean HDL levels between treatments using simple linear regression analysis, and the simple linear regression model was

$$\hat{y} = 39.21 + 0.95x,$$

where $\hat{y}$ is the estimated HDL level and x is a dichotomous (or indicator) variable reflecting the assigned treatment (1 = new drug and 0 = placebo). We know that there is no significant difference in mean HDL levels by treatment and thus we would fail to reject $H_0: \beta_1 = 0$ and that investigators are concerned about the small—and statistically insignificant—difference in mean HDL levels by treatment and question whether the effect of the treatment might be related to participant gender.

In Table 9.9, we showed that there was an important difference in the efficacy of the new drug depending on the participant's gender. We described this as effect modification by gender. Multiple regression analysis can be used to assess effect modification. This is done by estimating a multiple regression equation relating the outcome of interest (y) to independent variables representing the treatment assignment, gender, and the product of the two (called the treatment by gender interaction variable). For the analysis, we let T = the treatment assignment (1 = new drug and 0 = placebo), M = male gender (1 = male and 0 = female), and TM = T × M, the product of treatment and male gender. The multiple regression model is

$$\hat{y} = 39.24 - 0.36T - 0.18M + 6.55TM.$$

In this model, the regression coefficient associated with the interaction term, b_3, is statistically significant (i.e., $H_0: \beta 3 = 0$ versus $H_1: \beta 3 \neq 0$). The details of the test are not shown here.

The significance of this test indicates that there is a different relationship between treatment and outcome by gender.

The model shown here can be used to estimate the mean HDL levels for men and women who are assigned to the new medication and to the placebo. To use the model to generate these estimates, we must recall the coding scheme (i.e., T = 1 indicates new drug, T = 0 indicates placebo, M = 1 indicates male gender, and M = 0 indicates female gender). The expected or predicted HDL for men (M = 1) assigned to the new drug (T = 1) can be estimated as

$$\hat{y} = 39.24 - 0.36(1) - 0.18(1) + 6.55(1)(1) = 45.25.$$

The expected HDL for women (M = 0) assigned to the new drug (T = 1) is

$$\hat{y} = 39.24 - 0.36(1) - 0.18(0) + 6.55(1)(0) = 38.88.$$

The expected HDL for men (M = 1) assigned to the placebo (T = 0) is

$$\hat{y} = 39.24 - 0.36(0) - 0.18(1) + 6.55(0)(1) = 39.06.$$

The expected HDL for women (M = 0) assigned to the placebo (T = 0) is

$$\hat{y} = 39.24 - 0.36(0) - 0.18(0) + 6.55(0)(0) = 39.24.$$

Notice that the expected HDL levels for men and women on the new drug and on the placebo are identical to the means shown in Table 9.9.

Because there is effect modification, separate simple linear regression models can be estimated to assess the treatment effect in men and women:

$$\text{Men: } \hat{y} = 39.06 + 6.19T.$$

$$\text{Women: } \hat{y} = 39.24 - 0.36T.$$

In men, the regression coefficient associated with treatment ($b_1 = 6.19$) is statistically significant but in women, the regression coefficient associated with treatment ($b_1 = -0.36$) is not statistically significant (details not shown).

Multiple linear regression analysis is a widely applied technique. We showed here how multiple regression analysis can be used to assess and account for confounding and to assess effect modification. The techniques we described can be extended to adjust for several confounders simultaneously and to investigate more complex effect modification (e.g., three-way statistical interactions). There are many other applications of multiple regression analysis. A popular application is to assess the relationships between several predictor variables simultaneously and a single, continuous outcome. For example, it may be of interest to determine which predictors in a relatively large set of candidate predictors are most important or most strongly associated with an outcome. It is always important in statistical analysis, particularly in the multivariable arena, that statistical modeling is guided by biologically plausible associations.

9.5   MULTIPLE LOGISTIC REGRESSION ANALYSIS

Logistic regression analysis is similar to linear regression analysis except that the outcome is dichotomous (e.g., success/failure, yes/no). Logistic regression is very popular in biostatistical analysis. Simple logistic regression analysis refers to the regression application with one dichotomous outcome and one independent variable, and multiple logistic regression analysis applies when there is a single dichotomous outcome and more than one independent variable. Here again we present the general concept. Hosmer and Lemeshow provide a very detailed description of logistic regression analysis and its applications.[3]

The outcome in logistic regression analysis is often coded as 0 or 1, where 1 indicates that the outcome of interest is present and 0 indicates that the outcome of interest is absent. If we define p as the probability that the outcome is 1, the multiple logistic regression model can be written as

$$\hat{p} = \frac{\exp(b_0 + b_1 x_1 + b_2 x_2 + \ldots + b_p x_p)}{1 + \exp(b_0 + b_1 x_1 + b_2 x_2 + \ldots + b_p x_p)},$$

where $\hat{p}$ is the expected probability that the outcome is present, x_1 through x_p are distinct independent variables, and b_0 through b_p are the regression coefficients.

The multiple logistic regression model is sometimes written differently. In the following form, the outcome is the expected log of the odds that the outcome is present:

$$\ln\left(\frac{\hat{p}}{1-\hat{p}}\right) = b_0 + b_1 x_1 + b_2 x_2 + \ldots + b_p x_p.$$

Notice that the right side of the preceding equation looks like the multiple linear regression equation. The technique for estimating the regression coefficients in a logistic regression model is different from that used to estimate the regression coefficients in a multiple linear regression model. (Details can be found in Hosmer and Lemeshow.[3]) The interpretation of the regression coefficients in the multiple logistic regression model is as follows. b_1 is the change in the expected logs odds relative to a one-unit change in x_1, holding all other predictors

constant. The antilog of an estimated regression coefficient, $\exp(b_i)$, produces an odds ratio. In Example 9.6, we estimate a multiple logistic regression model and discuss the interpretation of the regression coefficients.

Example 9.6. In Example 9.1, we analyzed data from a study designed to assess the association between obesity (defined as a BMI greater than 30) and incident CVD. Data were collected from participants who were between the ages of 35 and 65 and free of CVD at baseline. Each participant was followed for 10 years for the development of cardiovascular disease. A summary of the data are contained in Table 9–1.

In Example 9.1, we estimated the association between obesity and incident CVD. The unadjusted or crude relative risk was $\hat{RR} = 1.78$, and the unadjusted or crude odds ratio was $\hat{OR} = 1.93$. We also determined that age was a confounder, and using the Cochran-Mantel-Haenszel method we estimated an adjusted relative risk of $\hat{RR}_{CMH} = 1.44$ and an adjusted odds ratio of $\hat{OR}_{CMH} = 1.52$. We now use logistic regression analysis to assess the association between obesity and incident cardiovascular disease adjusting for age.

The following simple logistic regression model relates obesity to the log odds of incident CVD:

$$\ln\left(\frac{\hat{p}}{1-\hat{p}}\right) = -2.367 + 0.658(\text{Obesity}).$$

Obesity is an indicator variable in the model, coded as $1 =$ obese and $0 =$ not obese. The log odds of incident CVD is 0.658 times higher in persons who are obese as compared to not obese. If we take the antilog of the regression coefficient, $\exp(0.658) = 1.93$, we get the crude or unadjusted odds ratio. The odds of developing CVD are 1.93 times higher among obese persons as compared to non-obese persons.

In Example 9.1, we determined that age was a confounder. The following multiple logistic regression model estimates the association between obesity and incident CVD, adjusting for age. In the model, we again consider two age groups (less than 50 years of age and 50 years of age and older). For the analysis, age group is coded as $1 = 50$ years of age and older and $0 =$ less than 50 years of age.

$$\ln\left(\frac{\hat{p}}{1-\hat{p}}\right) = -2.592 + 0.415(\text{Obesity}) + 0.655(\text{Age group}).$$

If we take the antilog of the regression coefficient associated with obesity, $\exp(0.415) = 1.52$, we get the odds ratio adjusted for age. The odds of developing CVD are 1.52 times higher among obese persons as compared to non-obese persons, adjusting for age. In Section 9.2, we used the Cochran-Mantel-Haenszel method to generate an odds ratio adjusted for age and found $\hat{OR}_{CMH} = 1.52$.

Multiple logistic regression analysis is a widely applied technique. We showed here how multiple logistic regression analysis can be used to account for confounding. The models can be extended to account for several confounding variables simultaneously. Multiple logistic regression analysis can also be used to assess confounding and effect modification, and the approaches are identical to those used in multiple linear regression analysis. Multiple logistic regression analysis can also be used to examine the impact of multiple risk factors (as opposed to focusing on a single risk factor) on a dichotomous outcome. An example of the latter is a risk function predicting incident cardiovascular disease on the basis of age, gender, blood pressure, cholesterol, smoking, and so on. These types of models have been published extensively in the Framingham Heart Study.[4,5] Similar modeling approaches have been used to evaluate risk factors for other conditions such as breast cancer and diabetes.[8–10]

9.6   SUMMARY

Multivariable methods include a number of specific procedures to simultaneously assess the relationships between several exposure or risk factor variables and a single outcome. The methods are computationally complex and generally require the use of a statistical computing package. Multivariable methods can be used to assess and adjust for confounding, to determine whether there is effect modification or to assess the relationships of several exposure or risk factors on an outcome simultaneously. Multivariable analyses are complex and should always be planned to reflect biologically plausible relationships. Whereas it is relatively easy to consider an additional variable in a multiple linear or multiple logistic regression model, only variables that are clinically meaningful should be included.

We described how multivariable methods can be used to assess and account for confounding. It is worth repeating that multivariable methods should not be relied upon to "correct" problems in a study. Multivariable models are used for statistical adjustment of confounding, whereas careful study design can provide much more in the way of minimizing confounding. Randomization is the most effective means of minimizing confounding. Unfortunately, randomization is not always possible. Matching participants in the comparison groups is another option. The objective of matching is to distribute potential confounding variables equally among the comparison groups. However, if matching is employed, then analyses

must be tailored to appropriately account for matched (or dependent) samples.

It is important to remember that multivariable models can only adjust or account for differences in confounding variables that were measured in the study. In addition, multivariable models should only be used to account for confounding when there is some overlap in the distribution of the confounder in each of the risk factor groups. For example, in Example 9.1, there was an imbalance in the age distribution in obese as compared to non-obese persons. If the imbalance was extreme (e.g., suppose that all of the obese persons were 50 years of age and older and all of the non-obese persons were less than 50 years of age), then it would not be appropriate to use multivariable techniques to account for confounding. The data would simply not be suitable for the analysis.

With regard to effect modification, a major issue is the fact that analyses must be stratified to appropriately convey associations in the data. This can present issues with regard to lack of precision or low power. Stratified analyses are informative but if the samples in specific strata are too small, the analyses may lack precision. In planning studies, investigators must pay careful attention to potential effect modifiers. If there is a suspicion that an association between an exposure or risk factor is different in specific groups, the study must be designed to ensure sufficient numbers of participants in each of those groups. Specifically, the sample size formulas in Chapter 8 must be used to determine the numbers of subjects required in each strata to ensure adequate precision or power in the analysis.

Multivariable methods are very powerful. In this chapter, we discussed only a few specific applications. Practicing biostatisticians must understand multivariable methods broadly to work effectively in investigative teams, and therefore we encourage students to pursue more coursework in multivariable analysis. That being said, it is critically important to appropriately describe data (using the methods we presented in Chapter 4) and to investigate relationships among variables carefully (using the methods and techniques described in Chapter 6 and Chapter 7). Mastery of the principles and techniques presented in previous chapters will provide a solid foundation.

In the opening paragraph of the textbook, we stated that implementing and understanding biostatistical applications is a combination of art and science. This is probably most evident in this chapter. Successful biostatisticians must not only understand the theory and principles of statistics, they must also understand the substantive nature of research problems to effectively implement them.

9.7 PRACTICE PROBLEMS

1. A study is conducted to estimate the association between exposure to lead paint in childhood and attention-deficit hyperactivity disorder (ADHD). Data on $n = 400$ children are collected, and data on exposure and ADHD diagnosis are shown in Table 9–13.
   a. Estimate the crude or unadjusted relative risk.
   b. Estimate the crude or unadjusted odds ratio.

2. In the study described in Problem 1, data were also available reflecting whether or not the child's father had ADHD. The relationship between the father's diagnosis, the child's exposure to lead paint, and the child's diagnosis are shown in Table 9–14.
   a. Estimate the relative risks and odds ratios for a child's diagnosis of ADHD relative to exposure to lead paint, stratified by the father's diagnosis of ADHD (i.e., for fathers with and without the diagnosis).
   b. How do the results in Part (a) of this problem compare to the results in Problem 1?

3. Use the data in Problem 1 and Problem 2 to conduct tests of hypothesis to determine whether the father's diagnosis of ADHD is a confounder. (Hint: Test if there is a relationship between the father's diagnosis and the child's exposure, and between the father's diagnosis and the child's diagnosis.) Is the father's diagnosis of ADHD a confounder? Justify your conclusion.

4. Use the data in Problem 2 to estimate the relative risk and odds ratio for a child's diagnosis of ADHD relative to exposure to lead paint, adjusted for the father's diagnosis using the Cochran-Mantel-Haenszel method.

5. The data presented in Problem 1 and Problem 2 are analyzed using multiple logistic regression analysis and the models are shown here. In these models, the data are coded as p = the proportion of children with a diagnosis of ADHD, and *Child Exposed* and *Father's Diagnosis* are coded as 1 = yes and 0 = no.

$$\ln\left(\frac{\hat{p}}{1-\hat{p}}\right) = -2.216 + 1.480(\text{Child exposed}) \quad (1)$$

Father with diagnosis: $\ln\left(\frac{\hat{p}}{1-\hat{p}}\right) =$
$$-1.665 + 1.297(\text{Child exposed}) \quad (2)$$

Father without diagnosis: $\ln\left(\frac{\hat{p}}{1-\hat{p}}\right) =$
$$-2.343 + 0.823(\text{Child exposed}) \quad (3)$$

$$\ln\left(\frac{\hat{p}}{1-\hat{p}}\right) = -2.398 + 1.056\,(\text{Child exposed}) +$$
$$0.906(\text{Father's diagnosis}) \quad (4)$$

   a. Which model produces the unadjusted odds ratio? Compute the unadjusted odds ratio using the regression coefficient from the appropriate model.
   b. Which model produces the odds ratio in fathers without a diagnosis of ADHD? Compute the unadjusted odds ratio using the regression coefficient from the appropriate model.
   c. What is the odds ratio adjusted for the father's diagnosis?

6. A study is conducted in patients with HIV. The primary outcome is CD4 cell count, which is a measure of the stage of the disease. Lower CD4 counts are associated with more advanced disease. The investigators are interested in the association between vitamin and mineral supplements and CD4 count. A multiple regression analysis is performed relating

TABLE 9–13 Exposure to Lead Paint and ADHD

Exposure to Lead Paint	ADHD	No ADHD
Yes	34	71
No	29	266

TABLE 9–14 Exposure to Lead Paint and ADHD by Father's Diagnosis

Father with ADHD		
Exposure to Lead Paint	ADHD	No ADHD
Yes	27	39
No	7	37

Father without ADHD		
Exposure to Lead Paint	ADHD	No ADHD
Yes	7	32
No	22	229

CD4 count to the use of supplements (coded as 1 = yes and 0 = no) and to the duration of HIV in years (i.e., the number of years between the diagnosis of HIV and the study date). For the analysis, y = CD4 count:

$$\hat{y} = 501.41 + 12.67(\text{Supplements}) - 30.23(\text{Duration of HIV}).$$

a. What is the expected CD4 count for a patient taking supplements who has had HIV for 2.5 years?

b. What is the expected CD4 count for a patient not taking supplements who was diagnosed with HIV at study enrollment?

c. What is the expected CD4 count for a patient not taking supplements who has had HIV for 2.5 years?

d. If we compare two patients and one has had HIV for 5 years longer than the other, what is the expected difference in their CD4 counts?

7. A clinical trial is conducted to evaluate the efficacy of a new medication to relieve pain in patients undergoing total knee replacement surgery. In the trial, patients are randomly assigned to receive either the new medication or the standard medication. After receiving the assigned medication, patients are asked to report their pain on a scale of 0 to 100, with higher scores indicative of more pain. Data on the primary outcome are shown in Table 9–15. Because procedures can be more complicated in older patients, the investigators were concerned about confounding by age. For analysis, patients were classified into two age groups, less than 65 years old and 65 years of age and older. The data are shown in Table 9–16. Is there a statistically significant difference in mean pain scores between patients assigned to the new medication as compared to the standard medication? Run the appropriate test at $\alpha = 0.05$. (Ignore age in this analysis.)

8. Use the data in Problem 7 to determine whether age is a confounding variable. Use the two age groups and run the tests of hypothesis to determine whether the age is related to treatment assignment and whether there is a difference in mean pain scores by age group. Is age a confounder? Justify your conclusion.

9. The data presented in Problem 7 are analyzed using multiple linear regression analysis and the models are shown here. In the models, the data are coded as 1 = new treatment and 0 = standard treatment, and age greater than 65 is coded as 1 = yes and 0 = no.

$$\hat{y} = 53.85 - 23.54(\text{Treatment})$$

$$\hat{y} = 45.31 - 19.88(\text{Treatment}) + 14.64(\text{Age} > 65)$$

$$\hat{y} = 45.51 - 20.21(\text{Treatment}) + 14.29(\text{Age} > 65) + 0.75(\text{Treatment} \times \text{Age} > 65)$$

Patients < 65: $\hat{y} = 45.51 - 20.21(\text{Treatment})$

Patients 65 +: $\hat{y} = 59.80 - 19.47(\text{Treatment})$

Does it appear that there is effect modification by age? Justify your response using the preceding models.

TABLE 9–16 Pain Scores by Treatment and Age

Age < 65	Sample Size	Mean Pain Score	Std Dev of Pain Score
New medication	40	25.30	2.46
Standard medication	25	45.51	1.83
Total	65	33.07	10.16

Age 65+	Sample Size	Mean Pain Score	Std Dev of Pain Score
New medication	20	40.33	2.16
Standard medication	35	59.80	2.49
Total	55	52.72	9.74

TABLE 9–15 Pain Scores by Treatment

	Sample Size	Mean Pain Score	Std Dev of Pain Score
New medication	60	30.31	7.52
Standard medication	60	53.85	7.44

10. Based on your answers to Problem 8 and Problem 9, how should the effect of the treatment be summarized? Should results be reported separately by age group or combined? Should the effect of treatment be adjusted for age? Justify your response using the models presented in Problem 9.

11. Generate a plot to display the mean pain scores by treatment and age group. (Hint: Use Figure 9.4 as an example.)

REFERENCES

1. Kleinbaum, D., Kupper, L.L., and Muller, K.E. *Applied Regression Analysis and Other Multivariable Methods* (2nd ed.). Boston: PWS-Kent, 1988.

2. Jewell, N.P. *Statistics for Epidemiology.* New York: Chapman and Hall/CRC, 2004.

3. Hosmer, D. Lemeshow, S. *Applied Logistic Regression.* New York: John Wiley & Sons, 1989.

4. Anderson, M., Wilson, P.W., Odell, P.M., and Kannell, W.B. "An updated coronary risk profile: A statement for health professionals." *Circulation.* 1991; 83: 356–362.

5. Wilson, P.W.F., D'Agostino, R.B., Levy, D., Belanger, A.M., Silbershatz, H., and Kannel, W.B. "Prediction of coronary heart disease using risk factor categories." *Circulation.* 1998; 97: 1837–1847.

6. SAS Version 9.1 (c) 2002–2003 by SAS Insitute, Cary, NC.

7. Aschengrau, A. and Seage, G.R. *Essentials of Epidemiology for Public Health.* Sudbury, MA: Jones & Bartlett Publishers, 2006.

8. Goldberg, J.I. and Borgen, P.I. "Breast cancer susceptibility testing: Past, present and future." *Expert Review of Anticancer Therapy.* 2006; 6(8): 1205–1214.

9. Meigs, J.B., Hu, F.B., Rifai, N., and Manson, J. "Biomarkers of endothelial dysfunction and risk of Type 2 diabetes mellitus." *Journal of the American Medical Association.* 2004; 291: 1978–1986.

10. Stern, M.P., Williams, K., and Haffner, S. "Identification of persons at high risk for Type 2 diabetes mellitus: Do we need the oral glucose tolerance test?" *Annals of Internal Medicine.* 2002; 136(8): 575–581.

Appendix

APPENDIX STATISTICAL TABLES

All table entries generated in SAS©. SAS Institute Inc. *SAS® User's Guide: Basics,* v 9.1. Cary, NC: SAS Institute Inc., 2002–2003.

TABLE 1. Probabilities of the Standard Normal Distribution Z

Table entries represent $P(Z < Z_i)$

e.g., $P(Z < -1.96) = 0.0250$, $P(Z < 1.96) = 0.9750$

Z_i	.00	.01	.02	.03	.04	.05	.06	.07	.08	.09
−3.0	0.0013	0.0013	0.0013	0.0012	0.0012	0.0011	0.0011	0.0011	0.0010	0.0010
−2.9	0.0019	0.0018	0.0018	0.0017	0.0016	0.0016	0.0015	0.0015	0.0014	0.0014
−2.8	0.0026	0.0025	0.0024	0.0023	0.0023	0.0022	0.0021	0.0021	0.0020	0.0019
−2.7	0.0035	0.0034	0.0033	0.0032	0.0031	0.0030	0.0029	0.0028	0.0027	0.0026
−2.6	0.0047	0.0045	0.0044	0.0043	0.0041	0.0040	0.0039	0.0038	0.0037	0.0036
−2.5	0.0062	0.0060	0.0059	0.0057	0.0055	0.0054	0.0052	0.0051	0.0049	0.0048
−2.4	0.0082	0.0080	0.0078	0.0075	0.0073	0.0071	0.0069	0.0068	0.0066	0.0064
−2.3	0.0107	0.0104	0.0102	0.0099	0.0096	0.0094	0.0091	0.0089	0.0087	0.0084
−2.2	0.0139	0.0136	0.0132	0.0129	0.0125	0.0122	0.0119	0.0116	0.0113	0.0110
−2.1	0.0179	0.0174	0.0170	0.0166	0.0162	0.0158	0.0154	0.0150	0.0146	0.0143
−2.0	0.0228	0.0222	0.0217	0.0212	0.0207	0.0202	0.0197	0.0192	0.0188	0.0183
−1.9	0.0287	0.0281	0.0274	0.0268	0.0262	0.0256	0.0250	0.0244	0.0239	0.0233
−1.8	0.0359	0.0351	0.0344	0.0336	0.0329	0.0322	0.0314	0.0307	0.0301	0.0294
−1.7	0.0446	0.0436	0.0427	0.0418	0.0409	0.0401	0.0392	0.0384	0.0375	0.0367
−1.6	0.0548	0.0537	0.0526	0.0516	0.0505	0.0495	0.0485	0.0475	0.0465	0.0455
−1.5	0.0668	0.0655	0.0643	0.0630	0.0618	0.0606	0.0594	0.0582	0.0571	0.0559
−1.4	0.0808	0.0793	0.0778	0.0764	0.0749	0.0735	0.0721	0.0708	0.0694	0.0681
−1.3	0.0968	0.0951	0.0934	0.0918	0.0901	0.0885	0.0869	0.0853	0.0838	0.0823
−1.2	0.1151	0.1131	0.1112	0.1093	0.1075	0.1056	0.1038	0.1020	0.1003	0.0985
−1.1	0.1357	0.1335	0.1314	0.1292	0.1271	0.1251	0.1230	0.1210	0.1190	0.1170
−1.0	0.1587	0.1562	0.1539	0.1515	0.1492	0.1469	0.1446	0.1423	0.1401	0.1379
−0.9	0.1841	0.1814	0.1788	0.1762	0.1736	0.1711	0.1685	0.1660	0.1635	0.1611
−0.8	0.2119	0.2090	0.2061	0.2033	0.2005	0.1977	0.1949	0.1922	0.1894	0.1867
−0.7	0.2420	0.2389	0.2358	0.2327	0.2296	0.2266	0.2236	0.2206	0.2177	0.2148
−0.6	0.2743	0.2709	0.2676	0.2643	0.2611	0.2578	0.2546	0.2514	0.2483	0.2451
−0.5	0.3085	0.3050	0.3015	0.2981	0.2946	0.2912	0.2877	0.2843	0.2810	0.2776
−0.4	0.3446	0.3409	0.3372	0.3336	0.3300	0.3264	0.3228	0.3192	0.3156	0.3121
−0.3	0.3821	0.3783	0.3745	0.3707	0.3669	0.3632	0.3594	0.3557	0.3520	0.3483
−0.2	0.4207	0.4168	0.4129	0.4090	0.4052	0.4013	0.3974	0.3936	0.3897	0.3859
−0.1	0.4602	0.4562	0.4522	0.4483	0.4443	0.4404	0.4364	0.4325	0.4286	0.4247
−0.0	0.5000	0.4960	0.4920	0.4880	0.4840	0.4801	0.4761	0.4721	0.4681	0.4641

TABLE 1. Probabilities of the Standard Normal Distribution Z (Continued)

Table entries represent $P(Z < Z_i)$

e.g., $P(Z < -1.96) = 0.0250$, $P(Z < 1.96) = 0.9750$

Z_i	.00	.01	.02	.03	.04	.05	.06	.07	.08	.09
0.0	0.5000	0.5040	0.5080	0.5120	0.5160	0.5199	0.5239	0.5279	0.5319	0.5359
0.1	0.5398	0.5438	0.5478	0.5517	0.5557	0.5596	0.5636	0.5675	0.5714	0.5753
0.2	0.5793	0.5832	0.5871	0.5910	0.5948	0.5987	0.6026	0.6064	0.6103	0.6141
0.3	0.6179	0.6217	0.6255	0.6293	0.6331	0.6368	0.6406	0.6443	0.6480	0.6517
0.4	0.6554	0.6591	0.6628	0.6664	0.6700	0.6736	0.6772	0.6808	0.6844	0.6879
0.5	0.6915	0.6950	0.6985	0.7019	0.7054	0.7088	0.7123	0.7157	0.7190	0.7224
0.6	0.7257	0.7291	0.7324	0.7357	0.7389	0.7422	0.7454	0.7486	0.7517	0.7549
0.7	0.7580	0.7611	0.7642	0.7673	0.7704	0.7734	0.7764	0.7794	0.7823	0.7852
0.8	0.7881	0.7910	0.7939	0.7967	0.7995	0.8023	0.8051	0.8078	0.8106	0.8133
0.9	0.8159	0.8186	0.8212	0.8238	0.8264	0.8289	0.8315	0.8340	0.8365	0.8389
1.0	0.8413	0.8438	0.8461	0.8485	0.8508	0.8531	0.8554	0.8577	0.8599	0.8621
1.1	0.8643	0.8665	0.8686	0.8708	0.8729	0.8749	0.8770	0.8790	0.8810	0.8830
1.2	0.8849	0.8869	0.8888	0.8907	0.8925	0.8944	0.8962	0.8980	0.8997	0.9015
1.3	0.9032	0.9049	0.9066	0.9082	0.9099	0.9115	0.9131	0.9147	0.9162	0.9177
1.4	0.9192	0.9207	0.9222	0.9236	0.9251	0.9265	0.9279	0.9292	0.9306	0.9319
1.5	0.9332	0.9345	0.9357	0.9370	0.9382	0.9394	0.9406	0.9418	0.9429	0.9441
1.6	0.9452	0.9463	0.9474	0.9484	0.9495	0.9505	0.9515	0.9525	0.9535	0.9545
1.7	0.9554	0.9564	0.9573	0.9582	0.9591	0.9599	0.9608	0.9616	0.9625	0.9633
1.8	0.9641	0.9649	0.9656	0.9664	0.9671	0.9678	0.9686	0.9693	0.9699	0.9706
1.9	0.9713	0.9719	0.9726	0.9732	0.9738	0.9744	0.9750	0.9756	0.9761	0.9767
2.0	0.9772	0.9778	0.9783	0.9788	0.9793	0.9798	0.9803	0.9808	0.9812	0.9817
2.1	0.9821	0.9826	0.9830	0.9834	0.9838	0.9842	0.9846	0.9850	0.9854	0.9857
2.2	0.9861	0.9864	0.9868	0.9871	0.9875	0.9878	0.9881	0.9884	0.9887	0.9890
2.3	0.9893	0.9896	0.9898	0.9901	0.9904	0.9906	0.9909	0.9911	0.9913	0.9916
2.4	0.9918	0.9920	0.9922	0.9925	0.9927	0.9929	0.9931	0.9932	0.9934	0.9936
2.5	0.9938	0.9940	0.9941	0.9943	0.9945	0.9946	0.9948	0.9949	0.9951	0.9952
2.6	0.9953	0.9955	0.9956	0.9957	0.9959	0.9960	0.9961	0.9962	0.9963	0.9964
2.7	0.9965	0.9966	0.9967	0.9968	0.9969	0.9970	0.9971	0.9972	0.9973	0.9974
2.8	0.9974	0.9975	0.9976	0.9977	0.9977	0.9978	0.9979	0.9979	0.9980	0.9981
2.9	0.9981	0.9982	0.9982	0.9983	0.9984	0.9984	0.9985	0.9985	0.9986	0.9986
3.0	0.9987	0.9987	0.9987	0.9988	0.9988	0.9989	0.9989	0.9989	0.9990	0.9990

TABLE 1A. *Z* Values for Percentiles

Percentile	Z
1st	−2.326
2.5th	−1.960
5th	−1.645
10th	−1.282
25th	−0.675
50th	0
75th	0.675
90th	1.282
95th	1.645
97.5th	1.960
99th	2.326

TABLE 1B. *Z* Values for Confidence Intervals

Confidence Level	Z
99.99%	3.819
99.9%	3.291
99%	2.576
95%	1.960
90%	1.645
80%	1.282

TABLE 1C. *Z* Values for Hypothesis Tests

Lower-Tailed Test α	Z
0.10	−1.282
0.05	−1.645
0.025	−1.960
0.010	−2.326
0.005	−2.576
0.001	−3.090
0.0001	−3.719

Upper-Tailed Test α	Z
0.10	1.282
0.05	1.645
0.025	1.960
0.010	2.326
0.005	2.576
0.001	3.090
0.0001	3.719

Two-Tailed Test α*	Z
0.20	1.282
0.10	1.645
0.05	1.960
0.010	2.576
0.001	3.291
0.0001	3.819

*α is the total tail area, α/2 in each tail

TABLE 2. Critical Values of the *t* Distribution

Table entries represent values from *t* distribution with upper-tail area equal to α.

e.g., $P(t_{df} > t) = \alpha$, e.g., $P(t_6 > 1.943) = 0.05$

Condence Level	80%	90%	95%	98%	99%
Two-Sided Test α	.20	.10	.05	.02	.01
One-Sided Test α	.10	.05	.025	.01	.005
df					
1	3.078	6.314	12.71	31.82	63.66
2	1.886	2.920	4.303	6.965	9.925
3	1.638	2.353	3.182	4.541	5.841
4	1.533	2.132	2.776	3.747	4.604
5	1.476	2.015	2.571	3.365	4.032
6	1.440	1.943	2.447	3.143	3.707
7	1.415	1.895	2.365	2.998	3.499
8	1.397	1.860	2.306	2.896	3.355
9	1.383	1.833	2.262	2.821	3.250
10	1.372	1.812	2.228	2.764	3.169
11	1.363	1.796	2.201	2.718	3.106
12	1.356	1.782	2.179	2.681	3.055
13	1.350	1.771	2.160	2.650	3.012
14	1.345	1.761	2.145	2.624	2.977
15	1.341	1.753	2.131	2.602	2.947
16	1.337	1.746	2.120	2.583	2.921
17	1.333	1.740	2.110	2.567	2.898
18	1.330	1.734	2.101	2.552	2.878
19	1.328	1.729	2.093	2.539	2.861
20	1.325	1.725	2.086	2.528	2.845
21	1.323	1.721	2.080	2.518	2.831
22	1.321	1.717	2.074	2.508	2.819
23	1.319	1.714	2.069	2.500	2.807
24	1.318	1.711	2.064	2.492	2.797
25	1.316	1.708	2.060	2.485	2.787
26	1.315	1.706	2.056	2.479	2.779
27	1.314	1.703	2.052	2.473	2.771
28	1.313	1.701	2.048	2.467	2.763
29	1.311	1.699	2.045	2.462	2.756
30	1.310	1.697	2.042	2.457	2.750

TABLE 2. Critical Values of the t Distribution (Continued)

Table entries represent values from t distribution with upper tail area equal to α.

e.g., $P(t_{df} > t) = \alpha$, e.g., $P(t_6 > 1.943) = 0.05$

Condence Level	80%	90%	95%	98%	99%
Two-Sided Test α	.20	.10	.05	.02	.01
One-Sided Test α	.10	.05	.025	.01	.005
df					
31	1.309	1.696	2.040	2.453	2.744
32	1.309	1.694	2.037	2.449	2.738
33	1.308	1.692	2.035	2.445	2.733
34	1.307	1.691	2.032	2.441	2.728
35	1.306	1.690	2.030	2.438	2.724
36	1.306	1.688	2.028	2.434	2.719
37	1.305	1.687	2.026	2.431	2.715
38	1.304	1.686	2.024	2.429	2.712
39	1.304	1.685	2.023	2.426	2.708
40	1.303	1.684	2.021	2.423	2.704
41	1.303	1.683	2.020	2.421	2.701
42	1.302	1.682	2.018	2.418	2.698
43	1.302	1.681	2.017	2.416	2.695
44	1.301	1.680	2.015	2.414	2.692
45	1.301	1.679	2.014	2.412	2.690
46	1.300	1.679	2.013	2.410	2.687
47	1.300	1.678	2.012	2.408	2.685
48	1.299	1.677	2.011	2.407	2.682
49	1.299	1.677	2.010	2.405	2.680
50	1.299	1.676	2.009	2.403	2.678
51	1.298	1.675	2.008	2.402	2.676
52	1.298	1.675	2.007	2.400	2.674
53	1.298	1.674	2.006	2.399	2.672
54	1.297	1.674	2.005	2.397	2.670
55	1.297	1.673	2.004	2.396	2.668
56	1.297	1.673	2.003	2.395	2.667
57	1.297	1.672	2.002	2.394	2.665
58	1.296	1.672	2.002	2.392	2.663
59	1.296	1.671	2.001	2.391	2.662
60	1.296	1.671	2.000	2.390	2.660

(Continued)

TABLE 2. Critical Values of the *t* Distribution (Continued)

Table entries represent values from *t* distribution with upper tail area equal to α.

e.g., $P(t_{df} > t) = \alpha$, e.g., $P(t_6 > 1.943) = 0.05$

Condence Level	80%	90%	95%	98%	99%
Two-Sided Test α	.20	.10	.05	.02	.01
One-Sided Test α	.10	.05	.025	.01	.005
df					
61	1.296	1.670	2.000	2.389	2.659
62	1.295	1.670	1.999	2.388	2.657
63	1.295	1.669	1.998	2.387	2.656
64	1.295	1.669	1.998	2.386	2.655
65	1.295	1.669	1.997	2.385	2.654
66	1.295	1.668	1.997	2.384	2.652
67	1.294	1.668	1.996	2.383	2.651
68	1.294	1.668	1.995	2.382	2.650
69	1.294	1.667	1.995	2.382	2.649
70	1.294	1.667	1.994	2.381	2.648
71	1.294	1.667	1.994	−2.380	2.647
72	1.293	1.666	1.993	2.379	2.646
73	1.293	1.666	1.993	2.379	2.645
74	1.293	1.666	1.993	2.378	2.644
75	1.293	1.665	1.992	2.377	2.643
∞	1.282	1.645	1.960	2.326	2.576

TABLE 3. Critical Values of the Chi-Square Distribution

Table entries represent values from X^2 distribution with upper tail area equal to α.

$$P(X^2_{df} > X^2) = \alpha, \text{e.g., } P(X^2_3 > 7.81) = 0.05$$

df α	.10	.05	.025	.01	.005
1	2.71	3.84	5.02	6.63	7.88
2	4.61	5.99	7.38	9.21	10.60
3	6.25	7.81	9.35	11.34	12.84
4	7.78	9.49	11.14	13.28	14.86
5	9.24	11.07	12.83	15.09	16.75
6	10.64	12.59	14.45	16.81	18.55
7	12.02	14.07	16.01	18.48	20.28
8	13.36	15.51	17.53	20.09	21.95
9	14.68	16.92	19.02	21.67	23.59
10	15.99	18.31	20.48	23.21	25.19
11	17.28	19.68	21.92	24.72	26.76
12	18.55	21.03	23.34	26.22	28.30
13	19.81	22.36	24.74	27.69	29.82
14	21.06	23.68	26.12	29.14	31.32
15	22.31	25.00	27.49	30.58	32.80
16	23.54	26.30	28.85	32.00	34.27
17	24.77	27.59	30.19	33.41	35.72
18	25.99	28.87	31.53	34.81	37.16
19	27.20	30.14	32.85	36.19	38.58
20	28.41	31.41	34.17	37.57	40.00
21	29.62	32.67	35.48	38.93	41.40
22	30.81	33.92	36.78	40.29	42.80
23	32.01	35.17	38.08	41.64	44.18
24	33.20	36.42	39.36	42.98	45.56
25	34.38	37.65	40.65	44.31	46.93
26	35.56	38.89	41.92	45.64	48.29
27	36.74	40.11	43.19	46.96	49.64
28	37.92	41.34	44.46	48.28	50.99
29	39.09	42.56	45.72	49.59	52.34
30	40.26	43.77	46.98	50.89	53.67
40	51.81	55.76	59.34	63.69	66.77
50	63.17	67.50	71.42	76.15	79.49
60	74.40	79.08	83.30	88.38	91.95
70	85.53	90.53	95.02	100.4	104.2
80	96.58	101.9	106.6	112.3	116.3
90	107.6	113.1	118.1	124.1	128.3
100	118.5	124.3	129.6	135.8	140.2

TABLE 4. Critical Values of the F Distribution with Upper Tail Area = 0.05

$$P(F_{df1, df2} > F) = 0.05,$$

$$\text{e.g., } P(F_{3,20} > 3.10) = 0.05$$

df1

df2	1	2	3	4	5	6	7	8	9	10	20	30	40	50
1	161.4	199.5	215.7	224.6	230.2	234.0	236.8	238.9	240.5	241.9	248.0	250.1	251.1	251.8
2	18.51	19.00	19.16	19.25	19.30	19.33	19.35	19.37	19.38	19.40	19.45	19.46	19.47	19.48
3	10.13	9.55	9.28	9.12	9.01	8.94	8.89	8.85	8.81	8.79	8.66	8.62	8.59	8.58
4	7.71	6.94	6.59	6.39	6.26	6.16	6.09	6.04	6.00	5.96	5.80	5.75	5.72	5.70
5	6.61	5.79	5.41	5.19	5.05	4.95	4.88	4.82	4.77	4.74	4.56	4.50	4.46	4.44
6	5.99	5.14	4.76	4.53	4.39	4.28	4.21	4.15	4.10	4.06	3.87	3.81	3.77	3.75
7	5.59	4.74	4.35	4.12	3.97	3.87	3.79	3.73	3.68	3.64	3.44	3.38	3.34	3.32
8	5.32	4.46	4.07	3.84	3.69	3.58	3.50	3.44	3.39	3.35	3.15	3.08	3.04	3.02
9	5.12	4.26	3.86	3.63	3.48	3.37	3.29	3.23	3.18	3.14	2.94	2.86	2.83	2.80
10	4.96	4.10	3.71	3.48	3.33	3.22	3.14	3.07	3.02	2.98	2.77	2.70	2.66	2.64
11	4.84	3.98	3.59	3.36	3.20	3.09	3.01	2.95	2.90	2.85	2.65	2.57	2.53	2.51
12	4.75	3.89	3.49	3.26	3.11	3.00	2.91	2.85	2.80	2.75	2.54	2.47	2.43	2.40
13	4.67	3.81	3.41	3.18	3.03	2.92	2.83	2.77	2.71	2.67	2.46	2.38	2.34	2.31
14	4.60	3.74	3.34	3.11	2.96	2.85	2.76	2.70	2.65	2.60	2.39	2.31	2.27	2.24
15	4.54	3.68	3.29	3.06	2.90	2.79	2.71	2.64	2.59	2.54	2.33	2.25	2.20	2.18
16	4.49	3.63	3.24	3.01	2.85	2.74	2.66	2.59	2.54	2.49	2.28	2.19	2.15	2.12
17	4.45	3.59	3.20	2.96	2.81	2.70	2.61	2.55	2.49	2.45	2.23	2.15	2.10	2.08
18	4.41	3.55	3.16	2.93	2.77	2.66	2.58	2.51	2.46	2.41	2.19	2.11	2.06	2.04
19	4.38	3.52	3.13	2.90	2.74	2.63	2.54	2.48	2.42	2.38	2.16	2.07	2.03	2.00
20	4.35	3.49	3.10	2.87	2.71	2.60	2.51	2.45	2.39	2.35	2.12	2.04	1.99	1.97
21	4.32	3.47	3.07	2.84	2.68	2.57	2.49	2.42	2.37	2.32	2.10	2.01	1.96	1.94
22	4.30	3.44	3.05	2.82	2.66	2.55	2.46	2.40	2.34	2.30	2.07	1.98	1.94	1.91
23	4.28	3.42	3.03	2.80	2.64	2.53	2.44	2.37	2.32	2.27	2.05	1.96	1.91	1.88
24	4.26	3.40	3.01	2.78	2.62	2.51	2.42	2.36	2.30	2.25	2.03	1.94	1.89	1.86
25	4.24	3.39	2.99	2.76	2.60	2.49	2.40	2.34	2.28	2.24	2.01	1.92	1.87	1.84
26	4.23	3.37	2.98	2.74	2.59	2.47	2.39	2.32	2.27	2.22	1.99	1.90	1.85	1.82
27	4.21	3.35	2.96	2.73	2.57	2.46	2.37	2.31	2.25	2.20	1.97	1.88	1.84	1.81
28	4.20	3.34	2.95	2.71	2.56	2.45	2.36	2.29	2.24	2.19	1.96	1.87	1.82	1.79
29	4.18	3.33	2.93	2.70	2.55	2.43	2.35	2.28	2.22	2.18	1.94	1.85	1.81	1.77
30	4.17	3.32	2.92	2.69	2.53	2.42	2.33	2.27	2.21	2.16	1.93	1.84	1.79	1.76

TABLE 4. Critical Values of the F Distribution with Upper Tail Area $= 0.05$ (Continued)

$P(F_{df1, df2} > F) = 0.05,$

e.g., $P(F_{3,20} > 3.10) = 0.05$

df1

df2	1	2	3	4	5	6	7	8	9	10	20	30	40	50
31	4.16	3.30	2.91	2.68	2.52	2.41	2.32	2.25	2.20	2.15	1.92	1.83	1.78	1.75
32	4.15	3.29	2.90	2.67	2.51	2.40	2.31	2.24	2.19	2.14	1.91	1.82	1.77	1.74
33	4.14	3.28	2.89	2.66	2.50	2.39	2.30	2.23	2.18	2.13	1.90	1.81	1.76	1.72
34	4.13	3.28	2.88	2.65	2.49	2.38	2.29	2.23	2.17	2.12	1.89	1.80	1.75	1.71
35	4.12	3.27	2.87	2.64	2.49	2.37	2.29	2.22	2.16	2.11	1.88	1.79	1.74	1.70
36	4.11	3.26	2.87	2.63	2.48	2.36	2.28	2.21	2.15	2.11	1.87	1.78	1.73	1.69
37	4.11	3.25	2.86	2.63	2.47	2.36	2.27	2.20	2.14	2.10	1.86	1.77	1.72	1.68
38	4.10	3.24	2.85	2.62	2.46	2.35	2.26	2.19	2.14	2.09	1.85	1.76	1.71	1.68
39	4.09	3.24	2.85	2.61	2.46	2.34	2.26	2.19	2.13	2.08	1.85	1.75	1.70	1.67
40	4.08	3.23	2.84	2.61	2.45	2.34	2.25	2.18	2.12	2.08	1.84	1.74	1.69	1.66
41	4.08	3.23	2.83	2.60	2.44	2.33	2.24	2.17	2.12	2.07	1.83	1.74	1.69	1.65
42	4.07	3.22	2.83	2.59	2.44	2.32	2.24	2.17	2.11	2.06	1.83	1.73	1.68	1.65
43	4.07	3.21	2.82	2.59	2.43	2.32	2.23	2.16	2.11	2.06	1.82	1.72	1.67	1.64
44	4.06	3.21	2.82	2.58	2.43	2.31	2.23	2.16	2.10	2.05	1.81	1.72	1.67	1.63
45	4.06	3.20	2.81	2.58	2.42	2.31	2.22	2.15	2.10	2.05	1.81	1.71	1.66	1.63
46	4.05	3.20	2.81	2.57	2.42	2.30	2.22	2.15	2.09	2.04	1.80	1.71	1.65	1.62
47	4.05	3.20	2.80	2.57	2.41	2.30	2.21	2.14	2.09	2.04	1.80	1.70	1.65	1.61
48	4.04	3.19	2.80	2.57	2.41	2.29	2.21	2.14	2.08	2.03	1.79	1.70	1.64	1.61
49	4.04	3.19	2.79	2.56	2.40	2.29	2.20	2.13	2.08	2.03	1.79	1.69	1.64	1.60
50	4.03	3.18	2.79	2.56	2.40	2.29	2.20	2.13	2.07	2.03	1.78	1.69	1.63	1.60
75	3.97	3.12	2.73	2.49	2.34	2.22	2.13	2.06	2.01	1.96	1.71	1.61	1.55	1.52
100	3.94	3.09	2.70	2.46	2.31	2.19	2.10	2.03	1.97	1.93	1.68	1.57	1.52	1.48

Index